CURE *for* CANCER
A National Goal

CURE *for* CANCER
A *National Goal*

By SOLOMON GARB, M.D., F.A.C.P.
*Professor of Pharmacology; Associate Professor
of Community Health and Medical Practice,
University of Missouri School of Medicine*

 SPRINGER PUBLISHING COMPANY, INC.,
NEW YORK

Preface

The theme of this book is that the time has come for a closer look at cancer research and for a new consolidation of effort aimed at cure or control of cancer.

Current efforts are good and many, but, as I will try to show, we could and should be doing much better. We need to shift gears—in our attitude toward cancer research, in our organization of the research and our support of it. It is time that cure or control of cancer become a national goal to be reached with the least possible delay.

For the past several years, I have given guest lectures on cancer research to the nursing students at the University of Missouri. Their interest in this topic has been most impressive, as is their ability to understand the principles once the facts are explained. Similarly, medical and veterinary students have indicated an intense interest in this subject, and several dozens of tnem have spent summer vacations in my laboratory working on some phase of the cancer problem. All these students from the health professions have asked many questions which show a deep desire to learn more about cancer research and to contribute in whatever way they can to the solution of this important health problem.

In 1966, John Lear, Science Editor of the *Saturday Review,* invited me to contribute to that magazine's anniversary issue an article on plants as possible sources of anti-cancer medicines. The favorable public response convinced me that there are many people, laymen as well as health professionals, who would be interested in supporting a better national effort toward finding a cure or control for cancer.

The role of members of the health professions in educating the public and forming and mobilizing public support for programs relating to health is so vital that few such programs could succeed without this support. Accordingly, in trying to bring about general support for major improvements in our national cancer research effort, I decided to direct my efforts first toward the health professions. I invite them to examine the theme of this book critically. If members of the health professions who are caring for patients with cancer accept and support this theme, the support of the general public should follow.

I have concentrated on the scientific aspects of cancer research in order to demonstrate that we already have a substantial number of excellent leads which are not being pursued with appropriate vigor. Indeed, to the best of my knowledge, some of these leads are not being followed at all. However, I believe that many of them, if properly pursued, could result in practical, lifesaving discoveries within a few years. In Part IV, 12 leads are presented that appear to have enough promise to warrant much greater effort and financial support than they now receive. If even one of the suggested leads is successful, many lives would be saved and the cost of the program fully justified. Political, organizational, and fiscal matters are also discussed, since these have become important aspects of the cancer research problem.

A major hindrance to effective cancer research has been a chronic, severe shortage of funds—a situation that is not generally recognized. It is not enough, however, to point this out or to repeat it; it is also necessary to explain how any additional funds would be used, what projects they would pay for, why such projects deserve support, and where the skilled scientists and technicians to do the work would come from. This I have tried to do, recognizing that if these projects were undertaken, modifications and changes in the national program, as outlined here, would be needed as the work progressed.

SOLOMON GARB

Columbia, Missouri
January, 1968

Contents

Part V

Mobilization of Our National Resources against Cancer

Part VI

Organization of a National Goal Approach

PART I

GENERAL CONSIDERATIONS

Introduction

Many people assume that medical research programs that are sponsored and supported by the Federal Government proceed as rapidly and as efficiently as possible. This assumption is quite understandable but, like other assumptions, should not be accepted uncritically. In some fields of medical research, enormous strides have certainly been made. However, in one of the most important areas—cancer—little of practical importance has as yet developed from our present research program. It has been fairly successful in disclosing basic facts about cancer and about some cellular functions, but thus far, it has not resulted in the development of any major treatments that have significantly improved the survival rate in patients. Advances in the clinical treatment of cancer have come about largely from improvements in surgical and radiological techniques, and from the development by scientists of Eli Lilly and Company of anti-cancer drugs (from the periwinkle plant). Undoubtedly the Federally supported program has played an indirect role in helping with these advances.

Are we doing everything that is reasonably possible and practical to find a cure or control for cancer? Certain bits of information available to the general public may make it seem as if we were. For example, we occasionally hear statements about the "enormous" Federal funds being spent on research. Yet few people realize that less than 2 per cent of the Federal funds allocated for research are used for cancer research. The fact is that since 1962 there has been a decrease in the net amount of money available for cancer research, although this is not apparent in a cursory examination of government appropriations. This point will be considered in greater detail in Chapter 9.

Another factor, which may lead some people to think that our cancer research program is proceeding at a satisfactory rate, is the great number of newspaper stories about it. The newspaper reporter, who is just as eager as anyone else to see progress in this field, tends to stress the hopeful implications of research. The reader, in many cases, interprets the story in a still more optimistic fashion, and as a result may come to believe that discovery of a major treatment is imminent, whereas the particular treatment he reads about may actually be many decades away. The fact is that, for over the past decade, most of the hopes which were nourished by optimistic statements have not been realized.

Under these circumstances, it is appropriate to examine our national cancer research program. We ought to note its strengths and preserve them, to note the weak areas and strengthen them, and to look for any important gaps in the program and fill them.

The major strength of our current program lies in the support given to basic approaches from which an eventual cure could result. The major weakness and defect in the program, is a chronic lack of adequate financial support. As a consequence, in part at least, there have been inadequate follow-up studies of promising leads, and there has been an inadequate and inefficient use of personnel and facilities. In the following chapters, these points will be considered in more detail.

In all fairness, we should note that the deficiencies and weaknesses in our cancer research program are, to a degree, the result of its early successes. In the decade between 1952 and 1962, it was responsible for training large numbers of research scientists, constructing several research facilities, and developing several useful leads. Since 1962, however, the program has not kept up the pace. It seems that the present arrangement which worked so well in managing the program in the early phases, is not well suited for the next phase. If we continue as before, the prospect of finding a cure or a satisfactory control for cancer in the foreseeable future does not seem bright. The time has come to reorganize and strengthen our cancer research program, and to move into a new phase in our attack on this disease—a concerted, broad-front advance, backed by all of America's scientific ability and technology.

This can be done through a national commitment to make the cure, or the satisfactory control, of cancer a national goal, in the same way that putting a man into orbit around the earth was made a national goal, and then achieved.

Because of the accomplishments in the first phase of our national effort, we now have a solid foundation to build on. We have a much better concept than before of the nature of cancer. We have a substantial number of well-trained cancer researchers—more than twice as many as can be adequately supported by our current appropriations; we have a nucleus of excellent research institutions and facil-

PART I

ities; and we have many trained scientists in related cooperating fields. Above all, we have an impressive list of approaches to cancer which can be explored simultaneously, with a reasonably good chance of success. If even one of these approaches proves effective, a major part of our goal will have been achieved, and in time to help many of those living today.

The proposal to make a cure or control for cancer a national goal is not a proposal that we embark on an indiscriminate cancer-cure crash program. On the contrary, the proposal involves specific approaches, with the reasons for such approaches and the evidence supporting them given in some detail (Section IV).

It might be argued that before starting such a major new program, we ought to learn more about the basic biology of normal as well as cancer cells. This point of view, however, is not one that is supported by medical history. As Hiatt (1) has stated:

It is difficult to point to any drug whose mechanism of action was appreciated before its usefulness had been demonstrated. Indeed, recognition of the uniqueness of the metabolic pathway inhibited has almost always followed the discovery of the effectiveness of the agent.

To this we may add that there are drugs whose mechanisms of action are still unknown, but which have been used for generations with considerable benefit to patients. Digitalis glycosides have been the mainstay in the treatment of congestive heart failure for almost 200 years, and despite extensive, vigorous, and imaginative research we still do not know how the digitalis glycosides act on the heart.

A mathematician, Oliver Heaviside (2) is reported to have said, "Should I refuse my dinner because I don't understand the digestive process?" Surely the same sort of reasoning ought to govern our medical research program.

On the other hand, this reasoning does not in any way imply a lack of respect for basic cellular research. Perhaps such research will lead to important lifesaving discoveries some day. However, the likelihood that it will do so in the near future does not seem great enough to justify us in neglecting any other approaches that offer a reasonable chance of success.

Aspects of the proposed program that deserve careful evaluation and scrutiny include a definition of the two parts of the goal, the mechanics of achieving the goal, the resources available and those still to be developed, and the probable costs.

4

Cure for cancer, to be considered adequate in this program, must be a procedure or medication that will offer better than 95 per cent chance of complete obliteration of the cancer process, including metastases, without detriment to the patient, if it is instituted at a time when the signs and symptoms of cancer are sufficiently clear for a definite diagnosis by the general practitioner. This definition implies several things: that after being cured the patient will be able to live and work in a normal manner, and without any serious lessening of his life expectancy; and that the cure will be effective, not only in the very earliest small cancers in accessible locations, but also in the larger internal cancers that may not give any warning until they are far advanced. A cure for cancer might be achieved through surgery, medication, radiation, immunologic therapy, or any combination of these.

Control of cancer, to be considered adequate in this program, should be a procedure, medication or combination of these that although not destroying the cancer keeps it in check in a reliable fashion in at least 95 per cent of patients, so that by continuing the prescribed treatment the patient can live and work in a normal manner, and without any serious lessening of his life expectancy. Control should be effective if instituted at a time when the signs and symptoms of cancer are sufficiently clear for a definite diagnosis by the general practitioner. Some examples of other diseases that are now well controlled although not curable are diabetes which is controlled by insulin, diet and other general measures; and pernicious anemia which is controlled by cyanocobalamin (Vitamin B^{12}).

Let us keep these two aspects of the goal clearly in mind as we consider the mechanics of achieving them.

References

1. Hiatt, H. H. Cancer chemotherapy—present status and prospects. *New Eng. J. Med.* *276:*157, 1967.
2. Sellers, E. E. Early pragmatists (letter). *Science 154:*1604, 1966.

But You Can't Buy Brains

When this book was in its planning stages I discussed its theme with a person who has had an active interest in cancer for many years. One comment she made was: "But you can't buy brains." Others have expressed similar ideas using other words. Apparently some people feel that any major expansion of our cancer research program is not likely to be effective because we are already using all of the brain power available to us for cancer research.

Upon exploring this attitude, it seemed to me that there were two basic beliefs underlying it: the belief that finding a cure or control for cancer depends upon one or a few geniuses who will come up with the right answers through the exercise of a unique kind of brain power, somewhat in the manner in which Galileo, Newton and Einstein made their discoveries; and the belief that the number of top quality scientists who could make important contributions to the cancer problem is limited. As a corollary to these two assumptions, there appears to be another, namely, that all or almost all of the scientists, who could find or help find a cure or control for cancer, are already working in the field at close to their maximum efficiency.

The evidence does not support these assumptions; indeed, there is good reason to believe that they are completely inaccurate.

Let us consider the genius theory. It is true that there have been geniuses, with intellects that far surpassed those of their contemporaries. Some of them have made great contributions to science. Certainly we would all like to have a genius discover a cure or control for cancer quickly. It would not be wise, however, to base our hopes and plans on such rarities because, even if we have among us the rare geniuses who have the *ability* to find a cure or control for cancer relatively soon, we cannot, with any confidence, assume that these people are working in the cancer field, or that they are being given the financial support needed for such work. In the history of *medicine,* as distinct from pure science, we find that the men who made the major *practical* discoveries, which have saved many, many lives, were not necessarily geniuses but simply highly intelligent men who also possessed excellent powers of observation. Some examples are: Edward Jenner who developed vaccination; William Withering who discovered the effects of digitalis on the heart; James Lind who discovered the way to prevent scurvy; John Snow who discovered the role of contaminated water in causing cholera; Banting and Best who discovered insulin, and Fleming who discovered penicillin.

It is important, too, to ask whether all or almost all of the capable scientists who *could* make worthwhile contributions to the solution of the cancer problem are actually working on that problem with reasonable efficiency and speed. The answer is that many capable people who would like to work in this field have thus far been unable to do so for financial reasons. Others who have already demonstrated their abilities in cancer research are being forced out of the field because they cannot obtain adequate funds for their research (*see* Chapter 10).

Another part of the problem concerns the maximum usage of the abilities of people who are already in the field of cancer. In many laboratories, chronic shortage of funds for technicians' salaries have made it necessary for research scientists to spend much of their time on repetitive tasks which could be done just as well by assistants with lesser training.

There is also a marked under-utilization (for cancer research) of scientists in other fields, such as veterinary medicine, dentistry, botany, pharmacy and general biology, as described in greater detail in Chapters 29 and 30.

The disappointing results of our cancer research program to date cannot be reasonably attributed to any national shortage of brains to do cancer research; they must be attributed to other causes. One is our antiquated and unwieldy system of allocating research funds which results in much of our available brain power being lost to cancer research or diverted to other research areas. Also, the chronic, severe money shortage sharply reduces the effectiveness of scientists already doing cancer research. These points are discussed more fully in Chapters 8 and 9.

The origin of the phrase "but you can't buy brains" is of interest. Apparently, the statement originated several years ago in a congressional hearing on the national medical research programs. The Congressmen who, like most Americans, were eager to expand our medical research effort asked certain high-ranking officers of the National Institutes of Health (NIH) why they had not requested more funds with which to do a better job. The reply was that all the available brains were already engaged in medical research, and since extra money could not buy extra brains that there was no need for more funds. This seemed strange to the many cancer researchers whose work had been slowed for years because of a chronic fund shortage. It also seemed strange to the Congressmen who investigated and found that these statements had been made by the officers of the NIH under orders of higher executive authority and did not represent the personal opinions of the persons making them. In effect, it appears that the Bureau of the Budget had decided to stop any further increases in expenditures for medical research and had arranged to have the Secretary of Health, Education, and Welfare order the officers of the NIH to make the statement. The reasons for this action by the Bureau of the Budget are not clear. Subsequently, the Chairman of the Congressional Committee, when questioning officers of the NIH on their budget requests, followed a procedure of first examining the official request and official statement, and then asking the witness to forget the Bureau of the Budget and his superiors and be honest with the committee (1). This testimony is described further in Chapter 9.

Unfortunately, the phrase "but you can't buy brains" has been echoed by others and has been used as a partial justification for the lack of growth of our cancer research program. Ironically, and tragically, some brains are being bought away from cancer research by other programs, which are not hampered by fund shortages.

Perhaps the best example of brain-buying comes from the space program. At the time when the political decision was made to launch a national space program there were only a handful of rocket and space experts in the nation. The offer of high salaries and virtually unlimited research funds and assistance recruited many scientists from various fields and disciplines into the space program. Brain-buying has become a permanent feature of the space program; it starts with the student in high school (2) and continues at all levels. Its effectiveness is evident in the accomplishments of the space program, regardless of one's opinion of the importance of space explorations.

The University of Missouri Space Sciences Research Center furnishes an example that probably represents a rather widespread practice at major universities. The Center is supported partly by state appropriations and partly by funds from the National Aeronautical and Space Administration (NASA). The staff of the Center have faculty appointments at the University of Missouri, but their salaries are considerably higher than those of regular faculty. They train

Ph.D. candidates and can offer them scholarships and fellowships, which are usually not available to students in other areas of science.

Some time ago, while interviewing some scientists who were being considered for positions at the University of Missouri Space Science Research Center, I found that one of the men to be interviewed was an outstanding cancer researcher whose reports I had often referred to and whose studies have formed the basis for some of my own ideas in cancer research. He had published outstanding articles in leading research journals including several in *Cancer Research*. I asked him why he was changing from a field as important as cancer to a new area. His reply was direct and forthright. First, he explained that as a family man he found the salary he received for cancer research inadequate, and space research would involve a substantial increase. Of greater importance was the difficulty he was experiencing in getting adequate research funds to pursue his cancer research program properly. The Center had offered him funds adequate to conduct a sound research program and he would not have to spend a large portion of his time and energy in fruitless and repetitive applications for research grants. He felt that he would rather do a good job in space biology research than be forced by shortages of funds to do an inadequate job in cancer research. This outstanding scientist is now working at the University of Missouri Space Science Research Center. Fortunately the director of that center has given him permission to do cancer experiments in his spare time.

We have no way of knowing in what numbers scientists move away from cancer research to better supported areas. On the basis of informal conversations and correspondence, I believe that the movement has become substantial. There can be little doubt that, in some areas of research, brains are being bought, and some are being bought away from cancer research.

References

1. *Hearings before a Subcommittee of the Committee on Appropriations, House of Representatives, Eighty-Ninth Congress*—Part 4—Department of Health, Education, and Welfare Appropriations for 1967, U. S. Government Printing Office, Washington, 1966, p. 345.
2. Peter, H. J., Angus, S. F. and Fes-sells, J. J. *7 Steps to a Career in Space Science and Technology*. High School Edition. U. S. Government Printing Office, Washington, 1966.

Relationship of Cancer Research Program to Other National Research Programs

The relationship of our present cancer research program to other national research programs is a complex one. The various programs often compete with each other for funds and skilled personnel, but in some ways they may aid and supplement each other. Furthermore, some of the other programs may provide useful examples for the cancer program, in terms of organization and effectiveness.

Each year the United States Government spends approximately 12 to 16 billion dollars on research. Accurate figures cannot be obtained because some of the research is secret and because some of it which is carried on within departmental budgets, is not readily identifiable. The largest research expenditure is for military purposes; developing better weapons, defenses and tactics. The nature of this program, naturally, is secret and little is known about it.

The research programs that are of interest in terms of interaction with cancer research programs are those in space, those related to atomic energy, those supported by the National Science Foundation (NSF), those carried out by agencies of the United States Public Health Service (USPHS) other than the National Cancer Institute (NCI), and certain newly proposed programs.

Space Research

The National Aeronautical and Space Administration (NASA) has for several years appeared to be the most favored of all government-supported research programs. The yearly appropriations for this activity—over 5 billion dollars per year from 1963 on—have been about 35 times as large as the appropriations for cancer research and about four times as large as the funds for all health-related research, including private and governmental resources. The first question that arises is whether the space program has taken up funds that otherwise would have gone to cancer research. This point has been a matter of some dispute. When the space program was first under consideration by the Congress, approximately one of its opponents was invited to testify before the Congressional Committee for every three or four proponents of the program. A general theme of the testimony against the space expenditures was that they would tend to reduce the funds available for other more important programs, such as cancer research. On the other hand, the backers of the space program contended that this was not the case. They said that if the funds were not appropriated for space research they would not be appropriated for any other research either—Congress would just keep the research budget low.

There is, of course, no way to prove what Congress would have done if the expenditures for the space program had not been so enormous. However, Figure 3-1 is suggestive. It demonstrates the relationship between appropriations for space and appropriations for cancer research. Between 1956 and 1963 there was a slow but steady increase in the funds appropriated by Congress for cancer and all other health-related research. In 1962 and 1963, there were tremendous jumps in the space appropriations, and the growth in cancer and other health-related research came to an end. Next, the appropriations for space continued at a plateau and the funds for cancer and other health-related research programs began to climb again, although at a slower rate. It is reasonable to assume that most people would consider this pattern to be the result of more than just chance and would conclude that the vast expenditures for space have in fact taken funds that under different circumstances would have been appropriated for cancer and other health-related research.

Unfortunately, since 1962, there has been no testimony concerning this point before the space committees of Congress because these committees have followed the policy of inviting testimony only from proponents of the space program, about 90 per cent of them being employees of NASA or its contractors. The opponents of expenditures for the space program have not been heard; it has also become difficult for them to have their letters published in some leading magazines and newspapers that carry large volumes of advertising for NASA contractors.

The competition between space and cancer research for trained scientists has been described in Chapter 2. Of particular significance is the competition for gifted students. The average college graduate does not have enough financial resources to pay for the four years of graduate study necessary to get a Ph.D. He must have some sort of help. If he takes a job as a teaching assistant, his progress toward his degree will be slow; it might take seven years instead of four.

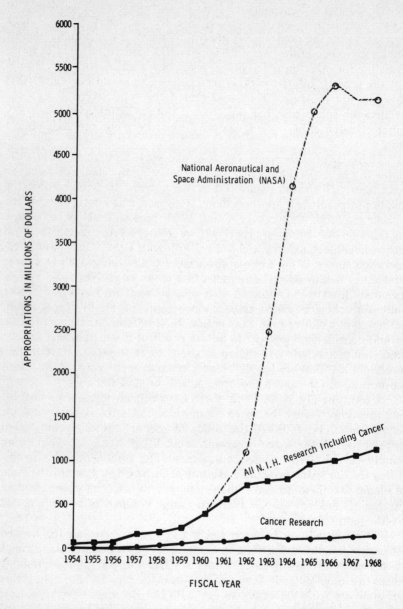

Figure 3–1. Appropriations for space and cancer research—1954–1968

Thus, he tries to get a fellowship that will pay his tuition and living expenses while he is studying. At this stage in his career he is rather easily influenced in his choice of research area if he is offered a fellowship. In 1965 NASA provided fellowships for over three thousand students working toward their doctoral degrees. In the same year the NCI was able to give financial support to only 181 students working toward their doctoral degrees (1). (It should be noted that the National Institute of General Medical sciences also supported 1,673 students working toward their doctorates. However, these were on the basis of discipline rather than disease-oriented programs, and the students on graduation, are at least as likely to go into space-related research as into cancer research.)

It seems important to determine why cancer research is at such a disadvantage compared to space research insofar as the Federal Government is concerned.

One reason for some of the difficulties encountered by the NCI is its status as a government agency. As of 1966, it is one of nine institutes within the National Institutes of Health (NIH) (2) which is one of four bureaus making up the Public Health Service (PHS). The PHS itself is one of seven divisions of the Department of Health, Education, and Welfare (HEW). Thus the NCI is rather far down on the list in terms of the interests of Secretary of HEW. Insofar as financial matters are involved, the NCI submits its proposed yearly budget which is based on the experience of its experts. This budget is routinely reduced at the next higher administrative level in the NIH. Then it is reduced again at the level of the PHS, and at the Department level a third reduction is made. Finally the mutilated budget proposal reaches the Bureau of the Budget where the biggest slash of all is made. If the leaders of the NCI wish to protest and argue against the cut by the Bureau of the Budget they must work their way up through the bureaucratic hierarchy and try to convince the Secretary of HEW to intercede for them. No one of lesser rank is likely to accomplish anything worthwhile in discussions with the Bureau of the Budget. Unfortunately the Secretary of HEW has not, in the past six years, shown much inclination to support the NCI. First, it is only one of many divisions for which he is responsible. Secondly, this office has never been held by a physician or a member of any group trained in or interested in medical areas or health. It has almost always been held by a lawyer whose major interest was in other areas of his domain. Some administrative changes are now being made in the Public Health Service structure, but they are far from adequate.

13

For years proposals have been made that the health functions of the Department be separated and put under a new cabinet member, a Secretary of Health. It has also been suggested that the Secretary of Health be a physician. The American Medical Association has supported these suggestions, but thus far, nothing constructive has been done about them.

By contrast, research missions of some other government agencies are in a far more favorable position. NASA is a separate, independent agency which is part of the Executive Office of the President. Thus the head of NASA does not have to work up through a bureaucratic overlay to get what he wants. He is not subordinate to any cabinet member and is on an equal footing, administratively, with the Director of the Bureau of the Budget. The only superiors of the Director of NASA are the President and Vice-President.

Figure 3-2 shows the comparison between NASA and the NCI in the administrative hierarchy as of the end of 1966. If the NCI en-

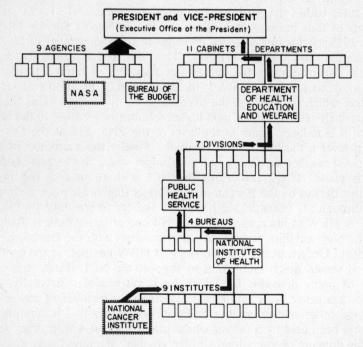

Figure 3–2. The relative positions of The National Cancer Institute and NASA in the Federal Government

joyed an administrative position comparable to NASA many of its problems would be lessened.

We must recognize, however, that only some of the difficulties encountered by the NCI have any relation to NASA. On the other hand, it may prove especially helpful to examine NASA not as an actual and potential rival for research funds and personnel, but as an example of a particularly successful organization, both in its relationship to the government and in its accomplishments. Such an examination may reveal much of importance not only to cancer research but to other medical research as well. Indeed, it is possible that enough of value may be learned from NASA to more than compensate for any deleterious effect that the space program has had on cancer research.

First, let us consider the relationship of NASA to the sources of power in the Federal Government.

The first and present administrator of NASA is a former Director of the Bureau of the Budget. It appears that appointing him to head NASA was a particularly brilliant move insofar as insuring sympathetic treatment for NASA's financial requests was concerned. It is hoped that in the future the leadership in any cancer research program will also include former officers of the Bureau of the Budget. The relationship of NASA to the President and Vice-President may be a bit more subtle. The practice of making the Vice-President directly responsible for the space program insures that program of a position favored above all others.

It would be helpful to know why Presidents and many Senators and Congressmen favor space research while paying so little attention to cancer research. Ostensibly, the reason would seem to be that we are in a space race with the Russians, and that our national interests require that we win that race in order to hold the respect of other nations. No doubt those who advance this argument are completely sincere in their support of it. In the 1967 NASA authorization hearings before the U. S. Senate Committee, discussion of and reference to the Russian space program appeared on over 40 pages scattered throughout the testimony. In contrast, there seems to have been virtually no consideration of the possible political impact of a Russian discovery of a cure for cancer. It should not be too difficult to imagine the reaction of people all over the world, including our friends and allies, to a future announcement that Russia had discovered a cure for cancer. One can also imagine the impact of the ensuing Russian propaganda, stating that while America concentrated on military and space research, Russia concentrated her resources on research designed to save life and promote health. This is not a particularly unlikely event, since Russian scientists are probably already ahead of ours in several areas of cancer research.

The preoccupation of American political leaders with space (and similar) research projects may be based on some psychologic considerations that have not yet been adequately aired. Since any speculation on psychologic motivations of public figures may be misleading, the hypothesis that I am offering is put forward in the most tentative fashion, largely in the hope of stimulating further discussion. I suggest that, in the minds of most people, major voyages and trips of exploration and discovery are associated with the heads of state to whom the explorers professed allegiance. For example, Columbus' explorations are readily associated with the rulers of Spain, Ferdinand and Isabella, and the Lewis and Clark expeditions with Thomas Jefferson. Yet it appears that chiefs of state are not usually identified with, or given a public share in the credit for, important medical discoveries. How many persons could identify the chief of state of France when Pasteur made his great discoveries? How many could identify the American President during whose term Joseph Goldberger, one of his subordinates in the Federal Government, discovered the cause and prevention of pellagra? In a sense, this situation is unfair to those heads of state and members of government in many nations who have encouraged and helped medical scientists. It is also unfortunate in terms of future governmental support for major medical research programs. When a President feels the need, whether because of external events or his own inner feelings, to set a major national research goal, he may be more likely to think in terms of physical exploration than medical research.

If this admittedly speculative hypothesis has any substance to it, the health professions ought to do what they can to give greater credit to government officials for medical discoveries made during their tenure of office. It would be helpful, as well as an acknowledgment of a real debt, if we named some of our medical and research institutions after political figures.

Effectiveness of NASA

The history of our national space program affords some excellent examples of vigorous, intelligent leadership, and of steady progress toward a clearly defined goal. When the space program was inaugurated, the United States had less than a dozen space scientists of international reputation and stature. We took some from Germany, converted other scientists to space work, and began to train new groups of scientists for space research. After less than 10 years, we have thousands of well-trained and qualified space scientists, and we are training thousands more. It was only a few years ago that there were many jokes and adverse comments about the failures of some of our rockets. Today, we expect each mission to succeed, and have become used to almost unbelievable precision and accuracy in orbital flights. These successes, however, did not just happen; they came from superior planning and utilization of resources.

A major factor in the progress of our space research has been the organization of the program into a series of projects, each directed by a full-time employee of NASA, and each having clearly defined goals. The code names of each project, such as Apollo, Gemini, Ranger, and Mariner, are widely recognized.

Although NASA does consider research projects suggested by individual scientists, and supports many of them, it does not depend on such suggestions for the direction and implementation of its primary goals. NASA utilizes what might be called the "task-force approach" to scientific problems, and has had great success with it. It is encouraging that the NCI is also beginning to utilize the task-force approach in certain aspects of its program.

Atomic Energy Research

When the atomic energy research program was inaugurated, great emphasis was placed on the potential value of such research in cancer. It was implied that since the radiation energies of certain radioactive materials were so much greater than those of x-rays, we could anticipate a tremendous increase in effectiveness of radiation therapy, with the consequent saving of many lives. Unfortunately, these implications turned out to be grossly exaggerated. A few institutions use radioactive cobalt to treat cancer patients and get reasonably good results. But few lives have been saved. Radioactive tracer materials have proven useful in certain aspects of cancer research, and it now appears that the atomic energy research program may make a real contribution to cancer and other medical research although the atomic energy program itself is still a military program.

National Science Foundation

The NSF was set up to help develop our national capacity in pure science. It sponsors and supports research in what might be called basic and intellectual areas. Thus it is likely to support a study on the reproduction of frogs, but would not ordinarily be expected to support

17

studies on experimental treatment of cancer in animals. The information obtained by NSF grantees may prove helpful to other scientists engaged in health research. The appropriations to NSF are quite small and the activities of this organization do not at this time compete significantly with cancer research for funds or personnel.

Other Institutes within the National Institutes of Health

There were, in 1966, eight other institutes within the NIH. They are operating in much the same way as the NCI. There is a certain degree of competition for funds and personnel, but this is more than compensated for by the mutual support and assistance that one Institute renders the others. In recent years, most of the other Institutes have also had their research programs held back by the Bureau of the Budget.

References

1. *Public Health Service Grants and Awards, Fiscal Year 1965 Funds, Part II. Training.* U. S. Dep't. of Health, Education, and Welfare, U. S. Gov't. Printing Office, Washington, p. 1.
2. *U. S. Gov't. Organization Manual, 1966-1967.* U. S. Gov't. Printing Office, Washington, 1966, p. 364, 360, 254.

Applied and Basic Research

There is a widespread concept that all research is worthwhile since it may, in some way, lead to future important discoveries. This concept contains an element of truth, but unfortunately that element is often exaggerated. It is appropriate to clarify some of the issues.

In the past, research has been divided into two general categories, applied research and basic research. Applied research involves an attempt to discover information of direct and immediate practical value. There is seldom much difficulty in recognizing applied research or in deciding how useful an applied research project has been.

In basic research, the results sought are not immediately practical, but instead knowledge is accumulated that may or may not be of value to future investigators. Unfortunately, anything can be called basic research if it does not produce immediately useful results, and usually that is what happens. It is frequently stated that no one can predict the eventual value of a piece of research; examples are given of basic research projects which seemed completely impractical when they were performed, but that later became the basis of some highly practical discovery. Although no one can accurately predict the eventual value of a single piece of basic research, it may be quite possible to predict with some degree of accuracy the eventual value of certain broad categories of basic research. For example, the chances seem good that basic research into the biology of viruses will eventually lead to important practical discoveries.

In other areas of science, basic astronomic studies of the moon or sun could be of considerable practical value in terms of understanding weather patterns on earth, and perhaps eventually learning to predict or even control hurricanes, tornadoes and so forth. By contrast, astronomic studies of quasars, which are millions of light years away from earth, are not likely to produce results of practical value for millions of years, no matter how exciting and challenging the quasars are to the astronomers.

One step in clarifying some of the confusion about research would be a new classification of research into three instead of two categories. The first category, *applied research,* would be the same as it is now.

The second category, *basic research,* would be used to describe studies having a reasonable chance of providing information that could help in or lead to an applied research project within a reasonable period, say 10 or 25 years.

The third category of research could be called *intellectual research.* This term would apply to research that has no immediate practical application and that does not seem likely to provide useful leads to future applied studies in a reasonable time. An example of intellectual research is research on high-energy physics. The high-energy particles to be studied do not ordinarily exist on earth and physicists who advocate studying them have no idea where such studies might lead them. It is, of course, possible that studies in high-energy physics might provide information useful to scientists a few hundred years from now. There is even a chance that high energy-physics research, like any other research project, would provide useful information within a reasonable period of time, but the chance is so small that it could hardly justify the expense involved.

In suggesting new categories for research, I am not unmindful of the difficulties that may arise when a particular project is to be put into a category. There will always be gray areas, but that is so in virtually any classification system. Furthermore, a project that is classified in one way at a particular time may be classified in another way at a different time. This too would not destroy the value of the system. Even our system of classifying animals changes over the years; several species of animals once put in one order have been reclassified into completely separate orders.

A new classification of types of research could clarify our thinking about the projects that merit support from taxpayers' funds. Elementary fairness requires that substantial expenditures of public funds, taken from people in all walks of life, should be used to benefit broad groups within the population rather than a few individuals.

Unfortunately, some scientists take a rather selfish (and shortsighted) view of the situation. One leading scientist is reported to have argued that . . . science was the highest flowering of civilization, and that it was not only the duty but the privilege of society to support scientists and their work. He is also reported to have regarded scientists as an elite class, with a privileged position. Since the common man was supposedly incapable of understanding what scientists were doing, he had no right to ask how his money was being spent (1).

Fortunately, most scientists are less extreme in their views, but according to Fischer (1):

. . . research for the sake of research alone is indeed what the scientist prizes most. In his ideal world, society would provide all competent scientists with all the money, equipment, and staff that they want; let them use these resources in any way they choose; and never ask what the payoff would be or when.

This may apply in certain branches of science, but it does not usually apply to medical scientists.

Let us note that no attempt is being made here to put a comparative *scientific* value on different kinds of studies. It is quite possible that a study classified as intellectual research could be so brilliant and elegant that most scientists would consider it a major intellectual achievement. This is quite another matter, however, than deciding to use large amounts of public funds to support such a project.

Nevertheless, proposals are being made by scientists in several areas for Federal support of research projects that would be classified as purely intellectual research. One such project, an enormous accelerator for study of high-energy physics, is already in the planning stage and will cost about $200 million for a single instrument—with total costs in the billions. It is difficult to see how this sort of project would benefit the taxpayer, and why some scientists and government officials consider it proper to use tax monies for such a project when other programs of great potential value to the citizen are hampered by fund shortages.

On the other hand, the use of large amounts of public funds for medical research seems fully justified since the major beneficiaries would be the people whose taxes are paying for the research.

References

1. Fischer, J. Why our scientists are about to be dragged, moaning, into politics. *Harpers Mag. 233:*19, 1966.

The Nature of Cancer

Cancer is a disease condition in which abnormal cells develop, multiply, and invade normal tissues, interfering with their function and eventually causing death unless, in some cases, adequate therapy is given early. There have been many misconceptions about cancer which have, in turn, probably led to errors in research approaches. It is therefore important to consider the cancer cell in some detail.

Kinds of Cancer

Cancer may develop in any type of tissue. In general, the term *carcinoma* is used to refer to a malignant growth that originates in cells that are epithelial in embryonic origin. This includes the cells of skin, mucous membranes, all glands, all outpocketings of the gastrointestinal tract (such as liver and lung), nerves, brain and some types of bone.

The term *sarcoma* is used to refer to a malignant growth that originates in cells of connective tissue origin. This includes the cells of cartilage, fatty tissue, some bone, nerve sheaths and so forth. Malignant tumors of muscle cell origin are also referred to as sarcomas. At times, the distinction between carcinoma and sarcoma is unclear; the terms are not always used in the classical sense. The appearance of a tumor may change, so that what was first thought to be a carcinoma later seems to be a sarcoma. In rare cases, both kinds of tumors may occur in a mixed form. Many forms of cancer have several names, and the terms carcinoma and sarcoma may or may not form part of the name.

Leukemias, which may be considered special types of cancer, are conditions in which the cells that produce the white blood cells (leukocytes) become malignant. The close relationship between leukemia and other cancers is brought out by the observation that in cattle some leukemias become lymphosarcomas, and that in mice one can produce either a leukemia or a lymphosarcoma by injecting malignant cells, depending on the site of injection.

Other, Related Terms

The word *tumor,* strictly speaking, merely means a swelling; thus, a boil or blister could be called a tumor. Cancers are a type of tumor, and sometimes the words are used synonymously, although this is confusing. There are many types of tumors that are benign, meaning that they do not invade normal tissues and do not metastasize.

A *neoplasm* is, strictly speaking, a new growth. This term is used to describe benign as well as cancerous growth.

The Causes of Cancer

The evidence available today indicates that cancer may be caused by any one of a number of agents. Many cancer-producing materials are found in the environment (1-11). Simple chemical elements, and their salts, produce cancer in man as well as animals (12-26). Many complex organic compounds are potent inducers of several kinds of cancer (27-65, 99). At least 500 different organic compounds have been shown to have cancer-producing properties. Radiation is another source of cancer—alpha rays, beta rays, gamma rays, x-rays, and some of the rays included in sunlight (66-73, 99). Some forms of cancer are believed by clinicians to result from chronic irritation. One type of cancer follows an infection with treponemas. Cancer of the bladder may be caused by infection with schistosomes (parasitic flat worms).

In recent years, there has been a growing interest in the theory that viruses may be possible cancer-inducing agents. In part, this interest has been sustained by the hope that if cancer is caused by one or more specific viruses, a vaccine might be produced to prevent cancer. It is known that viruses are the cancer-producing agents in several types of animal cancer (74-77) (*see also* Chapter 13). Since man is an animal, it would therefore not be surprising to find that viruses may produce cancer in man. In Burkitt's lymphoma, a type of cancer found in Africa, the epidemiologic patterns strongly suggest a viral cause, even though no virus has been definitely identified. There is some evidence that acute leukemias of children have a viral origin. For the vast majority of human cancers, however, there is no evidence of a viral cause. To be sure, this lack of evidence does not prove that viruses are not the cause of human cancers, but we must be guided by the facts available, and we do have rather convincing evidence that other agents besides viruses cause cancer. It might be argued that the other cancer-inducing agents act by making the host more susceptible to viruses. This would be stretching the facts to fit a theory, a procedure that usually is misleading.

There are cancers that are caused by the eating of certain nuts which grow on Guam (78-80), and others that are caused by contamination of food by fungi, or some chemicals used for processing foods (81, 82). Experimentally, some cancers can be produced in over 50 per cent of animals by imbedding smooth, intact, inert plastic films within the tissues (83-87). If the plastic has holes in it, cancers do not develop.

In all likelihood, there are other causes of cancer of which we are not yet aware.

Rate of Multiplication of Cancer Cells

Until recently, it was widely believed, in medical as well as in lay circles, that cancer cells multiplied at excessively rapid rates, significantly more rapid than the multiplication rate of normal body cells. It is easy to understand how this concept arose when we consider the feelings of patients, families and doctors who have watched the progressive growth of a cancer. Our increasing understanding of normal physiology has cast a new light on relative multiplication rates of normal and cancerous cells.

It seems valid to make two types of comparison of multiplication rates: first, between cancer cells and normal cells that are absolutely necessary to life; second, between cancer cells and the normal cells from which they are derived. The first comparison is important in order to evaluate the possible effects of drugs and procedures that kill young, rapidly multiplying cells. If cancer cells do in fact multiply more rapidly than all the kinds of cells that are necessary to life, then drugs designed to kill rapidly reproducing cells have a reasonable chance of curing cancer. However, if cancer cells do not multiply more rapidly than all the kinds of cells essential to life, then drugs that kill rapidly multiplying cells could not be given in a dose adequate to kill all cancer cells—such doses would also kill the patient.

Let us, therefore, consider the rates at which some normal cells multiply.

In an adult human being, the red blood cells are produced by the multiplication of certain progenitors in the bone marrow. There are approximately 5 million red blood cells in a cubic millimeter of blood. This comes to 5 billion per cubic centimeter, 5 trillion per liter, and 25 trillion in the 5 liters of blood present in an average adult. These red blood cells have an average life span of about 120 days. Therefore, since the blood count remains fairly uniform in health, the average healthy adult will, in a 120-day period, produce 25 trillion red blood cells to make up for the 25 trillion that die. As there are 10,368,000 seconds in 120 days the number of red blood cells produced *per second* in the normal adult body is $\dfrac{25,000,000,000,000}{10,368,000}$, or approximately 2,400,000! This means that every *second,* day and night, the normal body produces about 2,400,000 red blood cells. In a similar fashion, we can calculate that, in a year, the normal adult body produces approximately 18 pounds of red blood cells. (Some idea of the mass involved can be visualized by looking at an 18 pound turkey.) There are few, if any cancers that grow to a mass of 18 pounds in a year. This is not the entire story, however. The rates of red blood cell production presented above apply to the normal body, not the body under stress. Under certain circumstances, such as blood loss after an accident or operation, an adult may produce red blood cells at a rate of more than 5 times the normal resting rate. Few, if any cancers can approach such rates of cell production.

Another example of cells that normally multiply rapidly is found in the lining of the gastrointestinal tract, from mouth to rectum. In many areas of the tract, these cells multiply so rapidly that the entire lining is replaced in less than 24 hours, and this turnover continues throughout most of one's life-span. The cells of the bone marrow and those lining the gastrointestinal tract are both essential to life. Accordingly, it seems that medications and procedures aimed at killing young, rapidly multiplying cells will probably not kill all cancer cells before they kill the patient. A number of chemical agents that do kill young, rapidly multiplying cells have been tried, and some are still used for palliation of some cancers. However, the limiting factor in their use, as might have been predicted, is damage to bone marrow and the lining of the gastrointestinal tract, often resulting in serious internal bleeding.

A comparison between the multiplication rate of cancer cells and the normal cells from which they are derived is of interest since it helps provide some understanding of what cancer is and what it is not. There are some normal cells which do not multiply at appreciable rates in the adult—those of the brain, heart, and kidneys, for example; therefore, cancers of these organs consist of cells that do multiply at rates greater than those of the normal parent cells. Liver cells can multiply at fairly rapid rates in the adult, in response to injury. Cells of liver cancer multiply at rates that are roughly comparable to the rates of the normal parent cell. Finally, there are normal cells that multiply at quite rapid rates in the adult, such as those lining the intestine, and those of the skin. Many cancers that stem from intestinal and skin epithelium tend to multiply at rates that are much slower than the rate of multiplication of the normal parent cell; for example, the fairly common basal cell cancer of the skin of the face.

A rather unusual example of normal cells multiplying at extremely rapid rates can be seen in the antlers of the deer and elk. These antlers are true bone. In an adult male elk, a mass of 20 to 50 pounds of bone can be grown in a few months, and then shed (88). Microscopic sections of rapidly growing antlers have certain resemblances to cancer, but they are perfectly benign growths (89, 90). It is of some additional interest that deer and elk antlers have never been reported to develop into cancers; indeed, bone cancer of any sort is almost non-existent in deer or elk. As a result, we cannot state with certainty that the normal bone cells in the antler multiply more rapidly than the cells of bone cancers would multiply *in deer or elk*. However, we can state that the normal cells in antlers do multiply at rates which exceed any multiplication rates reported for bone cancer cells in any species including man.

In summary, the evidence suggests rather strongly that rapidity of growth and rate of multiplication are not the features that differentiate cancer cells from normal cells.

Invasion of Normal Tissues

Cancer cells differ from almost all normal cells in their ability to invade normal tissues (91-98). If a group of non-cancerous cells begins to multiply and form a mass, that mass may push against normal cells. This occurs with some benign tumors. But the non-cancerous cells do not, with exceptions to be noted, push *between* normal cells. The cancer cells do, and it is this characteristic that accounts for the fact that the crab, with its claws embedded in the host's tissues, represents cancer. The word "cancer," of course, means crab in Greek.

It is not yet clear just how the cancer cells manage to invade normal tissues. A commonly held theory is that they behave somewhat like amebae, pushing pseudopodia between normal cells, and then flowing through the gap (93, 95, 97). Perhaps this does occur, but if it does, the existence of an additional mechanism seems likely. Normal cells do not merely abut one another; they are attached to one another by a fairly strong intercellular cement and are imbedded in a gel-like matrix. If the cancer cell passes through this barrier, it must have some mechanism for dissolving this cement. A number of investigators (*see* Chapter 21) have reported finding an enzyme, liberated by cancer cells, that makes permeable the matrix in which the normal cells lie.

There are two types of normal cells that can pass through normal tissues. The white blood cells (leukocytes) move rapidly between normal cells in response to local infection or irritation; their remains constitute pus. However, the normal white blood cells in the blood stream and tissues do not have the ability to multiply. Therefore, they do not produce a situation similar to cancer. The ability of the white blood cells to pass through cellular barriers appears to be dependent on ameboid movement, but there is also some evidence that they secrete enzymes that dissolve tissue barriers. Here again, our research effort is moving slowly.

Other normal cells that invade normal tissue are the trophoblast cells of the placenta that invade the wall of the uterus. Their function is to develop an intimate link between mother and fetus, so that, when the blood vessels of the placenta proliferate, maternal nutrients and oxygen, and fetal wastes, can be exchanged. At the end of pregnancy, the trophoblast is cast off as part of the placenta or afterbirth. A major difference between trophoblast and cancer is that the trophoblast invades the uterus to a limited extent only. Some scientists have been impressed by the superficial resemblances of the trophoblast and cancer, and have postulated that cancers are derived from cells that have either regressed to a primitive trophoblastic stage, or that they are tiny remnants of the original trophoblast. This interpretation of the nature of cancer has serious flaws. The trophoblast is a structure that occurs only in mammals. Cancers, on the other hand, occur, and may even be quite common in such lower forms of life as reptiles, amphibia, and fish, which do not develop a trophoblast and have no need for one. There can be little doubt that there were cancer cells in animals hundreds of millions of years before there were trophoblast cells.

Metastasis

Cancer cells have the ability to migrate to other parts of the body through lymphatic and blood vessels and to grow in the new location. The process is called *metastasis,* and the secondary growths are called *metastases.* It is this property of cancer that makes it so difficult to treat.

The cancer cells have much less cohesiveness than normal cells, and tend to break away from the cancer mass. Some penetrate the lymphatic vessels, and are carried along the lymphatics until they reach the lymph nodes where all or most are, in effect, strained out. But some of them grow and multiply while in the lymph nodes and, after a period of time, new generations of cancer cells migrate from the lymph node to lymphatic channels that may then carry them to the various internal organs and tissues.

Cancer cells that invade the blood vessels in or near the cancer mass are carried along the blood stream until they lodge in a capillary at some distance from the original cancer. Some of them then grow and multiply, producing new masses of cancer cells in the new locations. At one time, it was believed that metastasis occurred rather late in the course of cancer, that only a small number of cancer cells metastasized, and that most of the migrating cancer cells multiplied and formed metastatic nodules. Recent evidence suggests that this is not the situation. Apparently, cells begin to leave the parent cancer and get into the blood stream and lymphatics when the original cancer is still quite small, often when it is too small to be diagnosed. There are large numbers of these migrating cancer cells, but almost all of them die; only a very small fraction of one per cent survive and produce a metastatic growth. When the parent cancer is small, the chances that any of the migrating cells will multiply seem to be quite small. But as the parent cancer grows larger, the chances that the circulating cancer cells will multiply and produce metastases apparently increase. The mechanism of this effect is not understood. It may be related to the total number of cancer cells released into the general circulation, or it may be based on other factors not yet determined.

The pattern of distribution of metastases to the various parts of the body depends to a large extent on the nature of the primary cancer. Some kinds of cancer metastasize mainly through lymphatic channels, while others metastasize through the blood vessels. Some tumors metastasize primarily to the lung, others to the brain, or liver, or bone. Often metastases are found in several different sites. There are some curious patterns to metastases. It is easy to understand why the lungs, through which all the blood flows, become a site of metastases when the cancer cells lodge in a capillary. However, it is not clear why certain other tissues and organs that have many blood vessels are so often spared by metastases. The mass of skeletal muscle and the volume of its blood and lymphatic supply are so large that, if the sites of metastases were based merely on the mechanical

28

factor of straining out, we would expect many more metastases to skeletal muscle than are actually found. Apparently, the pattern of metastasis depends not only on the anatomy of the blood and lymphatic vessels but also on the nature of the tissues and organs in which the migrating cancer cells lodge. Some seem to be "more fertile soil" than others.

The Blood Supply of Cancer

Our understanding of the blood supply of cancer has changed and expanded considerably in the past 20 years. However, it is interesting to note that some observations and suggestions made more than 50 years ago by Walker and Whittingham (Chapter 18) have since been confirmed, and may prove to be of vital importance in the treatment of cancer. At one time, it was generally believed that there were few blood vessels in cancers. This belief resulted from observations on large numbers of cancers that were removed at surgery or autopsy, fixed in formalin, stained, sectioned, and studied under a microscope. However, some subsequent studies by several scientists (Chapter 19) showed that cancers actually have a widespread system of blood vessels. Most of these vessels have extremely thin walls—one cell thick—and are much larger than capillaries in diameter. Such vessels are called sinusoids. In life, they are kept open by the pressure of the blood, but when the cancer is removed, the blood pressure within it, of course, falls to zero, and the sinusoids collapse. On microscopic examination of a fixed section, one sees only some thin cells, since the lumen of the vessel is gone. In recent years, studies of living cancers, still in the host, have been done with ingenious techniques (see Chapter 19), and these studies showed that within the cancers there was a large number of sinusoids filled with blood. Thus there is convincing evidence that, for most cancers, the number and volume of blood vessels is high in relation to the rest of the body, and that, during life, the cancers contain large volumes of blood. It might seem at first that this would mean that cancers are well supplied with oxygen and nutrients, but such is not the case. The sinusoids are irregular and tortuous, and there are many cross-channels between them; as a result, the blood flows through them sluggishly. Some studies show that a gram of cancer receives much less blood per minute than the normal internal organs in which the cancers grow. Thus, most of the cancer cells live at low oxygen levels (hypoxia).

The inefficient blood flow through cancers may account for the inability to cure most cancers with chemotherapeutic agents that are highly effective in the test tube. If the anti-cancer drug does not reach the cancer readily, it cannot be effective. On the other hand, methods have been suggested that might markedly increase the efficiency of blood circulation to cancers for a short time. This will be discussed further in Chapter 20.

Another aspect of the blood supply to cancers is the genesis of the blood vessels that supply the cancer. A number of scientists have observed a proliferation of these vessels by the host, and several have suggested that the cancer secretes some chemical that stimulates the formation of blood vessels. This, too, may prove to be a useful research approach (Chapter 19).

For many years, it was generally believed that cancers had a glycolytic metabolism different from normal cells, and that the difference had been experimentally established. More recent evidence (100, 101) suggests that the glycolytic metabolism of cancer cells may not be different from that of normal cells. This does not mean that cancer cells are the same as normal cells in their metabolism: it means that we have no convincing evidence as to what any difference may be. It would be prudent to assume that significant differences exist, but these differences may be too subtle for our present biochemical techniques to identify.

References

1. Lynch, K. M. and Smith, W. A. Pulmonary asbestosis: Carcinoma of lung in asbesto-silicosis. *Am. J. Cancer 24:*56, 1935.
2. Dobrovolskaia-Zavadskaia, N. The constitution and the outside causes in the origin of various cancers. *Acta Union Internat.* Contre Cancrum *5:*55, 1940.
3. Dobrovolskaia-Zavadskaia, N. Heredity and environmental factors in the origin of different cancers. *J. Genetics 40:*157, 1940.
4. Doll, R. Mortality from lung cancer in asbestos workers. *Brit. J. Industr. Med. 12:* 81, 1955.
5. Peacock, P. R. Carcinogenesis. In *Cancer*—vol. 1. Edited by Raven, R. W. Butterworth, London, 1957, pp. 32-75.
6. Doll, R. Occupational lung cancer; a review. *Brit. J. Industr. Med. 16:*181, 1959.
7. Hieger, I. *Carcinogenesis.* Academic Press, London, 1961.
8. Clayson, D. B. *Chemical Carcinogenesis.* Boston, Little, Brown and Co., 1962, p. 107.
9. Payne, W. W. Occupational factors in carcinogenesis. *Pub. Health Rep. 81:*777, 1966.
10. National Advisory Cancer Council—*Progress Against Cancer*—1966—U. S. Dep't. of Health, Education and Welfare, Washington, p. 44.
11. National Advisory Cancer Council—*Progress Against Cancer*—1966—U. S. Dep't. of Health, Education and Welfare, Washington, p. 56.

12. Neuman, D. A case of adeno-carcinoma of the left inferior turbinate body and perforation of the nasal septum in the person of a worker in chrome pigment. *Glasgow Med. J. 33:*469, 1890.
13. Barnes, J. M., Benz, F. A. and Sissons, H. A. Beryllium bone sarcomata in rabbits. *Brit. J. Cancer 4:*212, 1950.
14. Gardner, L. V. and Heslington, H. F. Osteo-sarcoma from intravenous beryllium compounds in rabbits. *Fed. Proc. 5:*221, 1946.
15. Heath, I. C. Cobalt as a carcinogen. *Nature 173:*822, 1954.
16. Hueper, W. C. Experimental studies in metal cancerogenesis. I. Nickel cancers in rats. *Texas Rep. Biol. and Med. 10:*167, 1952.
17. Hueper, W. C. Experimental studies in metal cancerogenesis. IV. Cancer produced by parenterally introduced metallic nickel. *J. Nat. Cancer Inst. 16:*55, 1955.
18. Oppenheimer, B. S., Oppenheimer, E. T., Danishefsky, I. and Stout, A. P. Carcinogenic effect of metals in rodents. *Cancer Res. 16:*439, 1956.
19. Hoagland, M. B., Grier, R. S. and Hood, M. B. Beryllium and growth. I. Beryllium-induced osteogenic sarcomata. *Cancer Res. 10:*629, 1950.
20. Oppenheimer, B. S., Oppenheimer, E. T., Danishefsky, I. and Stout, A. P. Carcinogenic effects of metals in rodents. *Cancer Res. 16:*439, 1956.
21. Hueper, W. C. and Payne, W. W. Experimental cancers in rats produced by chromium compounds and their significance to industry and public health. *Amer. Industr. Hyg. Assoc. J. 20:*274, 1959.
22. Payne, W. W. Production of cancers in mice and rats by chromium compounds. *AMA Arch. Industr. Health 21:*530, 1960.
23. Hueper, W. C. Experimental studies in metal cancerogenesis. IV. Cancer produced by parenterally introduced metallic nickel. *J. Nat. Cancer Inst. 16:*55, 1955.
24. Gilman, J. P. W. and Ruckerbauer, G. M. Metal carcinogenesis. I. Observations on the carcinogenicity of a refinery dust, cobalt oxide, and colloidal thorium dioxide. *Cancer Res. 22:*152, 1962.
25. Gilman, J. P. W. Metal carcinogenesis. II. A study of the carcinogenic activity of cobalt, copper, iron and nickel compounds. *Cancer Res. 22:*158, 1962.
26. Payne, W. W. Carcinogenicity of nickel compounds in experimental animals. *Proc. Amer. Assoc. Cancer Res. 5:*50, 1964.
27. Orr, J. W. The changes antecedent to tumour formation during the treatment of mouse skin with carcinogenic hydrocarbons. *J. Path. and Bact. 46:*495, 1938.
28. Maltoni, C. and Prodi, G. Studio istologico sulla sarcogenesi sperimentale da 20-metilcolantrene in ratto. (Histological study on experimental 20-methylcholanthrene carcinogenesis in the rat.) *Tumori 43:*455, 1957.
29. Falk, H. L., Kotin, P. and Mehler, A. Polycyclic hydrocarbons as carcinogens for man. *Arch. Environ. Health 8:*721, 1964.
30. Hendricks, N. V., Berry, C. M., Lione, J. G. and Thorpe, J. J. Cancer of the scrotum in wax pressmen. I. Epidemiology. *AMA Arch. Industr. Health 19:*524, 1959.
31. Van Duuren, B. L., et al. Carcinogenicity of epoxides, lactones and peroxy compounds. *J. Nat. Cancer Inst. 31:*41, 1963.
32. Videbaek, A. Chlornaphazin (Erysan) may induce cancer of the urinary bladder. *Acta. Med. Scand. 176:*45, 1964.
33. Andervont, H. B. and Dunn, T. B. Response of mammary-tumorfree strain of DBA female mice to percutaneous application of methylcholanthreme. *J. Nat. Cancer Inst. 10:*895, 1950.
34. Bao-Syan, Ou. Changes in connective tissue in the rabbit ear during development of tumours induced by 9:10-dimethyl-1:2-benzanthracene. *Byull, Eksper. Biol. I. Med. 55:*83, 1963.

35. Biancifiori, C., Giornelli-Santilli, F. E., Milia, U. and Severi, L. Pulmonary tumours in rats induced by oral hydrazine sulphate. *Nature 212:*414, 1966.
36. Ghadially, F. N. and Roy, S. Experimentally produced synovial sarcomas. *Cancer 19:*1901, 1966.
37. Wilson, R. H., DeEds, F. and Cox, A. J., Jr. The toxicity and carcinogenic activity of 2-Acethaminofluorene. *Cancer Res. 1:*595, 1941.
38. Fare, G. Rat skin carcinogenesis by topical applications of some azo dyes. *Cancer Res. 26:*2406, 1966.
39. Haddow, A. and Robinson, A. M. The association of carcinogenicity and growth-inhibitory power in the polycyclic hydrocarbons and other substances. *Proc. Roy. Soc.* Series B. *127:*277, 1939.
40. Ranadive, K. J. and Hakim, S. A. The chemical induction of mammary cancer in four inbred strains of mice. *Indian J. Med. Res. 47:*123, 1959.
41. Vol'fson, N. I. Influence of certain androgen preparations on development of mammary carcinoma in mice. *Prob. of Oncology* (Russ. Eng. transl.) *4:*571, 1958.
42. Weisburger, E. K. and Weisburger, J. H. Chemistry, carcinogenicity, and metabolism of 2-fluorenamine and related compounds. *Adv. Cancer Res. 5:*331, 1958.
43. Potter, J. S., Taylor, M. J. and MacDowell, E. C. Tumor-specific immunity to transplanted dibenz (a-h)-anthracene-induced sarcomas. *Cancer Res. 20:*1614, 1960.
44. Sabes, W. R., Chaudhry, A. P. and Gorlin, R. J. Effects of cortisone on chemical carcinogenesis in hamster pouch and submandibular salivary gland. *J. Dent. Res. 42:*1118, 1963.
45. Kennaway, E. L. and Hieger, I. Carcinogenic substances and their fluorescence spectra. *Brit. Med. J. 1:*1044, 1930.
46. Cook, J. W., Hieger, I., Kennaway, E. L. and Mayneord, W. V. The production of cancer by pure hydrocarbons. *Proc. Royal Soc.,* Series, B. *111:*455, 1932.
47. Cook, J. W., Hewett, C. L. and Hieger, I. The isolation of a cancer-producing hydrocarbon from coal tar. *J. Chem. Soc. 1:*395, 1933.
48. Shubki, P. and Hartwell, J. L. *Survey of Compounds that have been Tested for Carcinogenic activity.* PHS Publication No. 149, Supp. 1, U. S. Government Printing Office, Washington, D. C., 1957.
49. Hueper, W. C., Wiley, F. and Wolfe, H. D. Experimental production of bladder tumors in dogs by administration of betanaphthylamine. *J. Industr. Hyg. Toxicol. 20:*49, 1938.
50. Kotin, P. and Falk, H. Production of tumors. C57 black mice with atmospheric-extracted aliphatic hydrocarbons. *Proc. Amer. Assoc. Cancer Res. 2:*30, 1955.
51. Weisburger, E. K. Carcinogenicity of alkylating agents. *Public Health Rep. 81:* 772, 1966.
52. Magee, P. N. and Barnes, J. M. The production of malignant primary hepatic tumours in the rat by feeding dimethylinitrosamine. *Brit. J. Cancer 10:*114, 1956.
53. Argus, M. F. and Hoch-Ligeti, C. Comparative study of the carcinogenic activity of nitrosamines. *J. Nat. Cancer Inst. 27:*695, 1961.
54. Kelly, M. G., *et al.* Induction of hepatic cell carcinomas in monkeys with N-nitrosodiethylamine. *J. Nat. Cancer Inst. 36:*323, 1966.
55. Colburn, N. H. and Boutwell, R. K. The binding of β-propiolactone to mouse skin deoxyribonucleic acid *in vivo;* its correlation with tumor-initiating activity. *Cancer Res. 26:*1701, 1966.
56. Magee, P. N. and Farber, E. Toxic liver injury and carcinogenesis. Methylation of rat-liver nucleic acids by dimethylnitrosamine *in vivo. Biochem. J. 83:*114, 1962.
57. Liebelt, A. G. The carcinogenic effects of 3-methylcholanthrene (MC) fed to inbred mice. *Proc. Am. Assoc. Cancer Res. 3:*130, 1960.

58. Leiter, J. and Shear, M. J. Quantitative experiments on the production of sub-cutaneous tumors in strain A mice with marginal doses of 3,4-benzpyrene. *J. Nat. Cancer Inst. 3:*455, 1943.
59. Lewis, W. H. Dibenzanthracene mouse sarcomas. *Am. J. Cancer 37:*521, 1939.
60. Shimkin, M. B. and Bryan, W. R. Morphology and growth of subcutaneous tumors induced with carcinogenic hydrocarbons in strain C3H male mice. *J. Nat. Cancer Inst. 4:*25, 1943-1944.
61. Stewart, H. L. Tumors induced by subcutaneously injected carcinogens. *Bull. Hosp. Joint Dis. 12:*131, 1951.
62. Lacassagne, A., Zajdela, F., Buu Hoi, N. P. and Chalvet, M. H. Sur l'activité cancerogène du 3.4-9.10-dibenzopyrène et de quelques-uns de ses dérivés. *Compt. rend. Soc. de Biol. 244:*273, 1957.
63. Allen, M. J., Boyland, E., Dukes, C. E., Horning, E. S. and Watson, J. G. Cancer of the urinary bladder induced in mice with metabolites of aromatic amines and tryptophan. *Brit. J. Cancer 11:*212, 1957.
64. Boyland, E. and Watson, G. 3-Hydroxyanthranilic acid, a carcinogen produced by endogenous metabolism. *Nature 177:*837, 1956.
65. Weil, C. S., Carpenter, C. P. and Smyth, H. F., Jr. Urinary bladder calculus and tumor response following either repeated feeding of diethylene glycol or calcium oxalate stone implantation. *Indust. Med. and Surg. 36:*55, 1967.
66. Cater, D. B., Baserga, R. and Lisco, H. Studies on the induction of bone and soft tissue tumours in rats by gamma irradiation and the effect of growth hormone and thyroxine. *Brit. J. Cancer 13:*214, 1959.
67. Lange, R. D., Moloney, W. C. and Yamawaki, T. Leukemia in atomic bomb survivors. I. General observations. *Blood 9:*574, 1954.
68. Folley, J. H., Borges, W. and Yamawaki, T. Incidence of leukemia in survivors of atomic bomb in Hiroshima and Nagasaki, Japan. *Am. J. Med. 13:*311, 1952.
69. Bizzozero, O. J., Jr., Johnson, K. G. and Ciocco, A. Radiation-related leukemia in Hiroshima and Nagasaki, 1946-1964. I. Distribution, incidence and appearance time. *New Eng. J. Med. 274:*1095, 1966.
70. MacMahon, B. Prenatal x-ray exposure and childhood cancer. *J. Nat. Cancer Inst. 28:*1173, 1962.
71. Simpson, C. L., Hempelmann, L. H., and Fuller, L. M. Neoplasia in children treated with x-rays in infancy for thymic enlargement. *Radiology 64:*840, 1955.
72. Court Brown, W. A. and Abbatt, J. D. Incidence of leukemia in ankylosing spondylitis treated with x-rays: preliminary report. *Lancet 1:*1283, 1955.
73. Blum, H. F. Relationships between spontaneous tumors of the lung and cutaneous tumors induced with ultraviolet radiation in strain A mice. *J. Nat. Cancer Inst. 5:* 89, 1944.
74. Rous, P. Transmission of a malignant new growth by means of a cell-free filtrate. *J.A.M.A. 56:*198, 1911.
75. Rous, P. A sarcoma of the fowl transmissible by an agent separable from the tumor cells. *J. Exp. Med. 13:*397, 1911.
76. Rous, P. Resistance to a tumor-producing agent as distinct from resistance to the implanted tumor cells. Observations with a sarcoma of the fowl. *J. Exp. Med. 18:* 416, 1913.
77. Dulbecco, R. Viral carcinogenesis. *Cancer Res. 21:*975, 1961.
78. Laqueur, G. L., Mickelsen, O., Whiting, M. and Kurland, L. T. Carcinogenic properties of nuts from Cycas circinalis L. Indigenous to Guam. *J. Nat. Cancer Inst. 31:*919, 1963.

79. Laqueur, G. L. Carcinogenic effects of cycad meal and cycasin, methylazoxy-methanol glycoside, in rats and effects of cycasin in germ-free rats. *Fed. Proc.* *23:*1386, 1964.
80. National Advisory Cancer Council—*Progress Against Cancer—1966*—U. S. Dep't. of Health, Education and Welfare, Washington, p. 58.
81. Kraybill, H. F. and Shimkin, M. B. Carcinogenesis related to foods contaminated by processing and fungal metabolites. *Adv. Cancer Res. 8:*191, 1964.
82. National Advisory Cancer Council—*Progress Against Cancer—1966*—U. S. Dep't. of Health, Education and Welfare, Washington, p. 57.
83. Oppenheimer, B. I., Oppenheimer, E. T., Stout, A. P., Willhite, M. and Danishefsky, J. The latent period in carcinogenesis by plastics in rats and its relation to the pre-sarcomatous stage. *Cancer 11:*204, 1958.
84. Oppenheimer, B. S., Oppenheimer, E. T., Stout, A. P., Willhite, M. and Danishefsky, I. The latent period in carcinogenesis by plastics in rats and its relation to the pre-sarcomatous stage. *Cancer 11:*204, 1958.
85. Oppenheimer, E. T., Willhite, M., Stout, A. P., Danishefsky, I. and Fishman, M. M. A comparative study of the effects of imbedding cellophane and polystyrene films in rats. *Cancer Res. 24:*379, 1964.
86. Bates, R. R. and Klein, M. Importance of a smooth surface in carcinogenesis by plastic film. *J. Nat. Cancer Inst. 37:*145, 1966.
87. Bates, R. R. and Klein, M. Importance of a smooth surface in carcinogenesis by plastic film. *J. Nat. Cancer Inst. 37:*145, 1966.
88. Personal communications—Fish and Game Bureaus—Idaho, Montana and Colorado.
89. Modell, W. and Noback, C. Histogenesis of bone in the growing antler of the cervidae. *Am. J. Anat. 49:*65, 1931.
90. Aub, J. C. and Wislocki, G. A comparison of the growth of deer antler and of osteogenic sarcoma. *Cancer Res. 3:*120, 1943.
91. Bierich, R. Über die Vorgänge beim Einwuchern der Krebszellen. (The invasiveness of tumor cells.) *Klin. Wschr. 6:*1599, 1927.
92. Willis, R. A. *The Spread of Tumours in the Human Body* (2nd Ed). Butterworth, London, 1952.
93. Hirono, I. Amoeboid motility of the ascites hepatoma cells and its significance for their invasiveness and metastatic spread. *Cancer Res. 18:*1345, 1958.
94. Vasilief, Ju. M. The role of connective tissues proliferation in invasive growth of normal and malignant tissues: A review. *Brit. J. Cancer 12:*524, 1958.
95. Willis, R. A. *Pathology of Tumours* (3rd Ed.). Butterworth, London, 1960.
96. Brennan, M. J. and Simpson, W. L. (Ed.) *Biological Interactions In Normal and Neoplastic Growth.* Churchill, London, 1962.
97. Cameron, E. *Hyaluronidase and Cancer.* Pergamon Press, Oxford, 1966, p. 16.
98. Coman, D. R. Mechanism of invasiveness of cancer. *Science 105:*347, 1947.
99. Mueller, G. C. Current aspects of cancer research. *Am. J. Pub. Health 51:*6, 1961.
100. Pitot, H. C. Some biochemical aspects of malignancy. *Ann. Rev. Biochem. 35:* 618, 1966.
101. Hiatt, H. H. Cancer chemotherapy—present status and prospects. *New Eng. J. Med. 276:*157, 1967.

Other Important Features of Cancer

In this chapter, we will consider certain aspects of cancer which may be less fundamental than those described in the preceding chapter. The potential importance of some of these characteristics is not known, but there is a definite possibility that one or more may be important in the search for an effective treatment for the disease.

The Growth Pattern of Cancer

Although the growth rates of cancers are not distinctive when compared to the growth rates of normal body cells, they are still of great importance and interest; a cancer that required 100 years to reach a substantial size would, of course, be harmless. Studies on the growth rates of cancers might provide clues which could enable us to find a way to slow or even stop such growth. It is well known that the growth rates of different kinds of cancers differ widely, and that the same general type of cancer often has a different growth rate in one patient than in another. There is convincing evidence that the growth rate of some types of cancers is influenced by hormones. Cancer of the prostate usually grows more rapidly when male hormones are circulating in the blood, and more slowly when female hormones are present. Some of the cancers of the female sex organs are also influenced by hormones, but the relationship is a complex one, and not always predictable in an individual patient. For most cancers, however, we do not know what factors stimulate or retard growth.

For many years, it was assumed that the growth rates of a particular cancer in an individual patient were fairly constant over the entire time-period of the cancer process. This assumption was based on the rate of multiplication seen in bacteria. If a single bacterium is placed in a large volume of the proper culture medium, it will divide into two bacteria in a unit of time, depending on the combination of such factors as temperature, nutrient mixture and so forth, which influence bacterial multiplication. If it takes one hour for a particular bacterium to multiply, there will be two in an hour, four in two hours, eight in three hours, 16 in four hours, 32 in five hours and so on,

35

until the external environment changes. Usually, in bacterial cultures, the change consists of either an exhaustion of a necessary nutrient, or excessive concentration of a toxic waste product, or both. At such a time, the multiplication rate suddenly falls abruptly. For a long time it was assumed that multiplication of cancer cells followed a similar geometric pattern, that this pattern remained essentially unchanged throughout the life of the cancer, and that it furnished a valid basis for calculating the probable time of origin of human cancers. Using this hypothesis as the basis for their calculations, scientists assumed that by the time cancers are large enough to be diagnosed, they have been present but too small to be found, for anywhere from five to eight years. Recently the studies of Laird have cast considerable doubt on the validity of such calculations (1, 2). She used some novel and powerful mathematical analyses to demonstrate that the rate of cancer growth is not steady, that at first it is high, but that it slows down as the cancer grows larger. Of particular importance are Laird's deductions that the pattern of slowing of growth rate in cancer cells is different from that of cells in bacterial cultures, and that the reduction in the growth rate of cancer cells is due to some form of host resistance. She brings out a most important point in terms of finding a control for cancer, stating (1):

> Search for natural growth-regulating mechanisms is of practical importance, because the clinical disease of cancer in both animals and humans, i.e., the systemic illness and death of the host, is limited to the time of the last two or three doublings of tumor size. Thus for most tumors a relatively small stimulation of growth-retarding factors might prevent a tumor from reaching the physiologic limit of host survival, with the consequence that the systemic illness might be delayed, or even in some cases eliminated, if the delay should exceed the normal life-expectancy of the host.

Other studies may also provide useful information on the growth rates of cancer (3-7). Of particular interest is the suggestion by Summers (7) that tumor growth depends upon and is limited by the available supply of fresh blood.

The Effects of Cancer on the Host

One of the mysteries of cancer is the manner in which it produces certain changes in the host. Repeatedly, and over long periods of time, clinical observations have been made of weight loss and anemia

36

(8) in cancer patients. At times, the cause and effect relationships are clear, as when the cancer invades the gastrointestinal tract. But in many cases it is not possible to correlate the observable effects on the patient with the presence of a small to moderate sized cancer. It has been suggested that the tumor takes up nutrients from the blood preferentially, thus starving the normal cells, but this does not agree with the known facts. First, the blood supply through cancers is so sluggish and inefficient (Chapter 19) that even if the cancer removed all the nutrients in the blood passing through it, it would not perceptibly change the body's nutrient balance. Second, although cancers do have a somewhat higher metabolic rate than most normal tissues, that rate is not nearly high enough to account for the general weight loss. Finally, in most conditions in which the body or one of its parts tends to utilize more nutrients than normal, the person's appetite and food intake tend to increase. In cancer this does not happen. Indeed, the appetite usually decreases.

The evidence today is not sufficient to allow us to do anything more than speculate about the mechanism responsible for the changes that cancer produces in the host. Nevertheless, such speculation can be valuable if it is in accord with other information, and if it leads to productive research projects. One explanation for the cancer's effect on the host that agrees with all the known facts, and for which scientists have obtained evidence, is that the cancer secretes or liberates some substance or substances that affect the host's functions (Chapter 22). (In the preceding chapter we noted that it is likely that cancers secrete a chemical that induces the host's blood vessels to proliferate; this point is considered in greater detail in Chapter 19.) This field of cancer research has been seriously neglected over the years and is fragmented and uncoordinated. We do not know whether a cancer secretes a single chemical, or a group of chemicals that affect the host, or whether each type of cancer secretes a specific material that is different from that secreted by other types. This aspect of cancer should be studied extensively because there is a good possibility that once the facts concerning it are known, a control for the disease may be found (*see* Chapter 22).

The Response of the Host to Cancer

It has been suggested that almost everyone develops several microscopic cancers during his lifetime, but that the body defenses cure them before they reach a noticeable size. According to this view, clinical cancer occurs only when the body defenses do not cope with

37

the early cancer. Thus far, we have no evidence that might support or disprove this hypothesis. Neither do we have a clear picture of the nature of the host's response to cancer. We surmise that there must be some host defenses, since most circulating cancer cells are destroyed without developing into metastases. Some scientists suspect that the effects of cancer may be much more widespread than it now seems.

It is not definitely known whether the body produces antibodies to cancers (*see* Chapter 23) although there is usually some evidence of body defense at the local site of a cancer. The connective tissue cells that grow around and within the cancer usually give it a hard, gritty texture. Perhaps the growth of these cells is a mechanism by which the body tries to wall off the cancer, but it is also possible that in some unknown way, the cancer cells are aided by this growth of connective tissue.

The recent studies of Wheatley and Ambrose in Britain (9) emphasize this aspect of tumor-host relations. These investigators noted that cancer cells initiate certain responses in the normal host tissues without having any actual contact with those tissues. This phenomenon is in accord with the findings of others on cancer cell secretions (Chapter 22) and cancer immunology (Chapter 23). However, Wheatley and Ambrose also found that these host responses made the host tissues *more* susceptible to cancer infiltration. They observed:

> The changes occurring in the host tissues by way of response create conditions which support the infiltration of tumour cells. Infiltration has not been found to occur where a host tissue shows no response to the tumour.

In other words, it appears that at least part of the host response to the cancer makes the host more rather than less vulnerable.

Spontaneous Remissions and Cures

Interest in spontaneous remissions and cures of cancer has been increasing in recent years. Such remissions, with the patient remaining in apparently excellent health for many years, appear to be not uncommon; spontaneous cures, in which all cancer cells disappear, seem to be quite rare in man. We must note, of course, that the term "spontaneous" may be quite misleading. In actuality, what we call spontaneous effects may result from external factors which are as yet unknown to us. In mice, untreated spontaneous mammary cancers regress at a rate of 8 per 100 cases. Woglom's studies (10) revealed no microscopic feature that distinguished regressing cancers from growing ones. He also noted that the regressing cancers had just as many mitotic figures as the growing cancers. After considering all possible factors, he suggested that the only one that explains the regression of cancer in mice is a change in the blood vessels.

Studies have also been made of the spontaneous remission and cure of cancer in man (11-29), but thus far they have produced little specific information. Observers feel that in some way, host resistance to the cancer increases suddenly, thus inhibiting the growth of the cancer. There is also a possibility that superimposed infection may trigger the improvement in some cases. Instances of spontaneous remissions and apparent cures in human cancers should of course be followed carefully, in the hope of discovering a useful method of controlling the disease.

Another point to consider is that spontaneous remissions and cures may be more common than is generally realized, but that they may be unrecognized as such because the patient is receiving some form of therapy. After all, most patients with cancer do receive some type of treatment; some of them may have what is really a spontaneous remission or cure, but the treatment receives the credit. This does not create a serious problem except when treatments are not based on any scientific evidence. A certain proportion of the patients who receive unorthodox therapies could develop spontaneous remissions and cures that are unrelated to the treatments. However, these patients and their families are likely to credit the improvement to the treatment and to tell others about it. Thus, a completely useless form of therapy may sometimes be touted as a "cure for cancer."

Mitosis

Mitosis is a type of cellular reproduction in which the chromosomal material is divided equally between the two daughter cells. Since the several phases in mitosis are well described in high-school and college biology texts, we will not repeat these descriptions here. Our concern is with the abnormalities of the mitosis seen in the cells of malignant tumor. At times the chromosomal material of cancer cells divides unevenly; for example, it may divide into three instead of two parts. The significance of this is not clear, except that it points to an abnormality in the multiplication process.

A second abnormality of mitosis seen in cancer is that a large number of its cells are in the process of mitosis at any given time. When a group of cells from normal tissue cells are examined under a microscope, only a small fraction will show the mitotic figures; that fraction, of course, varies with different tissues. For this reason, it was believed for years that cancer cells multiply rapidly. Recent studies have demonstrated, however, that the reason for the high proportion of mitotic figures in cancer cells is that the process of mitosis takes much longer in cancer cells than in normal tissue cells. Vladimirskaya and her colleagues in Russia (30) have described the mitosis in leukemia as being "frozen." This new information may require considerable change in our concept of the nature of cancer, and of the ways we seek to find a control for the disease. We do not know whether the "freezing" of mitosis is part of the malignant process, or whether it represents the operation of some host defense mechanism that partially interferes with the functioning of the cancer cells. Evensen and Iversen (31) have studied these problems too and have pointed out that a high mitotic count may not be evidence of a rapid rate of cell multiplication.

Adhesiveness of Cancer Cells

Most body cells adhere to neighboring cells with considerable tenacity. There is evidence that cancer cells display much less mutual adhesiveness than normal cells (32-36). The importance of this phenomenon is unclear, but since it might furnish a clue as to the reason that cancer cells affect the host in the way they do, it deserves further study.

The Morphology of Cancer

A cancer large enough to be clinically recognizable has millions of cells. Although there are differences in the cell arrangements of various cancers, there is one pattern that is consistent: All cancer cells can be divided into two groups; those in the outer layers of the cancer mass, and those on the inside. The layer of outer cells may be less than 1 mm thick. Thus, these outer cells constitute only a small fraction of the total number of cells in a cancer. They are the ones which affect the host directly, however, since they are in contact with, and invade the normal host tissues. They receive a substantial supply of blood, and live and multiply in an environment which furnishes them with as much oxygen and nutrients as most normal cells obtain. They are the cells most likely to reach lymphatic channels and travel via those channels to other parts of the body. They can be affected readily by blood-borne medications. Some of the outer cells leave the tumor mass and invade other tissues. Most of them, however, remain within the bulk of the cancer, and eventually become inner cells.

The inner cells do not ordinarily come in contact with *normal* host cells, although some dead and dying host cells may remain inside the tumor mass. Because a substantial number of the inner cells are in areas which are infarcted, they receive little or no blood. The cells in these areas, therefore, can hardly be affected by blood-borne drugs.

In untreated cancers, the inner cells probably have little or no effect on the course of the disease. However, they probably are of great importance in cancers that are treated with drugs. The reason for this lies in the ability of the inner cells (which were originally outer cells) to resume their invasion activities when conditions are ripe, even after a lapse of years. Let us assume that a patient with a cancer receives a cancerocidal drug for a period of several weeks, and let us further assume that this drug kills 100 per cent of the cancer cells it reaches. All the outer cells, and some of the inner cells which are near functioning blood vessels would be killed. However, the inner cells deep within the cancer—those without a functioning blood supply—would not be affected, since the drug would not have reached them.

As the dead cancer cells on the outside of the tumor are absorbed by the body, the cancer would shrink, and the patient would seem improved. However, the inner cells would gradually be exposed, become outer cells again, proliferate and resume the invasion.

This situation may account for the failure of cancerocidal drugs to cure most spontaneous cancers. However, if the morphology of cancer were properly evaluated, more effective control of cancer might be developed. Anti-cancer drugs might be given over a prolonged period, just as digitalis glycosides are administered in congestive heart failure, or quinine in malaria. Another possibility would be to administer the drugs intermittently at weekly or monthly intervals, so that successive layers of inner cancer cells reaching the periphery would be exposed to effective drug levels. However, for such treatment regimes to be effective, it would be necessary to first develop anti-cancer drugs of much less toxicity than those now available.

Another aspect of cancer morphology is its relationship to the biochemical characteristics of cancer cells. Since perhaps 99 per cent of the cells of a cancer are inner cells, biochemical studies can provide information about the metabolism and functioning of these cells that have been living in a hypoxic environment, but they do not necessarily provide information about the outer cells that live in the presence of relatively high oxygen tensions and are actively invading normal tissues. This fact demonstrates the difficulty in studying some vital aspects of cancer. For example, in studying secretion by cancer cells of enzymes that help these cells to invade normal tissues (Chapter 21), it has been customary for scientists to extract these enzymes from the total tumor mass. However, it is possible that the enzymes involved are secreted only by the outer cancer cells which are exposed to a relatively high oxygen tension and to a supply of nutrients. Since the outer cells form a small fraction of the cancer mass, it is quite possible that a relatively high concentration of enzyme in these cells could be diluted almost to the vanishing point in a specimen containing a large number of inner cells.

It is important to distinguish between the inner cancer cells and the frankly necrotic portions of the cancer. In all properly run studies on removed cancers it is customary either to discard those tumors with necrotic areas, or to trim off such areas. A point to be understood, however, is that in non-necrotic inner parts of the cancer, the cells have been surviving in a markedly hypoxic environment, and that they may be functioning quite differently than they would if they were located in the outer layer. Accordingly, when planning cancer research, one ought not assume that the cells of a cancer are homogenous. Instead, it would be prudent to assume, until proven otherwise, that the inner and outer cancer cells differ at a given moment, even though each has the ability to change into the other type over a longer period of time. If this precaution were taken, studies could be designed in which the outer rim of a cancer (including some normal tissues) is compared to the inner core. Small variations in findings might then provide useful insights into the differences between outer and inner cancer cells.

References

1. Laird, A. K. Dynamics of tumour growth. *Brit. J. Cancer 18:*841, 1964.
2. Laird, A. K. Dynamics of tumour growth: Comparison of growth rates and extrapolation of growth curve to one cell. *Brit. J. Cancer 19:*278, 1965.
3. Mayneord, W. V. On a law of growth of Jensen's rat sarcoma. *Amer. J. Cancer 16:* 841, 1932.
4. Schrek, R. A quantitative study of the growth of the Walker rat tumor and the Flexner-Jobling rat carcinoma. *Amer. J. Cancer 24:*807, 1935.

5. Klein, G. and Revesz, L. Quantitative studies on the multiplication of neoplastic cells *in vivo*. I. *J. Nat. Cancer Inst. 14:*229, 1953.
6. Steel, G. G. and Lamerton, L. F. The growth rate of human tumours. *Brit. J. Cancer 20:*74, 1966.
7. Summers, W. C. Dynamics of tumor growth: A mathematical model. *Growth 30:*333, 1966.
8. Betts, A., Rigby, R. G., Emerson, C. P. and Friedell, G. H. Experimental studies in the anemia of malignancy. *J. Lab. & Clin. Med. 58:*652, 1961.
9. Wheatley, D. N. and Ambrose, E. J. Tumour cell invasion from transplantable ascites tumours into host tissues. *Brit. J. Cancer 18:*730, 1966.
10. Woglom, W. H. The regression of spontaneous mammary carcinoma in the mouse. *J. Cancer Res. 7:*379, 1942.
11. Boyd, W. The spontaneous regression of cancer. *Canadian Cancer Conference 2:* 354, Academic Press, New York, 1957.
12. Brunschwig, A. Spontaneous regression of cancer. *Surgery 53:*423, 1963.
13. DeCourcy, J. L. The spontaneous regression of cancer. *Journ. Med. 14:*141, 1933.
14. Everson, T. C. Spontaneous regression of cancer. *Ann. N. Y. Acad. of Sci. 114:*721, 1964.
15. Everson, T. C. and Cole, W. H. Spontaneous regression of cancer. *Ann. Surg. 144:* 366, 1956.
16. Flesch, M. Zur Spontanheilung der Karzinome. *Münch. Med. Woch. 742:*1589, 1927.
17. Gaylord, H. R. and Clowes, G. H. A. On spontaneous cure of cancer. *Surg. Gyn. and Obst. 2:*633, 1906.
18. Godfrey, F. Spontaneous cure of cancer. *Brit. M. J. 2:*2027, 1910.
19. Hajek, O. Zur Frage der Spontanheilung des Karcinoms. *Med. Klin. 31:*1539, 1935.
20. Miller, H. C., Woodruff, M. W. and Gambacorta, J. P. Spontaneous regression of pulmonary metastases from hypernephroma. *Ann. Surg. 156:*852, 1962.
21. Rankin, G. B., Brown, C. H. and Crile, G., Jr. Spontaneous regression of hepatic metastases from a carcinoma of the colon: 10-year follow up of a patient with familial polyposis. *Ann. Surg. 162:*156, 1965.
22. Smith, J. L., Jr. and Stehlin, J. S., Jr. Spontaneous regression of primary malignant melanomas with regional metastases. *Cancer 18:*1399, 1965.
23. Stewart, F. W. Experiences in spontaneous regression of neoplastic disease in man. *Texas Rep. Biol. and Med. 10:*239, 1952.
24. Strauss, O. Über die Spontanheilung des Carcinoms. *Deutsch. med. Woch. 52:*1805, 1926. Also in *Zeitschr. f. Krebsf. 24:*367, 1927.
25. Strauss, O. Spontanheilung des Carcinoms in ihrer Beziehung zur Strahlentherapie. *Strahlentherapie 24:*672, 1927.
26. Strauss, O. Sur la guérison spontanée du cancer. *J. de. Chirurgie 29:*418, 1927.
27. Touraine, A. and Duperrat, R. Guérison spontanée ou medicale de quelques cas de cancers cutanes. *Bull. Soc. franc. de Derm. et Syph. 42:*1727, 1935.
28. Touraine, A. and Duperrat, R. Guérison spontanée de certains cancers cutanes. *Ann. Derm. et Syph. 7:*545, 1936.
29. Touraine, A. and Duperrat, R. La guérison spontanée du cancer. *Press Med. 46:* 59, 1938.
30. Vladimirskaya, E. B., Simonov, E. E., Balakhovskii, I. S. and Ivanova, I. E. Proliferative activity of leukemic cells in acute leukemia. *Fed. Proc.* (Trans. Suppl.) *25:*633, 1966.
31. Evensen, A. and Iversen, O. H. Rate of cell proliferation in a mouse squamous cell carcinoma. *Nature 196:*383, 1962.

PART I

32. Coman, D. R. Decreased mutual adhesiveness, a property of cells from squamous cell carcinomas. *Cancer Res. 4:*625, 1944.
33. Coman, D. R. Cellular adhesiveness in relation to the invasiveness of cancer: electron microscopy of liver perfused with a chelating agent. *Cancer Res. 14:*519, 1954.
34. Coman, D. R. Reduction in cellular adhesiveness upon contact with a carcinogen. *Cancer Res. 20:*1202, 1960.
35. Coman, D. R. and Anderson, T. F. A structural difference between the surfaces of normal and of carcinomatous epidermal cells. *Cancer Res. 15:*541, 1955.
36. Gatch, W. D. Degree of cohesion of cancer cells and its relation to cancer spread. *Arch. Surg. 74:*753, 1957.

PART II

CRITICAL EVALUATION OF THE OPERATION OF OUR CURRENT CANCER RESEARCH PROGRAM

There are advantages and disadvantages to the operation of our current research program. An understanding of both can be helpful in evaluating our present rate of progress, and in planning improvements. In this section some selected aspects of the operation of our cancer research program are considered.

Organization of Our Current Research Program

Our present national cancer research program is centered in the National Cancer Institute (NCI) of the United States Public Health Service (USPHS). About 90 per cent of the total national cancer research effort is supported by the NCI, about 8 per cent by the American Cancer Society (ACS) (from voluntary contributions), and from 1 to 2 per cent by other sources.

National Cancer Institute

The research program of the NCI is both intramural and extramural. The intramural research is carried on at the Institute's own laboratories in Bethesda, Maryland, a suburb of Washington. At one time, the intramural activities constituted the greater part of the total research program, but the extramural program is now larger. The scientists working in the intramural program are mainly career Public Health Service officers, together with Civil Service scientists. Arrangements are often made for other scientists to work at Bethesda also, usually for periods of a year or two.

Some of the investigators at Bethesda work on research projects which they themselves have planned. Others may be assigned to projects. If a particular intramural project seems important enough to the higher officials of the NCI, outside assistance or supplies may be purchased on a contract basis. For example, a project may need 1,000 mice of a particular strain each week; a contract will be given to a commercial mouse breeder to supply the animals. Many contracts are with drug companies which furnish large quantities of experimental drugs and chemicals. At times, universities and hospitals contract to carry out certain tests and studies needed for an intramural project.

Although the quality of the work done in the intramural program is considered to be uniformly high, certain problems related to it have come to public attention. The major one is the salary scale for established scientists. Salaries are lower than most of these men could earn at a university. Of course, they are far lower than salaries paid to industrial scientists. As a result, many of the outstanding research scientists retire after 20 years of service at the Institute and take other jobs while still in their late 40's. Furthermore, it has become increasingly difficult to recruit other leading scientists because of the low salaries paid.

The intramural program cannot be expanded substantially at its present location without uneconomic expenditures. Therefore, if the intramural program were to be enlarged several-fold, it would be advisable to build additional institutes in other parts of the country.

The Extramural Program

This program has grown until it now represents the major part of the total research effort. The extramural program is a means whereby the NCI, through a system of research grants, supports studies in other institutions throughout the nation. These grants are made to investigators who must take the initiative by applying for them; doing this they are competing with other investigators. The program is, therefore, investigator-centered. The Institute does not suggest projects to the investigators; indeed, it is apparently forbidden to do so. Each applicant must get an idea for a research project, write it up in a specified manner, and submit it to the National Institutes of Health (NIH). The decision as to who will be given a grant and who will be turned down is made by a series of "study sections" and committees. A study section consists of an executive secretary, who is a full-time professional employee of the NIH, and a group of selected, unpaid volunteer scientists (1). The number of scientists on a study section usually varies from 11 to 19 (1). (Any actual travel expense incurred by these scientists is reimbursed, and there is a modest per diem payment for meals and lodging when they are away from home, but this just covers out-of-pocket costs, and there are no direct payments made to these scientists in return for their efforts.) Each scientist member is appointed for a 3-year term, and the terms are staggered so that the composition of a study section changes each year. The chairman is appointed, and he, too, leaves after three years. Some scientists, after finishing a 3-year term on one section or committee are then appointed to another one, and a few may remain in similar positions for years. The selection of new members for a study section is done by the permanent professional staff of the NIH, often with the advice of retiring members of the section. In general, the persons chosen to serve on study sections are considered by the NIH to be mature, experienced scientists with a good grasp of their particular field.

When a new batch of applications is received by the executive secretary of a study section, he and the chairman of the section assign a copy of each application to two members of the section. These two review the application in detail, and then make their recommendations to the entire section. They may, if they wish, schedule a visit, called a site survey, to the investigator to inspect his facilities or to judge his capabilities. At a regular meeting of the study section, recommendations of the reviewers are considered and then the entire group, except the executive secretary, votes on each application. If a majority vote to reject it, the application has, for practical purposes, no further chance of being approved. If the majority votes to approve it, it is then given a priority rating. Each member of the section, except the executive secretary, assigns a priority number—from 100 to 500—to each approved application, and these numbers are averaged to determine the priority of the applications for the available funds.

It seems that study sections make decisions on whether a particular approach to cancer is more or less important than another one, and assign priorities on that basis. Unfortunately, they never tell the applicant which approaches they consider most promising; apparently they are forbidden to do so, lest they be accused of trying to "direct" research.

The decisions of the study sections are then transmitted to the Council of the NCI which must make the final decision. In theory, the Council members may vote to reconsider an application that has been turned down, but there is no evidence that this happens often. They are likely to scrutinize some of the large applications that were approved, but most applications are simply handled as recommended by the study section.

Next, the available funds are allocated according to priorities, and some approved applications are funded, while others are not.

The fate of the applications, considered in November 1965, is of interest. Of all those submitted to the NCI, less than half were approved. Of those approved, less than half were funded.

The investigator is notified, usually within six to eight months of sending in his application, about the decisions that have been made. If the application has been turned down, he may write to the Institute and ask why. One of the executive secretaries will then write him, explaining why the study section voted against his application. Perhaps they did not like his approach, or felt his techniques were not suitable, or thought that he had not quoted the proper references, or even felt that his background and experience were inadequate. In many cases, these comments are quite helpful to the applicant who then may rewrite and resubmit his application in a subsequent year.

If an investigator receives approval and funding of his application, he can start work on the day the grant is due to start. If his application is approved but not funded, he knows that the work he has done on it, including experimental design, literature research, and so forth has withstood intense critical scrutiny. However, since he has no funds with which to work, he cannot do the experiment. If he wishes, he may resubmit the application and hope that, because of the yearly change in study section personnel, he will encounter a group which will give his application a higher priority.

The scientist members of the various study sections and councils have an additional assignment at times. If it appears to them that an important area of investigation is being neglected, they are expected to stimulate interest in it by symposia and conferences throughout the nation. The extent to which this is done is not known. However, this seems to be the only mechanism whereby the nation's scientists are told just which research areas are considered by the study sections and councils as most important and likely to obtain a high priority.

The study section and committee system was set up in order to avoid, or at least minimize, any direction of the research effort by a central group. It is not clear whether it is necessarily a good system in all cases and there have been some serious criticisms of it (2). Undoubtedly the study sections have made some errors in judgment, but a certain proportion of errors can be expected in any complex affair requiring many difficult decisions. The sincerity, scientific standing, and willingness to work of the individual members of study sections have never, to my knowledge, been questioned. In all likelihood, the study section and committee members have done their jobs as well as they could be done within the framework of the system. Yet, when we consider the framework in relation to a national-goal program designed for practical results, we find several basic and serious flaws. First, there is no continuity. An investigator may receive a 3-year grant to do an experiment which a particular study section considers promising. At the end of the three years, having made good progress, he may apply for a renewal and be turned down because there has been a complete turnover in the membership of the study section, and because the new members think that another area of research is more important. This means that the effort and money already spent have been largely wasted. Secondly, under this system, responsibility for decisions is too diffuse. It is virtually impossible to find out who made what decisions about the kinds of research to be encouraged.

We must point out, however, that in the early years of the NIH, this arrangement worked reasonably well. And, with a view to the future, it has made a national-goal approach possible; it has provided a foundation of trained scientists, ideas, and facilities upon which a more effective structure can be built. But the present arrangement is hardly suitable for a substantially enlarged program directed at achieving practical results with a minimum of delay.

General Research Support Grants

The NIH also provides general research support grants to many qualifying universities and hospitals. This money, at the discretion of the head of the organization receiving it, may be used for any research purpose including paying for special, expensive equipment, research salaries, and the cost of small pilot studies. The general research support grant is based on the amount the institution is already receiving from other sources, so that the institutions receiving the most money in research grants also get the largest general research support grants. The extent to which these funds are used for cancer research is not known.

Construction

The NIH, which includes the NCI, sometimes helps provide funds for construction of research facilities. Such funds are usually given on a matching basis whereby the applying institution must provide half the cost of the construction and NIH will then provide the other half.

Fellowships

Finally, NIH provides fellowships and career research development awards to candidates who seem to have a good research potential. These awards, which start at the predoctoral level, help outstanding students obtain Ph.D. degrees in areas important to the national research program. Such fellowships, however, are not available to students enrolled for M.D., D.V.M., or D.D.S. degrees. Postdoctoral fellowships for research training are available to young scientists who have already received a doctorate degree, including Ph.D., M.D., D.V.M. and D.D.S. Postdoctoral awards are for no more than three years. For more experienced research scientists, there are two levels of career research development awards, one for training in research, and the other for independent research. The career research development awards are given for five years, and may be renewed for a second 5-year period.

The stipends of the predoctoral awards and the Career Research

Development Awards are generally close to the income that the individual would obtain from equivalent positions on a university staff or faculty. The postdoctoral stipends are somewhat smaller, and persons who take them receive less than they would in a regular faculty position. A regular university appointment for a scientist with the qualifications and experience of the average postdoctoral fellow usually provides from 20 to 40 per cent more real income, counting all family allowances and income tax features. A position in the pharmaceutical industry, which is actively seeking such persons, usually provides from 60 to 80 per cent more real income. Nevertheless, the number of candidates for postdoctoral fellowships exceeds by a good margin the number of fellowships available. Surely this is impressive testimony that our younger scientists are willing to accept personal sacrifices in order to contribute to medical research.

Voluntary Agencies

An important part of our present research effort in cancer is supported by various voluntary agencies, the American Cancer Society (ACS) in particular. Although the research funds provided by the ACS and smaller voluntary agencies are only a fraction of the amount provided by the NCI, they are highly effective for several reasons. The voluntary agencies provide fund sources for new ideas that are not yet considered sufficiently well-established for Federal support. They will provide funds for scientists who do not yet have a national reputation, but who show promise. They make a definite effort to develop cancer research programs in many institutions throughout the nation. This helps, to some extent, to develop our research potential on a sound foundation.

The ACS also makes moderate grants to universities which makes it possible for a faculty committee to provide pilot funds (usually not over $2,000 per year) for a scientist who wishes to try a small-scale experiment in order to see if the results would warrant his applying for funds for a full-scale study. Among scientists in the cancer field, there is a general feeling that the ACS has had a highly beneficial effect on cancer research because of its wise and imaginative use of the limited funds available to it.

References

1. *Roster of Members of PHS Public Advisory Groups,* October 1, 1965, U. S. Dep't. of Health, Education, and Welfare. Public Health Service Publication No. 262A.
2. Black, M. M. Letter to New York Times. March 16, 1968, Section 4, p. 10.

Applying for Research Grants

Since our present cancer research system is focussed primarily on the individual investigator who thinks of a research project and then tries to get financial support to work on it, it is helpful to try to see some of the procedures from his viewpoint. The initial steps may differ somewhat in different institutions, but are generally similar. For purposes of illustration, the practices at the University of Missouri will be described.

A member of the university faculty, almost always with a doctoral degree (M.D., Ph.D., D.V.M., or D.D.S.) gets an idea for an experiment in the field of cancer which he would like to perform, and for which he feels qualified. He usually discusses his idea with the chairman of his department and, if advisable, with colleagues in his own or other departments. Then he begins a search of the scientific literature to be sure that his experiment has not already been performed, and to accumulate all the relevant information on related past work and on exact technical laboratory procedures to be used. An adequate, but not absolutely complete, search and study of the literature may take about a month. Most of the time is spent searching—the number of really important papers to be studied seldom exceeds 15 for a particular experiment.

The scientist obtains a standard application form from the National Institutes of Health (NIH). He usually consults his department chairman and his colleagues about points to be included. In his application, he indicates the aim and general goals of his research and then describes in detail exactly how he intends to perform his experiments and interpret them. If experienced in making out grant applications, he includes every detail he can, since he knows that the application will be judged to a large extent by its completeness and clarity. For example, he does not say simply that he will do his studies on mice. He indicates which sub-line of mice he will use (such as C57/BL, DBA, IBR, A/Jax, and so forth); their sex, age, and numbers; how they will be caged, fed, watered, cared for, and so on. He indicates how he intends to measure changes and how he will accumulate and analyse the statistics. Then, he writes up a discussion of the possible significance of his proposed study in relation to the over-all field of cancer.

Next, the applicant reviews his past studies in the field of cancer giving enough detail to inform the reviewers of his qualifications to carry out the research. He also reviews the relevant work of others in fields related to his particular research proposal. This discussion is supposed to be complete, including references to all important contributions in the field (but not studies that do not bear directly on his proposal). He is expected to choose, from many thousands of published papers, the small number (generally 5 to 15 studies) that are most relevant to his proposal and to discuss them expertly.

Next, the applicant fills out the part of the form that shows his education, training, and experience in scientific and medical areas. If he expects to have associates or assistants at the professional level helping him, he includes a similar biographical sketch for each of them. In another form, he must indicate any other sources of financial support, whether governmental or private, that he is receiving for other research. In part, this is designed to make sure that no investigator obtains financial support for more research projects than he is considered capable of handling.

Finally, the applicant prepares a detailed budget for the first year of his study, and a less detailed one for any subsequent year up to a maximum of seven years. His budget must be clear, complete and accurate. If it appears too small or too large, his application may be turned down for that reason. If any special or unusual expenditures are included in the budget, they must be explained and justified fully. In the budget, the applicant must indicate (as a percentage) the time and effort that he and any other professional personnel will devote to the project.

The time required to prepare an application properly will usually vary between two and six months, depending upon the experience of the investigator in making out applications and the nature of the research to be conducted.

After completing his application, the investigator turns it over to his department chairman for review. The latter reads it carefully, and may make suggestions for changes and improvements. If he feels the project is unworthy, he may turn it down completely, but this is not likely to happen if the investigator has consulted him earlier, as is generally the case. It is not uncommon, however, for a department chairman to suggest that changes and improvements be made in the application and such suggestions are almost always accepted. After the department chairman has approved the application and indicated his approval by signing a university form, the application is reviewed carefully by the Assistant Dean for Research of the particular college with which the applicant is associated (Medicine, Veterinary Medicine, and so forth). He, too, may approve or reject, or may make suggestions for changes. If he approves, and signs the university form, the application is then read and reviewed again by the university's Vice-President for Research who also can approve, reject, or suggest changes. The budget pages are checked by the business office for accuracy, and conformity with Federal and university regulations. If all the university reviewers approve the research proposal, it is signed by the Comptroller and mailed to the NIH. If a proposal involves joint studies of investigators in two colleges of the university, such as Medicine and Veterinary Medicine, the application must be approved by each chairman and each assistant dean for research.

The reviews of the application are taken seriously and done meticulously. It is in the best interest of the university that applications from its staff be carefully prepared, professionally competent documents which will reflect favorably on the university. The review of an application within a university usually takes about two weeks, provided that no changes, except perhaps correction of a few typing errors, are involved.

Let us now consider the fate of the applications when they reach the NIH in Bethesda, Maryland.

First, each application is "logged in" and a postcard indicating receipt is sent to the applicant. Then many duplicate copies of the application are made and sent to staff members of the NIH to be examined. The applications are assigned to two separate categories of examiners. Those in one category correspond to the various Institutes within the NIH, such as Heart, Cancer, Mental Health, and so forth—we are here concerned only with applications assigned to the National Cancer Institute (NCI). The second category of examiners consists of members of a study section, which may, or may not, cross Institute lines. For example, the Allergy and Immunology Study Section might receive applications concerned with basic immunology, with asthma, with cancer immunology, or with allergic responses relating to heart disease. Some study sections have assignments that are less broad. It is in the study section that the application's fate is usually decided (*see* Chapter 7).

The applicant is notified of the decision within six to nine months after sending in his application. He has slightly less than a 25 per cent chance of receiving the funds needed for his project.

If he wishes, he can rewrite the application and resubmit it, hoping for a more favorable decision. However, compiling two sets of applications would take up two to three years of the applicant's time, and most of those who are unsuccessful turn to other fields of endeavor.

The Present Financial Support of Cancer Research

The financial support given to cancer research by the Federal Government involves certain complexities which we should understand in order to see clearly the general situation regarding funds available for cancer research. Some inaccurate and misleading statements have been made about the so-called enormous growth in cancer research funds. A careful analysis of the known facts shows that, during the fiscal years 1962-1966, there was a small increase in the amount of money appropriated for cancer research. Federal appropriations for the National Cancer Institute (in millions) follow:

1962—$143   (+5)
1963— 156
1964— 144
1965— 150
1966— 164
1967— 173

But in effect, there was a decrease in the net amount available for cancer research. There are several reasons for this. First, the cost of performing most studies has increased by about 10 to 15 per cent per year, largely because of higher costs of equipment, supplies, research facilities, and so forth. In addition, the new sophisticated types of equipment needed by investigators are expensive. Thus, if all other factors were equal, the $163 million appropriated in 1966 would have sufficed for a program about two-thirds as extensive as that supported by the 1962 appropriation of $143 million. Furthermore, there were changes in the fiscal management of the research grants that reduced the net amounts available for research still further.

Before 1962, most senior medical scientists on a university faculty received 100 per cent of their salary from the university's own funds and both teaching and research duties were considered part of their employment. The proportion of each type of work done varied from individual to individual and from school to school, but it seems fair to estimate that in the nation as a whole senior medical scientists on a full-time university salary exerted about half their efforts in teaching, and half in research. In the early 1960's, the universities took the position that if a faculty member received a research grant, part of his salary should be paid from that grant. The money that the university then saved could be used by the administration to defray other costs of running the university. This is a sound position to take, but one that must be remembered if the appropriations for 1966 and 1967 are to be compared with those of 1962.

A second set of changes involve the rates of overhead payments to the universities and hospitals; all these payments come out of the appropriations. Up to 1963, the universities and hospitals received as much as 15 per cent of the funds that were put at the disposal of the investigator; the funds for a few rare items of expensive equipment were excepted. The universities and hospitals also received almost all equipment as a gift, after the study was completed. In 1963, the overhead rate was raised to 20 per cent. The university and hospital administrators felt that this was inadequate and, in 1966, a new formula for computing the overhead charge was introduced. The universities and hospitals now receive overhead based on the amount of direct salary and wages paid by the grant. The rate of the overhead charged varies with the institution, but is approximately 50 per cent of salaries and wages paid by the grant to the researchers. As a result, a larger share of the appropriation for cancer research now goes to the university or hospital. This, of course, reduces the amount of money available for the actual research project. To see how these factors operate, let us consider a hypothetical research grant application made up in 1962, and in 1967, to do the same study. Let us assume that the principal investigator devotes 30 per cent of his energy to the project. Further, in order to simplify the matter, let us omit any consideration of increased costs of equipment and supplies, and assume that the two salaries involved were the same: $10,000 and $6,000 (Table 9-1). Note that in 1962, out of a total grant of $9,545, the investigator had $8,300 to spend on the research. By 1967, the total amount of grant needed to provide the investigator with $8,300 in direct funds had risen from $9,545 to $15,800. In 1962, the university or hospital received $1,245 of the total. By 1967, the university or hospital received $7,500 of the total; $4,500 as overhead and $3,000 as payment for part of the chief investigator's salary. It should be noted that the example given is a general one, and that with other grants, the proportions may vary. If

Table 9–1. Simplified Hypothetical Research Grant Applications Showing Differences between Funds Needed to Carry out the Same Research Project in 1962 and 1966 (Certain small items such as OASI are omitted)

Items	Funds	
	1962	1966
Personnel		
Principal investigator, Jones, A.B., M.D.—30% of effort	00	$3,000
Research assistant—100% of effort	$6,000	6,000
Equipment		
Centrifuge	800	800
Supplies		
Mice	800	800
Drugs and chemicals	400	400
Glassware and disposable items	300	300
Travel	00	00
Sub Total	8,300	11,300
Amount available for actual conduct of research	8,300	8,300
Overhead to university or hospital	1,245	4,500
Total amount of grant	9,545	15,800

a grant allows more money for supplies and equipment than for salaries and wages, the proportion for overhead will decrease; if more is stipulated as payment for the investigator's effort, or if a larger portion of the total goes into salaries and wages than is allowed for supplies and equipment, the overhead share will increase. Thus far it appears that only the new grants will be handled in this manner, and the annual renewals of old grants in the former way, at least for a while. Therefore, we can expect a gradual, rather than abrupt, rise in the portion of the research grants that are set aside as overhead.

Undoubtedly, the universities and hospitals need and deserve more support, and if this mechanism of obtaining it seems suitable one ought not object. The problem is that most citizens do not realize how the funds are being allocated. The statements released by the Federal Government, while accurate, do not convey the full picture to anyone other than those well versed in this particular area. The clear fact is that, because of changing policies on overhead and salaries, the 1967 appropriation provides about 30 per cent *less* funds for the actual research work than the 1962 appropriation did; because of the added effects of higher costs, the 1967 appropriation will provide funds that would have paid for only about one-half of the cancer research done in 1962.

Between 1962 and 1967, the number of cancer research grants awarded by the National Institutes of Health (NIH) dropped from 1,914 (1) to 1,525 (2). Thus, both in number of research grants and in net funds available for actual research, there has been a decrease since 1962.

The relationship of cancer research funds to the gross national product (9, 10) is revealing. Figure 9-1 demonstrates the fall in the proportion of cancer research funds to the gross national product since 1962. The index Gross National Product divided by Cancer Research Funds is a useful one since it provides two types of information. The effects of inflation are balanced out in this index, so that

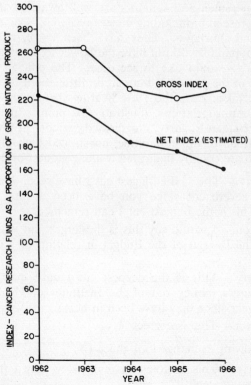

Figure 9–1. Relationship of cancer research funds to Gross National Product

we can readily see the true purchasing power of the dollars allocated to cancer research. Secondly, the index gives a good indication of the changing proportion of our national wealth being allocated to cancer research. In Figure 9-1 the gross index refers to the funds disbursed by the Federal treasury. The estimated net index is of more immediate concern, since it refers to the funds actually available for the research. The difference between the gross and (estimated) net indices consists of the funds that are kept by the grantee agencies such as universities and hospitals (*see* above). The funds kept by the grantee agencies are seldom, if ever, used directly to support cancer research. The estimated net index, therefore, is probably the most accurate available measure of the changes in the relative portion of our national income used directly for cancer research. An estimate, rather than exact figures, must be used, since each grantee agency now has a slightly different overhead rate, based on its estimated indirect costs.

Some congressmen and senators are well aware of the degree to which medical research, including cancer research, is being held back by chronic fund shortages. They have been trying to remedy the situation, but apparently do not have the power to do what they—and most Americans—would like to see done. The officials in the NIH are also aware of the problem, but can do little about it. Some of the exerpts below, taken from the 1966 hearings before the House Subcommittee on Appropriations, illustrate this point. In the hearings, the late Congressman Fogarty, a dedicated, wonderful public servant, who was chairman of the committee, questioned high officials of the NIH, men who are equally dedicated to the conquest of disease (3).

> Mr. Fogarty.—This is the biggest cut I have seen. Has there been any such severe cut since you have been at the Institutes of Health? This is the biggest cut I can remember.
>
> Dr. Shannon.—I would say this is the largest cut which has been made by the Bureau of the Budget in relation to a departmental request.
>
> Mr. Fogarty.—This is the deepest cut I have ever seen. They have cut more money out of the Institutes of Health this year than any year since they have been in being.
>
> Dr. Shannon.—That is correct.

Later, the following exchange took place (4):

> Mr. Fogarty.—This is going to really slow down the whole research program, isn't it?

Dr. Shannon.—I think the Bureau of the Budget is well aware that, in arriving at a political decision as to the funds that were to be made available, this would be well below the opportunities for supporting meritorious . . . .

Mr. Fogarty.—What kind of a decision did you call it—a political decision.

Dr. Shannon.—I think the budget is a political document.

Mr. Fogarty.—This kind of thing ought to be exempt from political decisions.

Dr. Shannon.—I am using "political" in a very broad sense.

Mr. Fogarty.—I understand.

In the testimony from Dr. Endicott, Director of the National Cancer Institute and Mr. Cardwell the Department Deputy Controller, the following was recorded (5):

Mr. Fogarty.—In the field of cancer, the whole program is going to be cut back under this budget because this $251,000 won't come anywhere near meeting your increased costs. We are going backward instead of ahead.

You did not fare very well, Dr. Endicott, you asked for $188 million and the Department and The Bureau of the Budget cut your request $24,177,000.

Dr. Endicott—Yes sir: There was a reduction.

Mr. Fogarty.—I thought we were supposed to be expanding this program of research in cancer. This is the biggest cut in the Institute's request I have seen since the Cancer Institute was formed in 1937. . . . This chart I have that is in the record, shows minuses everywhere down the line. As it developed yesterday, the Bureau of the Budget cut the Institutes of Health $308,860,000. This is the greatest cut by far that has ever been made in th NIH budget. No matter how you use your figures, you cannot get around it.

Do you still think you could use that $188 million if you had it?

Dr. Endicott.—Yes, sir.

Mr. Fogarty.—Things have not developed to indicate a cut should be made in your original estimates.

Dr. Endicott.—From the program standpoint the opportunities do exist, yes sir.

Mr. Fogarty.—And the problem is getting worse.

Dr. Endicott.—From the standpoint of the numbers of deaths, yes, sir.

Later, Mr. Fogarty questioned Dr. Shannon again (6):

Mr. Fogarty.—The big cut is in the cancer chemotherapy problem. . . . Where was this cut made?

Dr. Shannon.—That is a cut by the Bureau of the Budget.

Returning to Dr. Endicott, the following testimony was recorded (7):

Mr. Fogarty.—Getting back to research grants, I see minuses all the way down the line . . . and the table shows you will have to cut back by 58 the number of research projects you will be able to finance in 1967. Is that right?

Dr. Endicott.—That is what the table shows; yes.

Mr. Fogarty.—Forgetting the Bureau of the Budget and your superiors, be honest with us and tell us what, in your professional judgement, will be the immediate and long-range impact if Congress does not correct this situation that the Bureau of the Budget has presented to us.

Dr. Endicott.—The thing which concerns me most is the possible impact on the investigators in this field, and particularly the younger ones who are just getting a start in their research careers.

These statements speak for themselves; any comment on them would be superfluous.

Another way to evalute the adequacy of our current program is to compare the funds allocated to cancer research with the economic loss due to cancer. In the United States last year, the financial cost of treatment of cancer was over $1 billion and the total economic loss from cancer was over $12 billion (8). We are now spending less than 2 per cent of this figure per year on cancer research.

Role of Voluntary Agencies

Voluntary agencies, particularly the American Cancer Society (ACS), have played a vital role in our cancer research program, and with the help of the citizenry will continue to do so. It is essential that voluntary agencies continue their support of research, no matter how extensive a program is sponsored by the Federal Government. In the past, brilliant scientists have been denied financial support because their ideas seemed too far-fetched. In actuality, their ideas were too advanced for their day. These scientists have a greater chance of obtaining the needed support if they have more than one source to which to apply; in addition, voluntary agencies usually have somewhat more flexibility in their operations than government agencies.

The ACS, the major voluntary agency in this field, depends on public contributions for funding its projects. In recent years, it has been increasing the percentage of its funds allocated to research, with emphasis on the development of "seed" projects in various universities and hospitals. This important work deserves the fullest financial backing of every American. At times one hears some grumbling because the ACS conducts an independent fund raising campaign, instead of combining its efforts with the United Fund. However, this is a perfectly reasonable and proper position for the ACS to take. In the first place, it can raise much more money by an independent fund-raising effort than it can by combining with other groups. In addition, the functions of the ACS go beyond the functions of the community service groups that make up the United Funds. Although the Society does help the needy and disadvantaged who have cancer, it is much more than a charitable institution. The person who gives to the ACS is not merely helping the less fortunate in his community; he is making an investment in his own, and his family's, life and health.

However, the funds available to the ACS, and to all other voluntary agencies supporting cancer research, are limited. The ACS had slightly over $15 million available for research in 1965, about 10 per cent of the amount provided by the Federal Government; and, as we have seen, the latter is quite inadequate. Therefore, despite the great contributions of the voluntary agencies to cancer research thus far, it would be completely unrealistic to suppose that they could support a national-goal approach.

References

1. *Public Health Service Grants and Awards Fiscal Year 1962: Funds,* Part V, Summary Tables for the Extramural Programs. U. S. Dep't. of Health, Education, and Welfare, Public Health Service Publication No. 964, Part V., Washington, p. 2.
2. Hearings Before a Subcommittee of the Committee on Appropriations. House of Representatives, Eighty-Ninth Congress. Part 4. *Department of Health, Education, and Welfare Appropriations for 1967.* U. S. Government Printing Office, Washington, 1966, p. 364.
3. *Ibid.,* p. 26.
4. *Ibid.,* p. 44.
5. *Ibid.,* p. 324.
6. *Ibid.,* p. 325.

7. *Ibid.*, p. 345.
8. National Advisory Cancer Council, *Progress Against Cancer—1966,* U. S. Dep't. of Health, Education, and Welfare, Washington, p. 12.
9. *Statistical Abstract of the United States.* 87th ed. U. S. Gov't. Printing Office, Washington, 1966, p. 320.
10. *Readers Digest 1967 Almanac and Yearbook.* Pleasantville, New York, 1966, p. 417.

CHAPTER 10

Wasted Talent

One of the drawbacks of our present cancer research program is the waste of talent, ability, and energy that results from a lack of adequate coordination and central direction. There have been no studies of this phenomenon and many people do not realize that it exists. The author gradually became aware of this situation while working on this book and, in an effort to find out if and how certain studies were progressing, queried several scientists; their replies form the basis of this chapter. No claim is made that this is a statistically randomized sample, but the circumstances described are revealing. (In Chapter 8 the wasted time and energy involved in the application process are discussed.)

One reason for the great waste of research talent is the failure to utilize the services of all the capable scientists in many fields who could help find a solution to the cancer problem. (The potential contributions of these men and women are discussed in Chapters 28, 29, and 30.) In this chapter we will concentrate on another aspect of the problem—the waste that accompanies lack of financial support for continuing studies.

An outstanding example of waste incurred through failure to support continuing studies occurred at the University of Texas where McKenna and Taylor and their colleagues had carried out an impressive series of studies on plants (1). These pioneers in cancer research had tested 1,500 plant materials for anti-cancer effects, and had developed procedures and techniques as they went along. Their initial studies on crude extracts showed that a substantial percentage had significant anti-cancer effects. When McKenna and Taylor were asked (1966) whether any papers reporting their further studies on more purified extracts might soon be published, it was found that Taylor had retired, and that McKenna, unable to obtain financial support to continue the work, was no longer doing medical research. McKenna, who has given his permission to report this correspondence (2), stated that he had tried without success to obtain the funds to continue the work. To the best of his knowledge, no one, anywhere,

65

is following up their work on the crude extracts; no one is testing more purified extracts of the crude extracts that showed anti-cancer effects; no one is testing on spontaneous cancers the materials that were effective against transplantable cancers. Perhaps at some future time, someone will read the reports of these Texas scientists and be able to obtain the funds to follow them up—and perhaps not.

Another example of loss of scientific talent to fields other than cancer research, reported in Chapter 2, concerns a scientist whose studies of cancer immunology have been outstanding, and who has transferred to space research because of his inability to get the funds with which to continue his cancer work.

A basic and vitally important group of studies was reported from 1945 through 1956, when the results of the major research done by Algire (and his colleagues) on the blood supply of cancers was published (*see* Chapter 19). Attempts to find out if any follow-up was being done on these studies disclosed that Dr. Algire had died in 1956. Although some people are still working in related fields and using his techniques, the group of studies that he had started has not been expanded; the studies have not even kept up at the previous rate. Algire had written that there seemed to be a substance, secreted by cancers, that stimulated blood vessel proliferation by the host. The clarification of this point and the isolation and identification of the secreted substance would appear to be of major importance, but apparently no one at NCI is carrying on such a project; nor is there any evidence that any outside grantee is doing so.

Another distinguished American scientist suggested in a published report that the regression of cancers that he had observed in some animals may have resulted from bacterial infection. In his article, he indicated that he intended to do more studies to find out if bacteria could in fact be the cause of this regression, but on being questioned about what his later studies had shown, he stated that he had not been able to pursue the study because of a lack of specialized equipment.

Dr. Wooley, of Rockefeller University, published an article in 1961 that dealt with some important points in cancer research. The search for information concerning his subsequent findings revealed that Dr. Wooley had died in 1966, and that his work on tumors would probably be discontinued, because everyone else at the University was too busy with other important studies to take up Dr. Wooley's work.

Cancer researchers are sometimes forced by their institutions to retire at a particular age, even though they may be willing and able to continue their work (3). When this happens, their studies may, or may not, be continued by their former assistants.

In theory, it seems logical to expect that when one investigator discontinues an important line of research because of retirement, death, reassignment, or inability to obtain funds, other investigators will carry on his work. In practice, however, this occurs erratically. Most studies require the use of specialized equipment and trained assistants and technicians. These assets can seldom be acquired in a short period of time. A new investigator can seldom step in and take over the complete operation of another man's research project. Usually, he must laboriously build up his own research team and equipment pool. Furthermore, there may be a time lapse of a year or more before other researchers realize that one of their colleagues in another institution is no longer active.

Because of the lack of any effective central coordination of cancer research studies, projects that deserve to be followed through are often abandoned when the investigator leaves, or is forced to leave, active research. Herein lies a tremendous waste—waste of both ideas and leads to further studies which could conceivably achieve the practical goal of finding a cure for, or a method of controlling cancer.

There is, of course, always the hope that someone, in subsequent years, will do a literature search, come across the papers describing the abandoned studies, and take them up. This has occurred, occasionally. But what an inefficient way it is to conduct research!

References

1. See Chapter 18, references 13-23.
2. McKenna, G. F. Personal communication, 1966.
3. Davidsohn, I. Medical research (letter). *J.A.M.A. 160:*1092, 1956.

Accomplishments of Our Present System of Supporting Cancer Research

A balanced appraisal of our present cancer research program requires consideration of its positive accomplishments. Fundamentally, it has provided the foundation upon which a more effective program can be built. Cancer research scientists have been trained in large numbers. A large proportion, perhaps 90 per cent, of all the cancer research scientists in the United States have been supported at one time or another by fellowships or grants from the National Cancer Institute (NCI). It takes a long time to train competent scientists, and we are beginning to see the accomplishments of sections of the program started five and ten years ago.

Cancer research facilities have been built throughout the nation. A few are earmarked for cancer research only. Most, however, consist of areas within other university research buildings. Approximately half of the costs of such facilities have been borne by the NCI.

Above all, a series of research leads have been developed, which if properly followed up, could reach the goal of finding a cure or control for cancer within a relatively short time. Unfortunately the role of NCI in developing these leads has not always been acknowledged. When the actual work is done as part of the intramural program at Bethesda (as was the case in Algire's studies; *see* Chapter 19), the NCI did receive appropriate credit. But studies done in the extramural program have not always given a fair share of credit to the NCI. When important studies come to public attention, the newspaper and magazine articles usually play up the university or hospital in which the work was done. A typical story will start: "Two doctors at XYZ University announced today the discovery of. . . ." Sometimes the last sentence of the story may state: "Their work was supported by grants from the National Cancer Institute." However, for some unknown reason, many stories omit this credit.

Examination of the references to American cancer research studies, selected for the various chapters of this book, reveals that the great majority of the studies done after 1950 were supported by grants or fellowships from the NCI.

Another important accomplishment of our present program has been the development of standards of excellence for cancer research. Studies supported by the NCI are almost always well-controlled and accompanied by careful and accurate statistical analyses of the meaning of the results. The habits and standards of excellent research have been deeply impressed upon our scientists, and can be expected to be carried over into any future programs.

There is some evidence that the leaders of the NCI have planned to expand the present program into a national-goal type of program, with task forces directing their energies toward rapid exploitation of leads developed in the usual studies. Indeed, a few such task forces are already at work. However, the cutbacks in net cancer research funds from 1962 on, have probably prevented any great expansion of the task-force, goal-directed approach. The NCI operates on the basis of long-term commitments to research scientists at universities and hospitals. When a new program is developed, it must be financed by increased appropriations; as has been pointed out in Chapter 9, the appropriations since 1962 have not even kept up with the increased costs of a stationary program.

There is another accomplishment of our present program that, although quite abstract, may be the most important of all. It has been established beyond any doubt that the American people are solidly in favor of government-supported and financed programs in cancer (and other medical) research. There may be considerable controversy about government support of medical *care,* but there is little argument about support of medical research by the Government. Republicans and Democrats alike have given wholehearted support to the principle of tax-supported medical research programs. It is particularly noteworthy that the *elected* representatives of the American people, members of the Senate and the House of Representatives, have each year voted more funds for medical research than the Bureau of the Budget permitted the National Institutes of Health to request.

Accordingly, there are no major political or ideological obstacles to a properly financed and organized national-goal program for finding a cure or control for cancer as soon as possible. This is surely an important accomplishment.

PART III

CRITICAL EVALUATION OF SOME CURRENT RESEARCH APPROACHES TO CANCER

Many cancer research projects are under way at this time. Some of them consist simply of the efforts of a single research worker, using limited equipment and facilities. Others involve teams of researchers with assistants and technicians, and with extensive facilities and equipment. A review of some of the major projects in our present cancer research program reveals certain basic flaws and deficiences that make it unlikely that these projects will develop a useful treatment or prevention of cancer in the reasonably near future (5 generations). In some cases, the flaws seem correctable; in others the nature of the approach is such that the projects probably could not succeed before many decades, or even centuries, have elapsed.

The four areas of cancer research selected for discussion in this section were chosen because they illustrate why some of the present research projects are not succeeding and are not likely to succeed in a reasonable period of time, and why they do not, therefore, appear to warrant increased support in a national-goal program.

Screening for Anti-Cancer Materials

Probably the biggest cancer research projects presently under way are concerned with testing large numbers of chemicals against several types of cancer in mice. The hope is that, if enough materials are tested, at least one good anti-cancer drug will be discovered. The term "screening" is used for this kind of procedure since it implies that many useless materials must be tested to find a useful one.

The impetus for the screening procedure came from the results of screening studies in other areas of medicine. After penicillin had been discovered, several pharmaceutical companies set up programs in which they tested extracts made from various types of fungi, obtained from all over the world. These extracts were tested, or "screened," against several kinds of pathogenic bacteria, and those extracts that seemed to have antibacterial activity in the test tube were purified further and tested against infections in animals. As a result of these screening tests, we now have available a score of useful antibiotics.

A similar screening procedure of chemicals against malarial parasites has given us several excellent anti-malaria drugs. The fact that strains of malaria resistant to these new drugs have appeared in Vietnam does not denigrate the importance of the screening procedure for anti-malaria drugs.

With the past successes of screening so evident, it is quite understandable that a substantial effort should be put into screening chemicals for possible anti-cancer effects. The materials that have been screened come from several sources. Most are new chemical entities synthesized by chemists. Many are extracts of cultures of fungi and bacteria, and some are extracts made from plants of the higher orders.

Most of the actual screening is now done by commercial firms, operating under contracts from the National Cancer Institute (NCI). The screening program has been in existence for many years, and it seems appropriate to examine it carefully, and take note of its strengths and weaknesses.

The techniques used in the screening procedure have been changing in the light of previous experience. In general, there has been
a tendency to choose those screens that were most efficient in picking
up the presently available anti-cancer drugs. At once we can see a
potential weakness. If the screens are chosen on the basis of ability to
pick up the kinds of drugs now available (which are of limited
utility), there is a good chance that they will be most efficient in picking up new drugs that resemble the old ones, and we could end up
merely with a larger variety of drugs of limited utility, while perhaps
overlooking better materials with a completely different mode of
action. At this time, this is only a *potential* weakness; it may not
prove to be of practical importance.

The most common screening tests involve the injection of the
test material into mice bearing transplantable cancers. Studies are
also sometimes done on cancers growing in egg embryos or in tissue
culture. Promising materials are rarely tested in mice with spontaneous cancers. About 90 per cent of the screening tests have been
done on mice with one of three types of transplantable cancer; ordinarily, every new material being screened is tested against each of
these three types of malignancy. Some of the details of the procedure
are important, since they may indicate major weaknesses which should
be corrected.

In a typical procedure, a mouse with a cancer of moderate size
which has been transplanted through hundreds of generations (*see*
Chapter 14), is killed. The cancer is then removed aseptically, and
cut up into pieces small enough to pass through a large needle called
a trochar. With the trochar, pieces of the cancer are then put under
the skin of young inbred mice. The young mice are divided into
experimental and control groups. Each mouse in the experimental
group usually receives an injection of the test drug into the peritoneal
cavity every day for a predetermined period, usually either 10 or 14
days, beginning on the day the cancer is transplanted. Injection into
the peritoneal cavity is convenient, and also insures rapid absorption
of most materials, since drugs injected there are absorbed more
rapidly than those injected intramuscularly or hypodermically. In a
few cases, the test material may be injected every 12 hours, or in
even fewer cases, every 8 hours instead of every 24, but the usual
regimen is an injection every 24 hours. The control animals receive
injections of saline at the same times and in a similar manner.

At a predetermined time—usually on the eighth or the twelfth
day—all the mice are killed and the cancers removed and weighed.

The average weight of the cancers in the treated mice is compared to the average weight of the cancers in the control mice. If the cancers in the treated mice are less than 54 per cent of the weight of the cancers in the control mice (46 per cent inhibition), the material is retested. If there is less than 46 per cent inhibition, the test material is discarded, and not usually retested.

When the materials that pass the first screen are retested, they are required to show a still greater degree of cancer inhibition (55 to 58 per cent) in order to be studied further. These materials then may be given to mice with a wide variety of transplantable tumors, and perhaps to some mice with spontaneous tumors, before being scheduled for therapeutic trials in man. Thus far, there have been no intermediate tests on large animals with spontaneous cancers.

From the beginning of the screening program to the end of 1965, slightly over 250,000 different materials were tested on several million mice (1). Of these materials about 48 per cent were products of fermentation, about 44 per cent were synthetic compounds, and about 8 per cent were plant products. The current rate of screening is about 17,600 new materials per year, of which about half are synthetic, about 29 per cent are fermentation products, and about 21 per cent are plant products. Of all the materials tested, approximately one in 2,000 is selected for clinical trial. Thus, over 100 have been tried clinically.

In general, the results of the use of anti-cancer drugs (found through the screening) in treatment of human cancer have been disappointing, although a few have provided some patients with short periods of palliation. The anti-cancer drugs that do cure a few of the unusual cancers cannot be credited to the screening program as such. Methotrexate (Amethopterin), a folic acid antagonist which cures about half of the cases of choriocarcinoma, a cancer of the fetal placenta which metastasizes to the mother, really developed from the observation that folic acid made some cancers worse. Vinblastine (Velban) which also cures some cases of choriocarcinoma and some cases of Hodgkin's disease, and possibly some other related conditions, was discovered because of the wise decision on the part of some Canadian scientists to investigate further some unexpected actions of periwinkle plant extracts which were being tested for anti-diabetes effects. (The anti-diabetes testing was being done because natives of a Caribbean island had observed that the plant helped diabetics.)

It is appropriate to note an interesting point about choriocarcinoma, the one true cancer that is definitely curable by these

74

drugs: It is one of only two types of cancer known to be transplantable in man.

None of the anti-cancer drugs that were developed through the screening program have yet been reported as being able to cure or ✶ effectively control any solid cancers in man. Their major drawback seems to be a high index of toxicity; that is, doses that would kill all the cancer cells in a patient are larger than the doses that would kill the patient, usually through effects on bone marrow and gastrointestinal tract. Even the dosages that are used for palliation and to try to extend life often cause serious toxicity. A few patients with leukemia may have been cured by drugs.

In view of the disappointing results of our screening program, it seems proper to review some of its aspects, and see whether there are areas that should be improved. One criticism of the program is that the tests are started on the day of implantation of the cancer. Therefore, they could be considered tests of ability to affect early cancer, of a size much too small to be diagnosed, rather than tests of ability to affect moderately advanced cancer. The reply to this criticism has been that a system that picks out agents able to affect early cancer is less likely to miss an agent that would be useful for treating advanced cancer. In other words, although there may be more false positives— materials that affect only the earliest cancers—there will be fewer false negatives, that is, less chance of missing a material that could be generally useful in treating cancer. This seems a reasonable and logical position.

A second criticism is that all the initial screening is done on transplantable cancers, while the real interest is in materials able to affect spontaneous cancers. A fundamental assumption behind the screening procedure is that transplantable cancers are sufficiently similar to spontaneous cancers to be studied in place of them. There are some theoretical reasons to question this assumption, since the transplantable cancers have gone through so many generations that evolutionary processes have probably altered them significantly. More important, there is now definite evidence of important differences between the responses of transplantable and spontaneous cancers to drugs. Many drugs and chemicals that can cure transplantable cancers are ineffective against spontaneous cancers (see Chapter 14). Accordingly, there has been a gradual change in the assumptions underlying the screening tests. It is recognized that there will be false positives—that is, materials that affect transplantable but not spontaneous cancers. This is often attributed to the greater resistance of spontaneous cancers to chemotherapy. One aspect of this problem, however, is rarely discussed—the chances that some of the material being tested will work well against spontaneous cancers but not against transplantable cancers. The screening process may have produced false negatives, and we may have discarded an excellent drug against spontaneous cancers because it did not work well against transplantable cancers in mice. Unfortunately, we have no way to judge this possibility.

At times, it is argued that chances of false negatives are quite small because it is harder to treat spontaneous cancers than transplantable ones. According to such reasoning, it is unlikely that a drug would work on a hard-to-treat condition (spontaneous cancer) and not on a closely related easier-to-treat condition (transplantable cancer). However, such an argument overlooks the possibility that there may be qualitative as well as quantitative differences between the two kinds of cancer. Furthermore, in medicine there are several examples of drugs that are quite useful in treating severe, and hitherto hard-to-treat conditions, but much less effective in treating milder conditions that seem to be related. For example, drugs that are dramatically effective in treating severe psychoses have often been found to be of little, if any, value in treating psychoneuroses. Several drugs that can control grand mal epilepsy almost completely are much less effective, and are not often used in petit mal epilepsy. The fact is that we just do not know whether the screening program is discarding cures for spontaneous cancers.

Accordingly, there are suggestions that spontaneous mouse cancers as well as transplantable mouse cancers be used in the primary screen. Theoretically, this is a valid and logical plan and in a comprehensive, properly supported national program it should be followed. But with our present restricted program, this is virtually impossible. First of all, there are not nearly enough mice with spontaneous cancers available. (They could be made available in a properly designed and supported national program, as discussed further in Chapter 29). Secondly, the budget available for the screening program has not been sufficient to include the use of mice with spontaneous cancers in the primary screen.

However, there appears to be another defect in the screening program, just as serious as those mentioned above. It derives from the dosage schedule used in the testing program. To understand fully the significance of this point, it is helpful first to ask just what kinds of drugs we are seeking. The terms anti-cancer and chemotherapeutic are vague; it is necessary to go a bit deeper and ask what kind of pharmacologic action in a drug might make it useful in treating cancer patients.

The most obvious type of useful action is the direct cancerocidal effect, namely, a killing of cancer cells, without killing many normal cells. This is basically the "magic bullet" approach of Paul Ehrlich. Perhaps magic bullets for cancer exist, and we ought to keep looking for them. However, thus far, all chemicals that have been found to kill cancer cells also kill many normal cells. An added problem of a magic-bullet type of drug is that it should be 100 per cent effective. If it kills only 99 per cent of the cancer cells, the surviving cells will multiply, and as clinical experience indicates, they will usually be resistant to the cancerocidal drug, and pass this resistance on to their progeny. Therefore, a second course of treatment with a cancerocidal drug has much less effect, and a third course is often ineffective. Thus a drug that might kill 99.9 per cent of all malignant cells may frequently produce a remission of less than a year.

A second type of drug which could be useful would be a differential growth inhibitor—a drug that inhibits the growth and multiplication of cancer cells but not of normal cells vital to life. There is some evidence from other areas of biology to suggest that such differential growth inhibitors might be a reasonable target (*see* Chapter 20). Such a drug would not be used in the same way as a cancerocidal drug; it would have to be taken regularly, over a prolonged period of time, so that an effective level would be maintained in the patient's blood stream, at almost all times. Its action should be to keep the cancer from growing any further; in addition, there would be the hope that the body's defenses might be able to make the cancer regress. In other areas of medicine, there are several drugs that are given to patients in a dosage regimen that keeps an effective level in the blood at almost all times, and enables the patients to live virtually normal lives; for example, the anti-epilepsy drugs, the cardiac glycosides and thyroid hormone.

If a cancer-growth inhibiting drug (cancerostatic) were present in the blood stream less than 100 per cent of the time, it could still be a useful control for cancer. Let us assume that a particular cancer in a particular patient is growing at a rate that would cause death in one year. If a cancerostatic drug were present in adequate concentrations only 90 per cent of the time, the patient's life expectancy would be increased about ten years. If the inhibitor were present in adequate concentrations 95 per cent of the time, the patient's life expectancy could be expected to rise about 20 years. Thus, for drugs of this and related types of pharmacologic action, 100 per cent effectiveness is probably not necessary in every case.

A third type of potentially useful anti-cancer drug would be one that inhibits the proliferation of new blood vessels to the cancer (*see* Chapters 19 and 20). If the proliferation of blood vessels could be inhibited, there is good reason to believe that many cancers would stop growing. In an adult, this type of inhibition should cause no serious problems, but it might lead to stunted growth if used to treat children with cancer. Here, too, the object would not be to kill the cancer but to contain it and prevent its spread. We may hope, too, that some of the host defense mechanisms might cause the cancer to shrink; but even if this does not occur, the patient could live a relatively normal life even with his cancer. For this type of drug action to be effective, there should be an adequate level of the drug in the patient's blood at almost all times.

A fourth type of potentially useful anti-cancer drug would be one that in some way inhibits the ability of cancer cells to penetrate between normal cells. Such a drug, like those mentioned above, might effectively control cancer, provided adequate concentrations were present in the patient's blood stream at almost all times.

A fifth type of potentially useful anti-cancer drug would be one that in some manner improves host defenses against the cancer. Again, this type of action could be expected to be of significant value only if the drug is present in adequate concentrations for prolonged periods.

There are other types of potentially useful anti-cancer drugs, but those mentioned should be sufficient to illustrate the variety of pharmacologic actions that might be useful in an anti-cancer drug.

Let us now return to the details of the screening program and take note of two important points. The first point is that the cancer-bearing mice usually receive a single intraperitoneal injection of the test drug every 24 hours and, on that injection schedule, are required to show 45 to 58 per cent inhibition of the cancer if the test drug is not to be discarded. A regimen of this sort is probably reasonably effective in picking up cancerocidal drugs, since a drug of this type need not necessarily be present for prolonged periods to exert its effects. Some cancerocidal drugs—the nitrogen mustards—exert their effects in a few minutes. In actuality, all of the anti-cancer drugs chosen by our current screening process have been largely cancerocidal, although some may have other, secondary actions. These drugs all share the same disadvantages: a high level of host toxicity and usually an inability to control cancer for periods greater than a year.

However, the essence of this first point is that, thus far, the screening program has not picked up any drugs that selectively inhibit the growth of cancer cells, or that inhibit proliferation of host blood vessels to the cancer, or that inhibit the ability of cancer cells to invade normal cells or that improve host defenses. This is not surprising in view of the screening procedure used.

The second important point is that there are few drugs of any type that when given to man will exert an appreciable effect over a 24-hour period—and that mice tend to metabolize and excrete drugs from five to ten times faster than man. Thus, the proportion of drugs of any type that would show 45 to 58 per cent effectiveness in a mouse for 24 hours after a single intraperitoneal injection would be extremely small.

Since this point is so vital, it seems worthwhile to clarify and illustrate it. Let us assume that we actually had a highly effective drug which inhibited cancer growth completely in concentrations that were non-toxic to the host. What could be expected if this drug were put into the present screening program as an unknown? When injected into the mouse with cancer, it should completely stop cancer growth for the period when adequate concentrations of the drug were present in the mouse. If the drug is like most drugs, that period would be less than two hours. However, let us assume that this is a relatively long-acting drug, and that after a single intraperitoneal injection its action persists for four hours in the mouse. During that 4-hour period, cancer growth would cease (although an observer could not notice it), and during the remaining 20 hours, the cancer would grow at its normal rate. When the 10-day period of daily injections is over, there would have been 40 hours of no growth and 200 hours of growth of the cancer. This comes to approximately 17 per cent inhibition (a figure far lower than the minimum of 45 per cent required by the present procedure), and the drug would be discarded. Yet a drug of this type, taken every four hours by a human, might control his cancer completely.

Let us consider another illustration. Suppose we did not know how to relieve headache. Let us assume that a screening program were set up, using human volunteers having persistent headaches, and that each volunteer received a test drug once a day—either by mouth or by injection and, further, that each volunteer had to report on the percentage of inhibition of the headache over a 24-hour period. None of our present headache-relieving drugs would produce relief for more than 20 per cent of the 24-hour period if given once during that interval. If a minimum of 45 per cent inhibition over 24 hours were required, all of our useful anti-headache drugs, including aspirin and codeine (and even such potent narcotics as Demerol and morphine), would be discarded. The point to note here is that even if *man* were the experimental subject, the requirement of a minimum of a 45 per cent effect over a 24-hour period from a single injection of a drug would be quite unrealistic.

However, when mice, with their rapid metabolism, are used as experimental animals, the difficulties and the chances of false negatives are even greater. Let us consider what would happen if we did not know about barbiturates and set up a screening program in female mice to find a useful sedative. Let us assume that each mouse would receive, by intraperitoneal injection, a large dose of the barbiturate, defined as an amount equal to about one-half of a lethal dose. Let us further suppose that, immediately after the injection, each mouse is put into an opaque jiggle cage which is attached to recorders that measure the mouse's movements around the cage, and present the total on a 24-hour basis. When the mouse is sleeping, its movements would be virtually zero. After a large dose of pentobarbital (Nembutal), the mouse would sleep about 20 to 30 minutes (2), and the record for the 24 hours would show less than 5 per cent inhibition for the entire period. After a large dose of secobarbital (Seconal) a similar result would be obtained. After amobarbital (Amytal), the inhibition over the 24-hour period might be about 5 per cent, and after phenobarbital (Luminal), the animals would sleep about two to three hours, giving about 10 to 12 per cent inhibition of activity over the 24-hour period. Thus, if a minimum of 45 per cent inhibition of activity were required, all these useful drugs would be discarded. In man, the effects of equivalent doses of these barbiturates last eight to ten times as long.

Accordingly, it should be clear that in our present cancer screening program, the techniques and the selection criteria are such that drugs of several pharmacologic types that could provide control of cancer are not likely to be picked up. Indeed, it is not unreasonable to suggest that among the 250,000 materials discarded by the screen there may be several excellent drugs which could control cancer in many patients for many years, perhaps for their normal lifetimes.

This point of view may be disputed. One scientist engaged in a screening program reported on a list of materials that were discarded by the screen. He stated that in several cases he tried injections every 12 hours instead of every 24, and found no difference. From this he concluded that the usual procedure—one injection every 24 hours—was quite satisfactory. This argument has two flaws. First, unless the substances that were tested included an effective anti-cancer drug, negative results with more frequent injections would mean nothing. If a material does not affect cancer (and probably 1,999 out of 2,000 do not), a lack of effect with any regimen tells us nothing about that regimen. Secondly, injections every 12 hours would probably still not be frequent enough in mice to show which of the drugs being tested have anti-cancer actions other than the cancerocidal one.

It may seem puzzling to find that such a basic defect has been incorporated into a national screening program for so many years. There are probably several reasons for it. At the beginning of the program, hopes were high that a curative cancerocidal drug would be found soon. By the time the initial optimism had dissipated, the basis of the present procedure was probably well established. Undoubtedly, another problem was lack of funds. The chronic shortage of financial support for cancer research probably helped to make it impossible to conduct the screening program in the manner that would be considered best, and compromises had to be made. The tests would, of course, be much more costly if the mice were to receive more frequent injections. In retrospect, it may seem that it would have been worthwhile to screen fewer materials in a better manner. It would not be fair, however, to criticize those who had to make the decisions using the limited information and resources available then.

The important point is that these flaws be corrected in any future screening activities, since it seems vital that screening techniques and criteria be such that other useful anti-cancer drugs will be picked up along with cancerocidal ones. Several suggestions are appropriate.

If mice are to be the experimental animals, as seems highly likely, consideration should be given to their rapid metabolism and rapid excretion of drugs and chemicals. Perhaps it would be practical to give the mice an injection every four hours (as is done with many patients with varying disease conditions). Perhaps the test materials should be injected in a vehicle which prolongs absorption for a period of 18 to 24 hours. It would be unwise to try to guess which of these procedures would work better, or whether some other procedure would be best. However, in revising our screening program, more efficient use should be made of the training, experience and skills of those members of the scientific community who have not been given adequate opportunities to participate in the cancer research program. Veterinary pharmacologists who have a broad understanding of species differences in metabolism and excretion of drugs should play a greater role in deciding on schedules and routes of injections in experimental animals. The faculties of our colleges of pharmacy could probably provide invaluable help in finding ways of prolonging drug action in experimental animals since they have already developed ways of prolonging drug action in man.

We ought also to come to grips with the problem of spontaneous vs. transplantable cancers. The primary screen in any future screening program should include a significant group of spontaneous cancers. The difficulties in obtaining spontaneous cancers in adequate numbers could be resolved in a national-goal program (*see* Chapter 29).

Since there may be a substantial chance that one or more highly useful anti-cancer drugs have been discarded by our present screen, serious consideration should be given to retesting—in the improved screen—many of the 250,000 discarded materials. This would have to be done in such a way as to avoid interfering with the testing of new materials. A suggested plan is that retesting be done of all synthetic materials that showed more than 20 per cent inhibition of any kind of cancer in the old screen, and of all plant extracts or products of fermentation that showed more than 10 per cent inhibition. The reason for setting a lower limit on plant and fermentation products is that they are mixtures of many substances, and an active, potent ingredient might be concentrated and found to be highly effective. The synthetic chemicals, by contrast, are usually more than 90 per cent pure. These figures, of course, represent a compromise, and the limits suggested might have to be altered.

A well-designed screening program has a good chance of discovering a highly useful anti-cancer drug which could adequately control most cancers. The fact that errors and omissions have been pointed out in our present program is in no way a criticism of the screening concept. Few scientific programs are successful in the first round; they must be changed and corrected as sources of error are discovered. A corrected, expanded and adequately supported screening program should be a major component of a national-goal program to find a cure or control for cancer.

References

1. National Advisory Cancer Council, *Progress Against Cancer—1966,* U. S. Dep't. of Health, Education, and Welfare, Washington, p. 15.
2. Westfall, B. A., Boulos, B. M., Shields, J. and Garb, S. Sex differences in pentobarbital sensitivity in mice. *Proc. Soc. Expt'l. Biol. and Med. 115:*509, 1964.

Search for a Vaccine against Cancer

In recent years, the search for a cancer vaccine has caught and held the attention of many persons, including some scientists, numerous reporters, and a sizeable segment of the general public. A large and growing portion of our national cancer research program is concerned with the search for viral causes of cancer, with the ultimate aim of producing a vaccine to prevent cancer. The attractiveness of this approach is not difficult to understand. Vaccines have almost eradicated such diseases as smallpox, that in the past killed many millions. Furthermore, in the past decade we have seen the development of new and effective vaccines for such serious diseases as poliomyelitis and measles. The prevention of disease by means of a vaccine is about the simplest, least distressing, and most economical prophylactic measure available to the medical profession. If an effective vaccine for cancer could be developed within a reasonable period of time, it would be of the greatest value.

However, we cannot afford to let the intensity of our desire for a particular solution influence our judgment concerning its practicality. We must know whether it is likely that this approach could lead to prevention, control, or cure for cancer in the foreseeable future.

Since the pioneer work of Wade (1) and Rous (2-4), studies by many investigators have implicated viruses as causative agents in a wide variety of animal cancers (5, 79, 142-164). However, it is important to note that the cancer-inducing viruses do not belong to a single species.

Moore (80) in his preface to Koenig's review stated:

> More than a dozen different viruses have already been found to cause cancer in mice and they show a bewildering variety of behaviors. Tumor viruses are not restricted to a single class but are found in almost all of the different taxonomic divisions. There are both RNA and DNA-containing tumor viruses; there are lipid-containing and lipid-free tumor viruses; some have a definite spherical or polyhedral internal body covered with a loose-fitting membrane (Herpes type); some have a more amorphous internal

structure surrounded by a membrane (Rous sarcoma, Avian leukosis, Bittner virus); and some are polyhedral, with various numbers of capsomeres (Polyoma, wound tumor). Thus the number and complexity of tumor viruses and the enormous variety of approaches to discovering still more and to understanding the mechanisms of their operation have swollen the literature at an almost exponential rate.

Let us suppose that, as an early step in the attempt to develop a vaccine against human cancer, virologists try to make a vaccine to prevent cancer in mice. Since there are probably more than 12 viruses capable of causing cancer in mice, a separate vaccine would be needed for each one. The difficulty in making vaccines against all of these different strains would be very great.

Even if a vaccine were developed that could prevent all virus-induced cancers in mice, it would not completely solve the problem since there are many causes of mouse cancer besides viruses (Chapter 5). It might be argued that the fundamental cause of cancer is always a virus, and that other carcinogenic agents merely activate the virus or lower the host's resistance to it. However, the brilliant studies of Pollard (81-84) have virtually eliminated this line of reasoning from serious consideration. He used germ-free rats and mice, in which no virus of any sort had ever been found, and inoculated them with heat-sterilized carcinogenic chemicals. Despite the absence of viruses in the chemicals, the animals developed lung cancers, fibrosarcomas and breast cancers. These studies were repeated in at least four strains of mice and three strains of rats.

We have no reason to expect a cancer vaccine to prevent cancers that are not virus-induced. This brings up the question of the relative frequency of virus-induced cancers compared to those caused by other agents. Here, the data on mouse cancer can be misleading. The studies on viral causation of mouse cancer have been done mainly on highly inbred strains that have an hereditary susceptibility to a particular virus. Since virtually all cancers in experimental mice were deliberately produced by research scientists, these cancers gave no clue to the relative importance of different causal agents. Thus, if we were to find that 60 per cent of the research papers on mouse cancers referred to virus-induced cancers and only 10 per cent referred to chemically induced cancers, we could not conclude that virus-caused cancers were biologically more important than chemically induced cancers. We might logically conclude, however, that more funds were available for research into virus-induced than for research into chemically induced cancers.

When we turn to man, we find additional problems. First, despite intensive study, not a single type of human cancer has yet been definitely shown to be virus-induced. There is epidemiologic evidence that *suggests* that one type, Burkitt's lymphoma, may have a viral origin (85-87, 118-137). Furthermore, there is also some evidence that links certain human leukemias to viruses and mycoplasmas (88-98). However, for the vast bulk of human cancers—over 90 per cent of their total—there is no evidence of a viral etiology. Indeed, the available evidence points away from a viral cause of most human cancers. Virus diseases spread in patterns which are recognizable to epidemiologists. In effect, the evidence that points to the viral origin of Burkitt's lymphoma is primarily the difference between its patterns of geographic spread and the geographic patterns of other cancers. Therefore, to the extent that epidemiologic studies point to a viral cause of Burkitt's lymphoma, they point away from a viral cause of most cancers. Furthermore, there is convincing positive evidence that many human cancers are caused by agents other than viruses. Since the studies of Potts more than a century ago, it has been known that chimney sweeps are prone to develop cancer of the scrotum, caused by contact with soot containing carcinogenic chemicals. In other industries, too, cancer of the scrotum is found in workers who have contact with certain chemicals (99). Workers in the asbestos industry develop a characteristic type of cancer which is exceedingly rare elsewhere; its cause is almost certainly inhalation of asbestos dust (100, 101). Workers in other industries have developed lung cancer from inhaling materials used in these industries (102). Certain metals (103) and many chemicals produce cancer in man (104, 105). Certain foods tend to produce cancer (106), and there is strong evidence that some types of processing or contamination of foods cause cancer (107). A striking example is the high incidence of stomach cancer in Icelandic people, attributed to their high consumption of smoked goods contaminated by carcinogenic materials in the smoke. Also, we should all be aware that many cigarette smokers develop lung cancer.

There is, in addition, convincing evidence that radiation produces cancer and leukemia in man (108-112), and it has been known for years that cancer of the skin of the face may be the result of prolonged exposure to direct sunlight.

There is no reason whatever to suspect that there is any connection between all these cancers and viruses, and therefore, no reason to think that a vaccine would have any value in preventing such cancers.

Many of the common cancers in man are not as yet linked with any specific causative factors, nor do their patterns of distribution suggest, in any way, a viral etiology. With the increasing numbers of chemicals being added to the air we breathe, the food we eat, and the beverages we drink, it is a reasonable presumption that many human cancers are induced by chemicals.

Thus, even if a cancer vaccine were developed, there is no reason to believe that it would be effective in preventing more than a tiny fraction of human cancers.

Let us, however, for the sake of argument, assume that through some unknown mechanism it becomes possible to develop a vaccine against many human cancers. Still, there would be major difficulties, for many decades, in utilizing such a vaccine. To understand this point clearly, it is necessary to return temporarily to a consideration of the mouse cancers—the best models of virus-induced cancers available to us today. Mice can develop mammary cancers after swallowing a virus in their mother's milk (22, 24, 26, 80, 138-141), but the cancers do not develop until the exposed animals are well into middle age. Thus, the latent period between exposure to the virus and development of the cancer is approximately half of the animal's lifetime. With some other viruses, the latent period may be somewhat shorter, but, in general, it is a substantial part of the normal life expectancy of the species. If any of the common human cancers are virus-induced, it is likely that they, too, have a latent period that is a substantial part of the life span. This concept accords with our experiences in human cancer: most human cancers in man develop in people well past the age of 40. Even cancers that are known to be induced by non-viral agents usually have latent periods of many years between exposure and beginning of the cancer. The implications of this time factor warrant serious consideration. Let us assume that for a particular cancer, for which a vaccine is being developed, the latent period between exposure to the virus and onset of the cancer averages 40 years. In developing the vaccine, one step would be a testing of its effectiveness and safety on a sample population. This step cannot be omitted because it is possible that the vaccine would enhance the cancer rather than producing protection against it (*see* Chapter 23).

Let us assume that by 1975 a vaccine has been developed which the virologists hope will prevent a particular type of human cancer. To test the vaccine on a representative population sample, it would be necessary to give it to a group of infants and young children, and then follow them for more than 40 years—to the year 2015. Probably the follow-up would have to extend for at least another ten years so that one could be certain that the vaccine, in delaying the onset of the cancer, did not greatly increase its incidence a few years later. Let us now assume that by 2025 scientists are satisfied with the trial run, and able to produce enough vaccine for all the infants being born. The vaccine would be given to all of these infants. Thus, by the year 2065, when these people were 40 years old, the incidence of this kind of cancer would begin to drop, and by 2067, the death rate from it would also begin to fall gradually, coming down close to zero after another 30 to 40 years—around the year 2100. It is difficult to see any way of speeding up this process in view of the long latent period before development of cancer.

Of course, we are concerned about the welfare of our descendants 100 years from now, and thus it is appropriate to continue our efforts to find a vaccine for cancer. But even if such a vaccine were found tomorrow, there is very little chance of its helping anyone living today. It would seem unwise to devote too great a proportion of our resources and energies to this particular approach.

One further aspect of the relationship between cancer and viruses merits our consideration. It may be possible to find a virus that attacks cancer cells but not normal cells (113-117). This approach is analogous to the use of bacteria and bacterial products as anti-cancer agents (Chapter 25); it need not involve any long delays before an effective agent is found and tested, and deserves support.

The reasons for not being optimistic about development of a vaccine against most human cancers within a period of less than four generations are formidable. In summary, they are:

1. In animals subject to virus-induced cancers, many different types of viruses are involved, and a single vaccine could hardly be effective against all of them. If cancers in man are eventually shown to be virus-induced, the same problem will probably exist.

2. Most human cancers appear to be caused by agents other than viruses.

3. Thus far, not a single type of human cancer has been proven to be virus-induced, although two rather rare forms have epidemiological characteristics suggestive of a viral etiology.

4. If a viral cause of a common human cancer were identified and a vaccine developed, the long latent period between viral exposure and cancer development would probably mean that about 80 or more years would elapse before any benefits of the vaccine would become apparent.

References

1. Wade, H. An experimental investigation of infective sarcoma of the dog with a consideration of its relationship to cancer. *J. Path. and Bact. 12:384, 1908.*
2. Rous, P. A sarcoma of the fowl transmissible by an agent separable from the tumor cells. *J. Exp. Med. 13:*397, 1911.
3. Rous, P. Transmission of a malignant new growth by means of a cell-free filtrate. *J.A.M.A. 56:*198, 1911.
4. Rous, P. Resistance to a tumor-producing agent as distinct from resistance to the implanted tumor cells. Observations with a sarcoma of the fowl. *J. Exp. Med. 18:* 416, 1913.
5. Andervont, H. B. and Bryan, W. R. Properties of the mouse mammary-tumor agent. *J. Nat. Cancer Inst. 5:*143, 1944.
6. Andervont, H. B. Problems concerning the tumor viruses. In: F. M. Burnett and W. M. Stanley (eds.), *The Viruses,* New York, Acad. Press, 1959.
7. Aoki, T., Old, L. J. and Boyse, E. A. Serological analysis of leukemia antigens of the mouse. *J. Nat. Cancer Inst.* Monograph No. 22, p. 449, 1966.
8. Axelrad, A. A., McCulloch, E. A., Howatson, A. F., Ham, A. W., and Siminovitch, L. Induction of tumors in Syrian hamsters by a cytopathogenic virus derived from a C3H mouse mammary tumor. *J. Nat. Cancer Inst. 24:*1095, 1960.
9. Bang, F. B., Andervont, H. B. and Vellisto, I. Electron microscopic evidence concerning the mammary tumor inciter (virus). II. An electron microscopic study of spontaneous and induced mammary tumors of mice. *Bull. Johns Hopkins Hosp. 98:*287, 1956.
10. Bang, F. B., Vellisto, I. and Libert, R. Electron microscopic evidence concerning the mammary tumor inciter (Virus). I. A study of normal and malignant cells from the mammary gland of mice. *Bull. Johns Hopkins Hosp. 98:*255, 1956.
11. Bernhard, W. The detection and study of tumor viruses with the electron microscope. *Cancer Res. 20:*712, 1960.
12. Bittner, J. J. The influence of transplanted normal tissue on breast cancer ratios in mice. *Pub. Health Rep. 54:*1827, 1939.
13. Blair, P. B. Serologic comparison of mammary tumor viruses from 3 strains of mice. *Proc. Soc. Exptl. Biol. and Med. 103:*188, 1960.
14. Blair, P. B. Neutralization of the mouse mammary tumor virus by rabbit antisera against C3Hf tissue. *Cancer Res. 23:*381, 1963.
15. Bonar, R. A., Heine, U., Beard, D. and Beard, J. W. Virus of avian myeloblastosis (BAI strain A). XXIII. Morphology of virus and comparison with strain R (erythroblastosis). *J. Nat. Cancer Inst. 30:*949, 1963.

16. Dalton, A. J. An electron microscopic study of a virus-induced murine sarcoma (Moloney). *J. Nat. Cancer Inst.* Monograph, No. 22, p. 143, 1966.
17. DeHarven, E. and Friend, C. Further electron microscope studies of a mouse leukemia induced by cell-free filtrates. *J. Biophys. Biochem. Cytol.* 7:747, 1960.
18. DeHarven, E. and Friend, C. Structure of virus particles partially purified from blood of leukemia mice. *Virology 23:*119, 1964.
19. DeHarven, E. and Friend, C. Origin of the viremia in murine leukemia. *J. Nat. Cancer Inst.* Monograph, No. 22, p. 79, 1966.
20. DeOme, K. B. The mouse mammary tumor virus. *Fed. Proc. 21:*15, 1962.
21. De-The, G. Association of enzymes, adenosinetriphosphatase and alkaline phosphatase with the virions of murine leukemias. *J. Nat. Cancer Inst.* Monograph, No. 22, p. 169, 1966.
22. Dmochowski, L. The milk agent in the origin of mammary tumors in mice. *Adv. Cancer Res. 1:*103, 1953.
23. Dmochowski, L. and Grey, C. E. Subcellular structures of possible viral origin in some mammalian tumors. *Ann. N. Y. Acad. Sci. 68:*559, 1957.
24. Dmochowski, L., Grey, C. E., Pearson, L. O., Ward, D. N., Hulbert, R. B., Griffin, A. C. and Bresson, A. L. Studies on mammary tumor inducing virus in mice (Bittner Virus). *Proc. Soc. Exptl. Biol. and Med. 102:*174, 1959.
25. Dmochowski, L., Grey, C. E. and Magee, L. A. Studies on a virus ("Polyoma") inducing multiple tumors in animals. *Proc. Soc. Exptl. Biol. and Med. 102:*575, 1959.
26. Dmochowski, L. and Haagensen, C. D. The distribution of the mammary tumor-inducing agent in the various constituents of the cytoplasm of mammary tumor cells in mice. *Acta Unio Internat. Contra Cancrum 11:*646, 1955.
27. Dourmashkin, R. R. and Simons, P. J. The ultrastructure of Rous sarcoma virus. *J. Ultrastruct. Res. 5:*505, 1961.
28. Dunn, T. B., Moloney, J. B., Green, A. W. and Arnold, B. Pathogenesis of a virus-induced leukemia in mice. *J. Nat. Cancer Inst. 26:*189, 1961.
29. Fink, M. A., Cowles, C. A., Chirigos, M. A. and Messore, J. A comparison by several techniques of the antibody prepared in various species against the Rauscher murine leukemia virus. *J. Nat. Cancer Inst.* Monograph, No. 22, p. 439, 1966.
30. Fogel, M. and Sachs, L. The *in vitro* and *in vivo* analysis of mammalian tumor viruses. IV. Antibody response and tumor induction with polyoma virus in different species. *J. Nat. Cancer Inst. 24:*839, 1960.
31. Gotlieb-Stematsky, T., Karbi, S. and Allison, A. C. Increased tumour formation by polyoma virus in the presence of non-oncogenic viruses. *Nature 212:*421, 1966.
32. Graffi, A., Fey, F. and Schramm, T. Experiments on the hematologic diversification of viral mouse leukemias. *J. Nat. Cancer Inst.* Monograph, No. 22, p. 21, 1966.
33. Gross, L. Viral etiology of "spontaneous" mouse leukemia. A review. *Cancer Res. 18:*371, 1958.
34. Gross, L. Are the common forms of spontaneous and induced leukemia and lymphomas in mice caused by a single virus? *J. Nat. Cancer Inst.* Monograph, No. 22, p. 407, 1966.
35. Habel, K. Specific complement-fixing antigens in polyoma tumors and transformed cells. *Virology 25:*55, 1965.
36. Habel, K. Immunological determinants of polyoma virus oncogenesis. *J. Exp. Med. 115:*181, 1962.
37. Hartley, J. W., Rowe, W. P., Capps, W. I. and Huebner, R. J. Complement fixation and tissue culture assays for mouse leukemia viruses. *Proc. Nat. Acad. Sci.* (Wash.) 53:931, 1965.
38. Heller, J. R. Research on cancer viruses. *Public Health Rep. 75:*501, 1960.

PART III

39. Hoggan, M. D., Rowe, W. P., Black, P. H. and Huebner, R. J. Production of "tumor-specific" antigens by oncogenic viruses during acute cytolytic infections. *Proc. Nat. Acad. Sci.* (Wash.) *53:*12, 1965.

40. Huebner, R. J., Armstrong, D., Okuyan, M., Sarma, P. S. and Turner, H. C. Specific complement-fixing viral antigens in hamster and guinea pig tumors induced by the Schmidt-Ruppin strain of avian sarcoma. *Proc. Nat. Acad. Sci.* (Wash.) *51:* 742, 1964.

41. Huebner, R. J., Lane, W. T., Reynolds, J. and Turner, H. C. Replication of specific viral antigen in adenovirus type 12 tumor transplants. *Fed. Proc. 22:* 438, 1963.

42. Ida, N., Fukuhara, A. and Ohba, Y. Several aspects of vertical transmission of Moloney virus. *J. Nat. Cancer Inst.* Monograph, No. 22, p. 287, 1966.

43. Jonsson, N. and Sjogren, H. O. Further studies on specific transplantation antigens in Rous sarcoma of mice. *J. Exp. Med. 122:*403, 1965.

44. Kidd, J. G. The detection of a "masked" virus (the Shope papilloma virus) by mean of immunization. *J. Exp. Med. 74:*321, 1941.

45. Kidd, J. G. The enduring partnership of a neoplastic virus and carcinoma cells. Continued increase of virus in the V2 carcinoma during propagation in virus immune hosts. *J. Exp. Med. 75:*7, 1942.

46. Kirsten, W. H., Mayer, L. A. and Welander, C. W. Infective and noninfective viral murine leukemias. *J. Nat. Cancer Inst.* Monograph, No. 22, p. 369, 1966.

47. Klein, G. and Klein, E. Antigenic behavior of Moloney virus-induced lymphomas in mice. *J. Nat. Cancer Inst.* Monograph, No. 22, p. 481, 1966.

48. Kobayashi, H., Kodama, T. and Takeda, K. Electromicroscopy of Friend tumour cell with special reference to the influence of Friend virus immunity on Friend tumour cell. *Nature 212:*1260, 1966.

49. Law, L. W. Transmission studies of a leukemogenic virus, MLV, in mice. *J. Nat. Cancer Inst.* Monograph, No. 22, p. 267, 1966.

50. Levy, J. P., Boiron, M., Silvestre, D. and Bernard, J. The ultrastructure of Rauscher virus. *Virology 26:*146, 1965.

51. Lilly, F. Susceptibility to two strains of Friend leukemia virus in mice. *Science 155:*461, 1967.

52. Mayyasi, S. A., Schidlovsky, G., Bulfone, L. M. and Clifford, N. L. Antigenic study on the Friend, Moloney, and Rauscher viruses with the electron microscope agglutination test. *J. Nat. Cancer Inst.* Monograph, No. 22, p. 379, 1966.

53. Molomut, N. and Padnos, M. Inhibition of transplantable and spontaneous murine tumours by the M-P virus. *Nature 208:*948, 1965.

54. Moloney, J. B. A virus-induced rhabdomyosarcoma of mice. *J. Nat. Cancer Inst.* Monograph, No. 22, p. 139, 1966.

55. Mora, P. T., McFarland, V. W. and Luborsky, S. W. Isolation of the nucleic acid of Rauscher murine leukemia virus. *J. Nat. Cancer Inst.* Monograph, No. 22, p. 191, 1966.

56. O'Connor, T. E., Rauscher, F. J., De-The, G., Fink, M. A. and Gerber, P. Murine leukemia viruses: Rupture with ether and detergents to subviral constituents. *J. Nat. Cancer Inst.* Monograph, No. 22, p. 205, 1966.

57. Old, L. J. and Boyse, E. A. Antigens of tumors and leukemias induced by viruses. *Fed. Proc. 24:*1009, 1965.

58. Papparella, V., Cali, A. and Rossi, G. B. Studies on a virus isolated from a calf affected by lymphatic leukemia. *Acta Unio Internat. Contra Cancrum 19:*336, 1963.

59. Pasternak, G., Horn, K. H. and Graffi, A. Untersuchungen zur Frage der Isoimmunität gegen virus-induzierte Leukosen der Maus. *Acta Biol. Med. Germ. 9:* 314, 1962.
60. Pitelka, D. R., DeOme, K. B. and Bern, H. A. Virus-like particles in precancerous hyperplastic mammary tissues of C3H and C3Hf mice. *J. Nat. Cancer Inst. 25:*753, 1960.
61. Pluznik, D. H., Sachs, L. and Resnitzky, P. The mechanism of leukemogenesis by the Rauscher leukemia virus. *J. Nat. Cancer Inst.* Monograph, No. 22, p. 3, 1966.
62. Recher, L., Tanaka, T., Sykes, J. A., Yumoto, T., Seman, G., Young, L. and Dmochowski, L. Further studies on the biological relationship of murine leukemia viruses and on kidney lesions of mice with leukemia induced by these viruses. *J. Nat. Cancer Inst.* Monograph, No. 22, p. 459, 1966.
63. Rich, M. A. Murine leukemia and its viruses. *J. Nat. Cancer Inst.* Monograph, No. 22, p. 425, 1966.
64. Rowe, W. P., Hartley, J. W. and Capps, W. I. Tissue culture and serologic studies of mouse leukemia viruses. *J. Nat. Cancer Inst.* Monograph, No. 22, p. 15, 1966.
65. Sachs, L. The *in vitro* analysis of malignancy induced by polyoma virus. In: *Ciba Foundation Symp. on Tumor Viruses of Murine Origin.* London, Churchill, Ltd. 380 p., 1962.
66. Sachs, L. and Medina, D. *In vitro* transformation of normal cells by polyoma virus. *Nature 189:*457, 1961.
67. Sinkovics, J. G. Viral leukemias in mice. *Ann. Rev. Microbiol. 16:*75, 1962.
68. Sinkovics, J. G., Bertin, B. A. and Howe, C. D. Occurrence of low leukemogenic but immunizing mouse leukemia virus in tissue culture. *J. Nat. Cancer Inst.* Monograph, No. 22, p. 349, 1966.
69. Sjogren, H. O. Tumor specific antigens in viral neoplasms and in unrelated virus infected tumors. *Ann. Med. Exp. Fenn. 44:*227, 1966.
70. Stewart, S. E. and Eddy, B. E. Tumor induction by SE polyoma virus and the inhibition of tumors by specific neutralizing antibodies. *Am. J. Pub. Health 49:* 1493, 1959.
71. Stewart, S. E. and Eddy, B. E. The polyoma virus In *Advances Virus Res. 7:*61, 1960.
72. Tennant, J. R. and Snell, G. D. Some experimental evidence for the influence of genetic factors on viral leukemogenesis. *J. Nat. Cancer Inst.* Monograph, No. 22, p. 61, 1966.
73. Thiersch, J. B. Attempts to transmit leucaemia of man and of mice to the chick embryo and to the young chick by the amniotic and intravenous routes. *Australian J. Exper. Bio. and M. Sc. 22:*57, 1944.
74. Upton, A. C., Jenkins, V. K., Walburg, H. E., Jr., Tyndall, R. L., Conklin, J. W. and Wald, N. Observations on viral, chemical, and radiation-induced myeloid and lymphoid leukemias in RF mice. *J. Nat. Cancer Inst.* Monograph, No. 22, p. 329, 1966.
75. Winocour, E. and Sachs, L. Cell-virus interactions with the polyoma virus. I. Studies on the lytic interaction in the mouse embryo system. *Virology 11:*699, 1960.
76. Winocour, E. and Sachs, L. Tumor induction by genetically homogeneous lines of polyoma virus. *J. Nat. Cancer Inst. 26:*737, 1961.
77. Yumoto, T., Recher, L., Sykes, J. A. and Dmochowski, L. Morphology and development of some murine leukemia viruses. *J. Nat. Cancer Inst.* Monograph, No. 22, p. 107, 1966.

78. Zeigel, R. F., Tyndall, R. L., O'Connor, T. E., Tetter, E. and Allen, B. V. Observations on the morphology of a murine leukemia virus (Rauscher) propagated in tissue culture. *J. Nat. Cancer Inst.* Monograph, No. 22, p. 227, 1966.
79. Zilber, L. A. Progress in experimental virology of cancer. *Progr. Exp. Tumor Res. 1:1*, 1960.
80. Moore, D. H. in preface to Koenig, E. *Cancer and Virus* (A guide and annotated bibliography to monographs, reviews, symposia, and survey articles with emphasis on human neoplasm) 1950-1963. U. S. Dep't. of Health, Education, and Welfare, PHS Nat. Cancer Inst., 1965.
81. Pollard, M. Induction of tumors in germ-free rodents by methylcholanthrene. *Fed. Proc. 22:*314, 1963.
82. Pollard, M. Chemical induction of mammary cancer in germ-free rats. *Nature 200:* 1289, 1963.
83. Pollard, M. and Solomon, J. C. Oncogenic effect of methylcholanthrene in newborn germ-free mice. *Proc. Soc. Exptl. Biol. and Med. 112:*256, 1963.
84. Pollard, M. Germfree animals and biological research. *Science 145:*247, 1964.
85. Editorial-Etiology of Burkitt's lymphoma. *J.A.M.A. 198:*77, 1966.
86. Epstein, M. A., Henle, G., Achong, B. G. and Barr, Y. M. Morphological and biological studies on a virus in cultured lymphoblasts from Burkitt's lymphoma. *J. Exp. Med. 121:*761, 1965.
87. Hieger, I. Carcinogenesis and the biology of cancer generally. *Nature 212:*665, 1966.
88. Almeida, J. D., Hasselback, R. C. and Ham, A. W. Virus-like particles in blood of two acute leukemia patients. *Science 142:*1487, 1963.
89. Arnoult, J. and Haguenae, F. Problems raised by the search for virus particles in human leukemia. A study with the electron microscope of blood plasma, cerebrospinal fluid, and megakaryocytes from bone marrow. *J. Nat. Cancer Inst. 36:* 1089, 1966.
90. Burger, C. L., Harris, W. W., Anderson, N. G., Bartlett, T. W. and Kinseley, R. M. Virus-like particles in human leukemic plasma. *Proc. Soc. Exptl. Biol. and Med. 115:*151, 1964.
91. Dalton, A. J. In: Viral Etiology of Leukemia. Combined clinical staff conference of the National Institutes of Health. *Ann. Intern. Med. 62:*376, 1965.
92. Dmochowski, L., Taylor, H. G. and Grey, C. E. Viruses and mycoplasma (PPLO) in human leukemia. *Cancer 18:*1345, 1965.
93. Girardi, A. J., Hayflick, L., Lewis, A. M. and Somerson, N. L. Recovery of mycoplasmas in the study of human leukemia and other malignancies. *Nature 205:* 188, 1965.
94. Hummeler, K., Tomassini, N. and Hayflick, L. Ultrastructure of a mycoplasma (Negroni) isolated from human leukemia. *J. Bact. 90:*517, 1965.
95. Mathe, G. Virus et leucemies humaines. *Presse Med. 72:*2831, 1964.
96. Mettenleiter, M. W., Mannheim, J. H. and Borschardt, P. R. Isolation of viral agents from human blood and their relationship to lymphatic leukemia. *Oncologia 16:* 307, 1963.
97. Prince, A. M. and Adams, W. R. "Virus like" particles in human plasma and serum from leukemic, hepatitic and control patients. *Fed. Proc. 24:*175, 1965.
98. Smith, K. O., Benyesh-Melnick, M. and Fernbach, D. J. Studies on human leukemia. II. Structure and quantitation of myxovirus-like particles associated with human leukemia. *J. Nat. Cancer Inst. 33:*557, 1964.
99. Hendricks, N. V., Berry, C. M., Lione, J. G. and Thorpe, J. J. Cancer of the scrotum in wax pressmen. I. Epidemiology. *A.M.A. Arch. Indust. Health 19:*524, 1959.

100. Lynch, K. M. and Smith, W. A. Pulmonary asbestosis: Carcinoma of lung in asbesto-silicosis. *Am. J. Cancer 24:*56, 1935.
101. Doll, R. Mortality from lung cancer in asbestos workers. *Brit. J. Indust. Med. 12:* 81, 1955.
102. Doll, R. Occupational lung cancer; a review. *Brit. J. Indust. Med. 16:*181, 1959.
103. Neuman, D. A case of adeno-carcinoma of the left inferior turbinate body and perforation of the nasal septum in the person of a worker in chrome pigment. *Glasgow Med. J. 33:*469, 1890.
104. Falk, H. L., Kotin, P. and Mehler, A. Polycyclic hydrocarbons as carcinogens for man. *Arch. Environ. Health 8:*721, 1964.
105. Payne, W. W. Occupational factors in carcinogenesis. *Pub. Health Rep. 81:*777, 1966.
106. Laqueur, G. L., Mickelsen, O., Whiting, M. and Kurland, L. T. Carcinogenic properties of nuts from Cycas circinalis L. indigenous to Guam. *J. Nat. Cancer Inst. 31:*919, 1963.
107. Kraybill, H. F. and Shimkin, M. B. Carcinogenesis related to foods contaminated by processing and fungal metabolites. *Adv. Cancer Res. 8:*191, 1964.
108. Simpson, C. L., Hempelmann, L. H. and Fuller, L. M. Neoplasia in children treated with X-rays in infancy for thymic enlargement. *Radiology 64:*840, 1955.
109. MacMahon, B. Prenatal X-ray exposure and childhood cancer. *J. Nat. Cancer Inst. 28:*1173, 1962.
110. Folley, J. H., Borges, W. and Yamawaki, T. Incidence of leukemia in survivors of atomic bomb in Hiroshima and Nagasaki, Japan. *Am. J. Med. 13:*311, 1952.
111. Lange, R. D., Moloney, W. C. and Yamawaki, T. Leukemia in atomic bomb survivors. I. General observations. *Blood 9:*574, 1954.
112. Bizzozero, O. J., Jr., Johnson, K. G. and Ciocco, A. Radiation-related leukemia in Hiroshima and Nagasaki 1946-1964. I. Distribution, incidence and appearance time. *New Eng. J. Med. 274:*1095, 1966.
113. Moore, A. E. Viruses with oncolytic properties and their adaptation to tumors. *Ann. N. Y. Acad. Sci. 54:*945, 1952.
114. Moore, A. E. Effects of viruses on tumors. *Ann. Rev. Microbiol. 8:*393, 1954.
115. Moore, A. E. Oncolytic properties of viruses. *Texas Rep. Biol. Med. 15:*588, 1957.
116. Newman, W. and Southam, C. M. Virus treatment in advanced cancer. *Cancer 7:*106, 1954.
117. Southam, C. M. and Moore, A. E. Clinical studies of viruses as antineoplastic agents, with particular reference to Egypt 101 virus. *Cancer 5:*1025, 1952.
118. Burkitt, D. and Davies, J. N. P. Lymphoma syndrome in Uganda and tropical Africa. *Med. Press. 245:*367, 1951.
119. Burkitt, D. Sarcoma involving jaws in African children. *Brit. J. Surg. 46:*218, 1958-59.
120. Burkitt, D. A lymphoma syndrome in African children. *Ann. Roy. Coll. Surg.* (Eng.) *30:*211, 1962.
121. Burkitt, D. A tumour safari in East and Central Africa. *Brit. J. Cancer 16:*378, 1962.
122. Burkitt, D. Determining the climatic limitation of a children's cancer common in Africa. *Brit. Med. J. 2:*1019, 1962.
123. Burkitt, D. A children's cancer dependent on climatic factors. *Nature 194:* 232, 1962.
124. Burkitt, D. A tumour syndrome affecting children in tropical Africa. *Postgrad. Med. 38:*71, 1962.

93

125. Burkitt, D., Hutt, M. S. R. and Wright, D. H. The African lymphoma. Preliminary observations on response to therapy. *Cancer 18:*399, 1965.
126. Burkitt, D. and Wright, D. H. Geographical and tribal distribution of the African lymphoma in Uganda. *Brit. Med. J. 1:*569, 1966.
127. Bell, T. M., Massie, A., Ross, M. G. R. and Williams, M. C. Isolation of a reovirus from a case of Burkitt's lymphoma. *Brit. Med. J. 1:*1212, 1964.
128. Wright, D. H. Burkitt's tumor and childhood lymphosarcoma. *Clin. Ped. 6:*116, 1967.
129. Dalldorf, G., Bergamini, F. and Frost, P. Further observations of the lymphomas of African children. *Proc. Nat. Acad. Sci. 55:*297, 1966.
130. Epstein, M. A., Henle, G., Achong, B. G. and Barr, Y. M. Morphological and biological studies on a virus in cultured lymphoblasts from Burkitt's lymphoma. *J. Exp. Med. 121:*761, 1965.
131. Haddow, A. J. An improved map for the study of Burkitt's lymphoma syndrome in Africa. *East Afric. Med. J. 40:*429, 1963.
132. O'Conor, G. T. and Davies, J. N. P. Malignant tumours in African children. *J. Pediat. 56:*526, 1960.
133. O'Conor, G. T. Significant aspects of childhood lymphoma in Africa. *Cancer Res. 23:*1514, 1963.
134. Pulvertaft, R. J. V. Phytohaemagglutinin in relation to Burkitt's tumour. *Lancet 1:*238, 1964.
135. Stewart, S. E., Lovelace, E., Whang, J. J. and Ngu, A. Burkitt's tumour: tissue culture, cytogenetic and virus studies. *J. Nat. Cancer Inst. 34:*319, 1964.
136. Wright, D. H. Burkitt's tumour, a postmortem study of 50 cases. *Brit. J. Surg. 51:*245, 1964.
137. National Advisory Cancer Council—*Progress Against Cancer*—1966, U. S. Dep't. of Health, Education and Welfare, Washington, p. 39.
138. Bittner, J. J. Some possible effects of nursing on the mammary gland tumor incidence in mice. *Science 84:*162, 1936.
139. Green, R. G., Moosey, M. M. and Bittner, J. J. Antigenic character of the cancer milk agent in mice. *Proc. Soc. Exptl. Biol. and Med. 61:*115, 1946.
140. Axelrad, A. A. and Vander Gaag, H. C. Comparison of quantitative autologous and isologous transplantation of "spontaneous" (milk factor-induced) mammary tumors in C3H and DBA/2 mice. *Proc. Am. Assoc. Cancer Res. 3:*4, 1959.
141. Morton, D. L. Acquired immunological tolerance to spontaneous mammary adenocarcinomas following neonatal infection with mammary tumor agent (MTA. *Proc. Am. Assoc. Cancer Res. 5:*46, 1964.
142. Bases, R. Antigenic differences between normal and polyoma virus-transformed hamster cells. I. A quantitative study of the cytotoxic effect of antisera. *Cancer Res. 23:*811, 1963.
143. Burdette, W. J. *Viruses Inducing Cancer: Implications for Therapy.* Univ. of Utah Press, Salt Lake City, 1966.
144. Deichman, G. I. and Kluchareva, T. E. Immunological determinants of oncogenesis in hamsters infected with SV4O virus. *Virology 24:*131, 1964.
145. Duran Reynals, F. Immunologic factors that influence the neoplastic effects of the rabbit papilloma virus. *Cancer Res. 2:*343, 1942.
146. Fink, M. A. and Malmgren, R. A. Fluorescent antibody studies of the viral antigen in a murine leukemia (Rauscher). *J. Nat. Cancer Inst. 31:*1111, 1963.
147. Friend, C. Immunological relationships of a filtrable agent causing a leukemia in adult mice. I. The neutralization of infectivity by specific antiserum. *J. Exp. Med. 109:*217, 1959.

148. Gross, L. How many different viruses causing leukemia in mice? *Acta Haemat. 32:*44, 1964.
149. Gusev, A. I. Viral and tissue antigens of the Rous sarcoma. *Acta Uni. Int. Contra Cancr. 18:*151, 1962.
150. Habel, K. Common antigen in polyoma tumors. *Fed. Proc. 22:*438, 1963.
151. Harvey, J. J. An unidentified virus which causes the rapid production of tumours in mice. *Nature 204:*1104, 1964.
152. Harvey, J. J., Salaman, M. H., Chesterman, F. C., Gillespie, A. V., Harris, R. J. C., Evans, R. and Mahy, B. W. J. Studies on a murine sarcoma virus (MSV). *42nd Ann. Rep. Brit. Emp. Cancer Camp.* Part II, 185, 1964.
153. Herbut, P. A. Human leukemia virus in mice. *Arch. Path. 83:*123, 1967.
154. Klein, E. and Klein, G. Mouse antibody production test for the assay of the Moloney virus. *Nature 204:*339, 1964.
155. Klein, E. and Klein, G. Antigenic properties of lymphomas induced by the Moloney agent. *J. Nat. Cancer Inst. 32:*547, 1964.
156. Mahy, B. W. J., Harvey, J. J. and Rowson, K. E. K. Some physical properties of a murine sarcoma virus (Harvey). *Texas Rep. Biol. Med. 24:*620, 1966.
157. Moloney, J. B. Rodent leukemias: Virus-induced murine leukemias. *Ann. Rev. Med. 15:*383, 1964.
158. Sachs, L. Transplantability of an X-ray-induced and a virus-induced leukemia in isologous mice inoculated with a leukemia virus. *J. Nat. Cancer Inst. 29:*759, 1962.
159. Sachs, L., Fogel, M., Winocour, E., Heller, E., Medina, D. and Krim, M. The *in vitro* and *in vivo* analysis of mammalian tumour viruses. *Brit. J. Cancer 13:*251, 1959.
160. Sachs, L. and Heller, E. The *in vitro* and *in vivo* analysis of mammalian tumor viruses. Experiments on the epidemiology of the polyoma virus. *Brit. J. Cancer 13:*452, 1959.
161. Spjut, H. J., Van Hoosier, G. L. and Trentin, J. J. Neoplasms in hamsters induced by adenovirus type 12. *Arch. Path. 83:*199, 1967.
162. Wahren, B. Cytotoxic assays and other immunological studies of tumors induced by Friend virus. *J. Nat. Cancer Inst. 31:*411, 1963.
163. Zeigel, R. F. and Rauscher, F. J. Electron microscopic and bioassay studies on a murine leukemia virus (Rauscher). I. Effects of physiocochemical treatments on the morphology and biological activity of the virus. *J. Nat. Cancer Inst. 32:*1277, 1964.
164. National Advisory Cancer Council—*Progress Against Cancer*—1966. U. S. Dep't. of Health, Education and Welfare, Washington, p. 4.

Spontaneous, Induced and Transplanted Cancers

The experimental cancers used in research programs are of three general types.

Spontaneous cancers are those that arise in the animal without any known causative action. They correspond to the cancers which arise in man without known cause.

Induced cancers are those that are deliberately produced in animals through the use of such carcinogenic chemicals as benzpyrene, or by physical agents. The chemically induced cancers appear to correspond to occupational cancers in man, such as chimney sweeps' cancer.

Transplanted cancers are growths that originate in one animal, either spontaneously or following deliberate induction, and are then transplanted into other animals where they continue to grow. With one or two possible exceptions, transplanted cancers have no known counterpart in man. The main exception is choriocarcinoma, a cancer of the fetal part of the placenta which can grow within the mother. In a sense this is a transplanted cancer, although there are some important differences between it and the transplanted cancers used in research.

Most cancer research today is done on transplanted cancers. There has been increasing criticism, however, of the degree to which the national research effort is based on studies involving transplanted cancers. Primarily, the criticism results from the fact that scores of drugs and chemicals have been found that produce a high incidence of complete cures in mice with transplanted cancers, but none of these agents cure spontaneous cancers in mouse or man. There is also a suspicion that there may be drugs that could cure spontaneous cancers in mice and men, but which have little effect on the transplanted cancers. If this suspicion is well-founded, it is possible that materials that might have been effective anti-cancer agents in man have been discarded because they were ineffective in the transplanted cancers.

Accordingly, a careful evaluation of the advantages and disadvantages of each type of experimental cancer is a necessary prerequisite to planning a cancer research program aimed at curing or controlling cancer in man. Let us consider the advantages and disadvantages of studies on the three main types of experimental cancer.

Spontaneous Cancers

Spontaneous cancers in animals appear to have one major advantage as a research tool. They seem in their behavior to be quite similar to human cancers. Consequently, if a treatment were found that cured or controlled spontaneous cancers in mice, we would, in general, expect that treatment to be useful in man. However, there is one proviso that should be mentioned. Spontaneous cancers in non-inbred animals probably are similar to spontaneous cancers in man (who is a random-bred animal). But it is quite another matter whether spontaneous cancers in highly inbred (syngeneic) animals respond like spontaneous human cancers. We shall defer until later consideration of spontaneous cancers in inbred animals. Thus, in the following discussion, when we refer to spontaneous cancers we will be referring to spontaneous cancers in non-inbred animals.

Spontaneous cancers were used in early cancer studies, but after the development of transplanted cancers and inbred strains of animals, most studies were done on the latter. There are several disadvantages and inconveniences to the use of spontaneous cancers in non-inbred animals, but most of these can be overcome by good planning.

A major disadvantage to the use of the spontaneous cancers is their relative rarity and the high cost of the mice. In most strains of mice, spontaneous cancers do not develop until the mice reach middle or old age—usually 10 months or more. Most commercial breeders kill their mice before they reach the age at which tumors become fairly frequent. There are a few strains of mice in which the incidence of spontaneous cancers is high—reaching 90 per cent. However, these strains are difficult to breed, expensive, and the supply is limited. In most strains of mice, the incidence of spontaneous cancers is between 10 and 50 per cent, if the mice are allowed to live long enough. But commercial breeders whose business depends mainly on sales of mice under two months old do not find it profitable to keep breeding females beyond the age of eight to ten months. Even at these relatively young ages, some of the mice develop spontaneous cancers. A few breeders charge high prices ($3 to $5 each) for animals with such cancers because it is costly for them to ship a few special mice at a time. Others breeders will charge a more reasonable price (60¢

per mouse), if the investigator will adjust his orders to fit their business operations. However, the total number of mice with spontaneous cancers available in the nation at present is far too small to supply a major research program.

On the other hand, if the veterinary schools were asked to help provide mice with spontaneous cancers, as described further in Chapter 29, enough could be made available for really important studies.

Another disadvantage of using spontaneous cancers is their lack of chronologic uniformity. When using transplanted cancers, one arranges the experiment so that all the mice receive the cancer on the same day; thus, if the experimental design requires, say, 100 mice each with a 4-day-old transplanted cancer, it is a simple matter to supply them. This is impossible with spontaneous cancers. One never knows exactly when a spontaneous cancer begins to develop. As a result, experimental planning becomes more difficult and complex. This problem can be solved by using some techniques developed for clinical pharmacologic studies in human patients. When a physician wishes to test a new treatment in a group of patients, and compare it to the old treatment, he does not expect that 20 or 30 patients who have had the same disease for the same duration of time will come to the clinic on the same day. Instead, the physician can use a method of sequential pairing, with random assignment of each member of the pair to either an experimental group or a control group. It is not necessary to match members of each pair exactly: if true randomization has been used, the chances are that when the number of patients is large enough, the control and treated groups will be quite similar. A similar method of sequential pairing could be used for mice having spontaneous cancers. Of course, the number in each group must be larger than the number in each group of animals with transplanted cancers. Experience has shown that in studies using transplanted cancers, 15 treated and 15 control animals are almost always enough to give statistical significance to the findings. With the more variable spontaneous cancers, a minimum of 25 animals in the treated group and 25 in the control group are needed; in practice, I have used groups of 30.

Another disadvantage to the use of spontaneous cancers is the need for biopsy of each tumor. In working with transplanted cancers, it is assumed that a lump developing at the site into which cancer cells were transplanted is a cancer, and that assumption is right about 99.99 per cent of the time. Therefore a biopsy of every mouse with a transplanted cancer is unnecessary. When working with spontaneous growths, however, it is not always possible to distinguish by palpation between cancer and cyst or abscess. Even experienced observers are often in error, since mammary abscesses in the mouse often seem to be as hard as cancers. In an unpublished study, my associates and I evaluated this point: We found that in a series of 500 mice with breast tumors, which seemed on palpation to be cancer, only 75 per cent were actually cancer, and almost 25 per cent were abscesses or other nonmalignant swellings. When considering smaller numbers of mice, for example, those in a single shipment from a breeder, we found that from 11 to 50 per cent of a group of animals presumed to have mammary cancer actually had nonmalignant conditions.

Lewisohn *et al.* (1) who performed some outstanding studies with spontaneous cancers more than a quarter of a century ago found a similar situation. They reported:

> The great importance of a biopsy of spontaneous tumors is evident because it is impossible to establish the malignant or nonmalignant character of these tumors by palpation.

Many reports of studies on spontaneous cancers are unconvincing because it is not stated whether biopsy was done. Most of the time, a needle aspiration biopsy is preferable to an incisional biopsy. Usually, an experienced scientist can identify a tumor as cancer just by gross observation of the biopsy material, even before examining it microscopically.

Other features of spontaneous cancers are considered by some investigators to be disadvantages, but in the opinions of others they are, in the long run, advantages. For example, in a group of mice with spontaneous cancers each cancer is different from all the others, thus the cancers in this group are not homogenous. This means that it is more difficult to obtain clear-cut results and, consequently, a short-term goal of completing a particular study or writing a research paper is much harder to achieve. On the other hand, in terms of the ultimate goal, finding a cure or control for human cancer, the variation in the spontaneous cancers appears to be an advantage, since it parallels the variation in human cancers.

Induced Cancers

Induced cancers are used for several purposes. For example, if it is suspected that a particular chemical is carcinogenic, the chemical may be applied to animals to see if it provokes a cancer. In other experiments, cancers may be induced by chemicals *known* to be carcinogenic in order to study the cancer (2-18) (*see also* Chapter 5). This procedure has advantages and disadvantages. The induced cancer is probably more closely related to spontaneous cancers than are transplanted cancers. It seems, therefore, that drugs that are effective in treating induced cancers should have a better chance of being effective against spontaneous cancers. Since several cancers in man are known to be chemically induced, the induced mouse cancers ought to be fairly good objects for testing therapeutic procedures. Thus far, however, comparatively little research has been done to prove or disprove this assumption. As yet, there is not enough evidence to give a clear picture of the relationship between the immunologic patterns of induced animal cancers and those of human cancers.

A major disadvantage of induced cancers is the time and labor needed to produce them. Sometimes a chemical must be painted on for many days, and the animal then kept for months before the cancer develops. Thus, the cost of inducing cancers is high. Also, since the latent period before the cancer develops will vary from mouse to mouse (even with syngeneic animals), it is always difficult and often impossible to obtain large numbers of animals with cancers of the same age. This, of course, is a disadvantage shared with the spontaneous cancers. Some cancers, however, can be induced rapidly with one or a few administrations of carcinogenic chemicals (7-9).

Transplanted Cancers

There are several broad categories of transplanted cancers, depending on the relationships of donor and recipient animals. Some of the transplanted cancers have originated spontaneously and some have been induced. However, after transplantation they quickly lose the characteristics of spontaneous or induced cancers. As the cancers are transplanted from host to host, a type of evolution occurs in which the most abnormal cells tend to crowd out the others and perpetuate themselves. Some transplanted cancers are still in existence decades after the deaths of the original hosts. These cancers have changed greatly in the intervening years, and some have gone through hundreds of transplantations. They appear to be a unique biological phenomenon, not found in nature. When a cancer is transplanted more than once, it is sometimes called serially transplanted. There are several useful reviews of transplanted cancers (19-28) and some reports of important basic studies on transplanted cancers in general (29-42).

The most common divisions between transplanted cancers are based on the relationship of the animal in which the cancer originated with the one into which it is transplanted. There are heterologous transplants (heterotransplants), homologous transplants (homotransplants), isologous transplants (isotransplants) and autologous transplants (autotransplants).

Heterologous Transplants

A heterologous cancer transplant is one that originates in one species of animal and grows in another (43-68). Usually, heterologous transplants do not "take" unless there are some special conditions, since most animals will develop an intense immune reaction to cells from a foreign species and reject them. There is at least one mouse tumor, sarcoma 180, which can grow in rats, and perhaps in other species. After passing through hundreds of generations, this tumor has developed an extreme degree of malignancy, and has also lost some of its antigenic markers. It is not often grown in rats, but is still widely used in mice.

In another type of heterologous transplantation, the host's resistance to foreign cells is reduced by drugs, such as cortisone, or by radiation. While high levels of such drugs are present in the host's body, the heterologous cancer grows, but when the drugs are stopped, the heterologous transplant is quickly destroyed.

Most heterologous transplants today involve the transplantation of the cancer to a "privileged" site in the host animal. A privileged site is one that does not ordinarily develop a strong immunologic reaction to foreign cells or protein, and, therefore, has much less of a tendency to reject such foreign materials. There are at least three such sites known: the brain, the anterior chamber of the eye, and the cheek pouch of the hamster. In the past, studies have been done in which the brains and eyes of laboratory animals were used as transplantation sites. For most studies, however, the hamster cheek pouch (69-86) has proven to be more convenient. Many cancers, including human cancers can grow in the hamster cheek pouch, but the privileged status of the cheek pouch is not absolute, and sometimes drugs are used to increase it. This, of course, is a definite disadvantage. It would be most helpful if our veterinary and dental scientists, working together, could develop a strain of hamsters whose cheek pouches would permit the growth of more kinds of human cancer without the need for drugs. The potential value of research studies of hamster cheek pouch heterologous transplants is considerable. They may prove to be a reliable way of testing the effects of some new drugs on human cancers. Also, if in the future we develop some effective anti-cancer drugs with narrow spectra of action, it might be possible to find out which drug is most suitable for a particular patient by growing fragments of that patient's cancer in several hamsters and treating each with a different drug. This procedure would roughly parallel the practice of selecting the best antibiotic by doing antibiotic sensitivity tests; it would be more difficult and expensive, but not prohibitively so. However, in addition to improved strains of hamsters, we still need more information about the functioning of the hamster cheek pouch and its relation to the animal's total physiology.

Homologous Transplants

A homologous cancer transplant is one that is transplanted to an animal belonging to the same species as the one in which it originated (87-96). Thus, a mouse cancer transplanted to a mouse, or a rabbit cancer transplanted to a rabbit are homologous transplants. Technically, the more restricted types of transplants—isologous and autologous (*see* below)—are types of homologous transplants. However, in practice, the term "homologous" is used to imply that the transplants are not isologous or autologous. Therefore, the definition ought to be understood as meaning that the animals, although belonging to the same species, do not belong to the same inbred strain. Several types of cancers are used for homologous transplants. Those most commonly used in mice are probably sarcoma 1, sarcoma 180, and Ehrlich ascites cancer.

In a sense, choriocarcinoma, a cancer of the fetal part of the placenta which invades maternal tissues, can be considered a type of homologous transplant. It differs from those used in research in that it can make one passage only. Nevertheless, the relationships are underlined by the fact that choriocarcinoma is thus far the only kind of human cancer known to be curable by a chemical that also cures transplanted cancers in animals. In recent years, the trend in mouse studies has been away from the use of homologous transplants and toward greater use of isologous transplants.

Isologous Transplants

An isologous cancer transplant is one that is transplanted to an animal that has essentially the same genetic makeup as the animal in which the cancer originated (97-99). In theory, a transplant between identical twins would be isologous, but in animal cancer experiments such transplants are not made. To obtain animals of identical or almost identical genetic constitution, at least 20 generations of brother-sister matings are needed, and most of the inbred strains in use have gone through many more generations of such matings (100). It has been estimated that the genetic makeup of these animals at the end of 20 generations is at least 99 per cent identical. Accordingly, these inbred strains are called *syngeneic*.

The syngeneic mouse strains were developed to provide animals that are virtually identical with one another. There is, however, another aspect of the syngeneic strains, and it is not clear whether this aspect is advantageous or harmful to research. In nature, the genes come in pairs. Sometimes two genes in a particular pair are identical and we refer to that condition as homozygous. Often two genes in a particular pair are different, and we refer to that condition as heterozygous. We don't know exactly how many genes there are in any species, since there are many genes on each chromosome, but in general, there are hundreds of known genes in mammals. Although animals in the natural state are frequently homozygous in regard to a single pair of genes, they are probably never homozygous for all, or for 99 per cent of their genes. The odds against the genes of any natural mammal being 99 per cent or more homozygous are of the order of 1 in 2^{200} or greater—a number far larger than the number of all mammals that have ever lived. In contrast, the syngeneic mice are at least 99 per cent homozygous, and therefore constitute a phenomenon that must be considered a departure from natural conditions. We ought not assume that this departure is without influence on the experiments for which these animals are used; nor can we assume that the syngeneic mice respond differently than normal animals. What is the evidence? Insofar as the response to general drugs is concerned, the syngeneic animals behave like non-syngeneic animals. However, the reproductive physiology of the syngeneic animals seems to be somewhat different from that of non-inbred mice. The details are not clear, but it is usually much harder to raise litters of syngeneic animals. The question remains, whether there is any difference in response to cancer, host resistance to cancer, or response to anti-cancer drugs? We do not know. Certainly the information currently available is not nearly enough to warrant any diminution in our use of syngeneic animals, but we ought to check all important findings on animals that more closely fit the natural genetic patterns.

There are now many different strains of syngeneic mice available from commercial breeders.

Recently, the F_1 generations of crosses between two differing syngeneic strains have been used for cancer transplantation studies. Females of one syngeneic strain are mated to males of another strain, and the offspring all have identical genetic patterns, one from each parent. However, the offspring are heterozygous. This affords several advantages. The hybrid offspring will usually accept cancers that grow in either of the parent strains. Also, the hybrid mice are usually hardier and easier to raise. However, the F_1 hybrids cannot themselves be used to breed other mice, since the genes will sort out in varying patterns. The potential value of these F_1 hybrids to cancer research is not yet clear, but they would not possess the disadvantages, if any exist, of complete homozygosity.

Advantages and Disadvantages of Homologous and Isologous Transplants

The homologous and isologous cancer transplants offer several advantages and two major disadvantages. One of the advantages is the ability to conduct experiments with almost any number of mice, all with the same cancer of the same age. This reduces greatly the problem of individual variation, and therefore fewer mice have to be used in an experiment. Also, experimental procedures can be described precisely and repeated by other investigators. For example, if an investigator reports that he made certain observations on C57/BL6 mice bearing six-day-old E0771 carcinomas, any other investigator can get the same strain of mouse, implant the same cancer and look for the same phenomenon on the sixth day. This sort of precision would be impossible with spontaneous cancers.

Another advantage is the variety of cancers available. One can obtain transplanted cancers of almost every kind—mammary gland, ovary, stomach, liver, thyroid, brain, and so forth—and can often choose the type of growth pattern desired. That is, one may use a mammary gland cancer that grows rapidly, or one that grows slowly, or an intermediate one, depending on the experimental design. This is not practical with spontaneous cancers. The only kinds of spontaneous mouse cancers that could be available in reasonable quantities, even with the help of the veterinary schools (Chapter 29), would probably be mammary gland cancers.

The first disadvantage of the serially transplanted cancers is the possibility or even probability of bacterial and viral contamination. Although the procedures used to remove a cancer from one mouse and transplant it to others are designed to minimize contamination,

104

they are not perfectly aseptic since they involve passage of the material through the skin of two animals. It is difficult, if not impossible, to maintain sterility in each of scores of such passages, and if contamination occurs in even one passage, it continues in all later transplants. Furthermore, contamination of a transplanted cancer can originate in the host mouse itself if a slight bacteremia or viremia deposits some viable microorganisms in the cancer. This contamination is then likely to be carried over into each succeeding transplant generation. Unfortunately, few scientists using serially transplanted cancers bother to check for bacterial contamination at each transplantation, and it would be impossible to check for viral contamination. We do not know what effects these contaminating microorganisms might have on the cancer itself, on the host's immune responses, on other aspects of the host's defenses, or on the response to drugs being tested. It has been pointed out that in some transplantable cancers the numbers of contaminating bacteria are enormous—as high as 10^9 per cc (101). Furthermore, some apparent actions of these tumors on the host may in actuality be actions of secretions of the contaminating bacteria. Viruses may also be passengers in successive transplantations (102).

The greatest disadvantage of the homologous and isologous transplants however, is their apparent difference from spontaneous human cancers in response to medication and therapeutic procedures. There are literally scores of test materials that produce close to 100 per cent cures in animals with transplanted cancers, but all of them so far have failed to cure patients—or mice—with spontaneous cancers. This point has been brought out by several distinguished scientists.

Furth has stated (103):

To my knowledge, cures of animal tumors are based on experimentation with transplanted tumors, and efforts to bring about regression of spontaneous tumors by similar means have thus far invariably failed.

In discussing experiments on host resistance to cancer, Brunschwig et al. (88) have stated:

Animal experiments on host resistance to cancer—involving implantation of a transplantable tumor, its subsequent excision and apparent restraint of growth or failure to grow following reimplantation should be disregarded because these long-transplanted lines of rodent tumors represent foreign cells to the host.

105

Hirsch who has studied problems of cancer immunity points out (104):

> In addition to the many objections that can be made to the use of transplanted tumor model systems and the extrapolation of such results to the question of immunity against spontaneous tumor development, it should be realized that immune defense reactions of an animal going through the process of spontaneous tumor formation may be entirely different from those occurring in an animal serving simply as a 'test tube' for growing a tumor which has developed spontaneously in a different animal.

Also,

> . . . by comparison with the tremendous literature on immunity against transplanted tumors, the studies on spontaneous tumors have been meager and modest.

In his summary, Hirsch states:

> The difficulties and possible fallacies in extrapolating from work on tumor immunity involving transplanted tumors, carcinogen-induced tumors and other model systems to immunity against spontaneous tumors were stressed.

Holland and Heidelberger (105) have commented in an editorial in *Cancer Research:*

> We doubt the wisdom of accepting biochemical information derived from transplanted tumors when the data apparently are not consistently applicable to spontaneous neoplasms in the same species.

Stern (106) points out that although certain immunologic procedures produce a high incidence of resistance to transplantable cancers:

> No resistance resulted from analogous treatment of spontaneous mammary carcinoma.

Smithers (107) indicates his dissatisfaction with current research approaches in these terms:

> Organisation being a question of wholes, cancer research units would be transformed if they were directed with man as the object of their interest. They too often appear to be dedicated to the study of the artificialities of transplanted tumours in mice. . . .

Hoag (108) has stated:

> In conclusion, I wish to state that the proposition I am concerned with emphasizing is that if we are to continue to use experimental animals for the study of cancer etiology, epidemiology, immunity, and therapy in man we should place stronger emphasis on the naturally occurring disease in such animals.

(Hoag's paper also contains the most comprehensive bibliography available on mouse cancers arranged by mouse strain.)

Holland (109) has called attention to the need for more intensive work on spontaneous (autochthonous) cancers:

> Continuing awareness of immunologic considerations, and the possible laboratory artifacts of the transplanted tumor, have prompted some to undertake the study of autochthonous tumors. Autochthonous neoplasms of other tissues and organs and species will be welcome additions and are deserving of intensive work.

Scholler and her colleagues performed some valuable studies comparing first- and second-generation transplants of cancers with cancers in the original host (110-112). They found that agents that were highly effective in inhibiting the growth of first- or second-generation transplants (cancers that had been transplanted only once or twice from the original host) had little or no influence on the growth of spontaneous mammary cancers. Thus, neither the cancers transplanted through many generations nor even the first-generation transplants can be considered adequate or reliable models for spontaneous cancers. These findings should also induce caution about interpreting the relevance to man of studies on human cancers growing in the hamster cheek pouch, although it would be premature to discount such studies.

Medawar (113), who won the Nobel prize in Medicine for his studies in immunology, summarized the situation concisely:

> Nearly everyone who supposed that he was using transplantation to study tumors was in fact using tumors to study transplantation.

This does not necessarily mean that all materials that in the future will be found to cure transplanted cancers will be ineffective against spontaneous cancers. Nevertheless, the history of the transplanted cancers thus far should cast doubt on the wisdom of basing a cancer research program almost entirely on these growths.

Autologous Transplants

An autologous cancer transplant is one that is transplanted to a different site in the same animal in which it originated. Autologous

107

transplants have a certain similarity to cancer contamination of surgical wounds, and to metastases. They are used to study factors that may influence these phenomena. The initial cancer must be either spontaneous or induced but not transplanted; therefore, the number of autologous transplants is restricted by the number of spontaneous and induced cancers available. Since the autologous transplant always involves a single animal, it does not offer any possibility of increasing the number of animals with cancer. By contrast, the heterologous, homologous and isologous transplants can be put into large numbers of animals, increasing the supply of animals with cancer.

In current studies, autologous transplants are used rather rarely and in special circumstances. They have been employed in selected patients (114-123). One important use is in experiments designed to elucidate the relationships between growth rates of primary and secondary cancers.

In general, autologous transplants may prove to be most useful when done in large animals, such as pigs and cattle, where it is possible to implant many cancer fragments in different areas and follow them individually.

Comparison of Spontaneous and Serially Transplanted Cancers

As we have seen, there are both advantages and disadvantages to each of the different types of animal cancers used in research. The serially transplanted cancers—homologous and isologous—are convenient and readily available. Unfortunately they seem, thus far, not to resemble spontaneous cancers, animal or human, in their response to drugs. Their predictive value in choosing certain kinds of drugs— the highly toxic types that are being tested today—seems high, but these drugs are not solving the cancer problem. On the other hand the predictive value of the serially transplanted cancers in finding drugs that will cure or control cancer in man without killing the patient is unknown. There is some suspicion that it may be quite low, certainly lower than the predictive value of spontaneous animal cancers. However, there is no reason to think that the response of serially transplanted animal cancers to *every* possible anti-cancer drug would differ from that of spontaneous cancers. It seems reasonable to assume that there will be some materials that are effective in both transplanted and spontaneous cancers. The question is what percentage of the materials that exist unknown to us and that could cure or control spontaneous cancers would be correctly identified in tests using transplanted cancers. We do not know, and we do not even have the basis for a good estimate. A prudent assumption, which would tend to maximize our gains if correct, and minimize our losses if incorrect, would be that at least 10 per cent of materials that could cure or control spontaneous cancers in man would be correctly identified in properly designed tests on serially transplanted cancers. This assumption is portrayed in Figure 14-1.

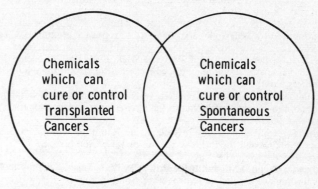

Figure 14–1.

Although the studies on spontaneous animal cancers have been few compared to those on transplanted tumors, there are some excellent basic studies that have been conducted on these naturally occurring cancers (124-138).

The similarity between spontaneous cancers in animals and man seems clear. We have no reason to doubt that the predictive values of these cancers in finding materials that would cure or control human cancers would be high, perhaps 90 per cent or more. It might even seem at first that all our studies should be done on these spontaneous cancers. But as has been pointed out, the supply of spontaneous animal cancers is limited, and even with the help of the veterinary colleges (Chapter 29) we could hardly obtain enough spontaneous cancers to maintain a major cancer research program without using the transplanted cancers also.

Accordingly, a balance should be struck. In many studies, serially transplanted cancers could be used, but there should be frequent checks in which spontaneous cancers are used. Above all, a major expansion in our use of spontaneous cancers seems essential. If our national resources were properly used (as described further in Part V), this could be a feasible, practical and economical step toward carrying out this research program.

References

1. Lewisohn, R., Leuchtenberger, C., Leuchtenberger, R. and Laszlo, D. The treatment of spontaneous breast adenocarcinomas in mice with extracts of spleen or yeast. *Am. J. Path. 17:*251, 1941.
2. Biedler, J. L., Old, L. J. and Clarke, D. A. Chromosomal lesion associated with carcinogen-induced tumors in mice. *Nature 192:*286, 1961.
3. Biedler, J. L. Chromosomal patterns in chemically-induced tumors in mice. *Proc. Am. Assoc. Cancer 3:*304, 1962.
4. Davis, A. P., Gropper, L. and Shimkin, M. B. Response of Wistar rats with breast cancer induced by 3-Methylcholanthrene to thirty-one compounds. *Cancer Res. 26:* 19, 1966.
5. Davis, A. P., Gruenstein, M. and Shimkin, M. B. Evaluation of chemotherapeutic agents in mammary carcinoma induced by 3-methylcholanthrene in Wistar rats. *Cancer Res. 26:*1, 1966.
6. Griswold, D. P., Skipper, H. E., Laster, W. R., Jr., Wilcox, W. S. and Schabel, F. M., Jr. Induced mammary carcinoma in the female rat as a drug evaluation system. *Cancer Res. 26:*2169, 1966.
7. Huggins, C., Briziarelli, G. and Sutton, H., Jr. Rapid induction of mammary carcinoma in the rat and the influence of hormones on the tumors. *J. Exper. Med. 109:*25, 1959.
8. Huggins, C., Grand, L. C. and Brillantes, F. P. Mammary cancer induced by a single feeding of polynuclear hydrocarbons, and its suppression. *Nature 189:*204, 1961.
9. Huggins, C., Moril, S. and Grand, L. C. Mammary cancer induced by a single dose of polynuclear hydrocarbons: Routes of administration. *Ann. Surg. 154:*315, 1961.
10. King, H. D. and Lewis, M. R. A study of inducement and transplantibility of sarcomata in rats. *Growth 9:*155, 1945.
11. Klein, G., Sjogren, H. O., Klein, E. and Hellstrom, K. E. Demonstration of resistance against methylcholanthrene-induced sarcomas in the primary autochthonous host. *Cancer Res. 20:*1561, 1960.
12. Medvedev, N. N. Spontaneous and induced lung tumors in CC57W and CC57BR mice and their F_1 hybrids. *Doklady Akad. nauk SSSR, Biol. Sci.* (Transl.) *130:* 90, 1960.
13. Mori, M., Miyaji, T., Murata, I. and Nogasuna, H. Histochemical observations on enzymatic processes of experimental carcinogenesis in hamster cheek pouch. *Cancer Res. 22:*1323, 1962.
14. Owens, A. H. and Busch, G. J. The utility of a carcinogen induced rat mammary cancer as a chemotherapeutic screening device. *Bull. Johns Hopkins Univ. School Med. 116:*249, 1965.
15. Salley, J. J. Experimental carcinogenesis in the cheek pouch of the Syrian hamster. *J. Dent. Res. 33:*253, 1954.
16. Shay, H., Aegerter, E. A., Gruenstein, M. and Komorov, S. A. Development of adenocarcinoma of the breast in the Wistar rat following the gastric instillation of methylcholanthrene. *J. Nat. Cancer Inst. 10:*255, 1949.
17. Teller, M. N., Stock, C. C., Stohr, G., Merker, P. C., Kaufman, R. J., Escher, G. C. and Bowie, M. Biologic characteristics and chemotherapy of 7, 12-dimethylbenz anthracene-induced tumors in rats. *Cancer Res. 26:*245, 1966.
18. Wodinsky, I., Helinski, A. and Kensler, C. J. Experimental tumorigenesis in the hamster cheek pouch. *Nature 207:*770, 1965.

19. Dunham, L. J. and Stewart, H. L. A survey of transplantable and transmissible animal tumors. *J. Nat. Cancer Inst. 13:*1299, 1953.
20. Crabb, E. D. Transplantable and transmissible tumours of animals. In: *Atlas of Tumor Pathology,* Sec. 12, Fasc. 40, Washington, D. C., 1959.
21. Hellstrom, K. E. and Moller, G. Immunological and immunogenetic aspects of tumor transplantation. *Progr. Allergy 9:*158, 1965.
22. Hirsch, H. M. Tumor immunity and tissue transplantation. *Journal-Lancet 79:* 340, 1959.
23. Klein, G. The usefulness and limitations of tumor transplantation in cancer research: A review. *Cancer Res. 19:*343, 1959.
24. Snell, G. D. The immunogenetics of tumor transplantation. *Cancer Res. 12:* 543, 1952.
25. Snell, G. D. "Transplantable tumors" in: Homburger, F. and Fishman, W. H. *The Physiopathology of Cancer,* Ch. 14. New York, Paul B. Hoeber, Inc. 1953.
26. Snell, G. D. Genetics of transplantation. *J. Nat. Cancer Inst. 14:*691, 1953.
27. Snell, G. D. Genetics of transplantation. *Ann. N. Y. Acad. Sci. 69:*555, 1957.
28. Stewart, H. L., Snell, K. C., Dunham, L. J. and Schlyen, S. M. Transplantable and transmissible tumors of animals. *Atlas of Tumor Pathology* Sec. 12, Fasc. 40. Washington, Armed Forces Institute of Pathology, 1959, p. 378.
29. Bullock, F. D. and Rohdenburg, G. L. Fluctuations in induced immunity to transplanted tumors. *J. Cancer Res. 5:*119, 1920.
30. Chambers, H., Scott, G. M. and Russ, S. On the action of x-rays upon the transplantation of a spontaneous carcinoma of the rat. *J. Path. and Bact. 23:*384, 1919-20.
31. Farpour, A., Agostino, D. V. and Cliffton, E. A transplantable lung cancer in rats. *Arch. Surg. 89:*942, 1964.
32. Handler, A. H., Sarris, T. G. and Wills, C. Chemotherapy studies on primary tumor grafts and metastases in hamsters and mice. *Acta Unio. Int. Contra. Cancr. 20:*176, 1964.
33. Hellstrom, K. E. Studies on allogeneic inhibition. I. Differential behavior of mouse tumors transplanted to homozygous and F$_1$ hybrid hosts. *Int. J. Cancer 1:*349, 1966.
34. Horn, K. H., Pasternak, G. and Graffi, A. Versuche zur Induktion von Immunität gegen methylcholanthren-Tumoren durch Vorbehandlung der Mäuse mit homologen und heterologen Tumortransplantaten. *Acta Biol. Med. Germ. 9:*309, 1962.
35. Koike, A., Moore, G. E., Mendoza, C. B. J. and Watne, A. L. Heterologous, homologous and autologous transplantation of human tumors. *Cancer 16:*1065, 1963.
36. Molomut, N., Spain, D. M., Kreisler, L. and Warshaw, L. J. The effect of an allergic inflammatory response in the tumor bed on the fate of transplanted tumors in mice. *Cancer Res. 15:*181, 1955.
37. Moppett, W. Substances controlling the growth of implanted tumours. *Med. J. Australia 2:*1065, 1937.
38. Schmidt, F. and Brada, Z. Eine Teilübersicht über in europäischen Laboratorien gehaltene tierische Transplantations tumoren. *Zschr. Versuchstierkunde 4:*122, 1964.
39. Sjogren, H. O., Hellstrom, I. and Klein, G. Transplantation of polyoma virus-induced tumor in mice. *Cancer Res. 21:*329, 1961.
40. Wexler, H., Minton, J. P. and Ketcham, A. S. A comparison of survival time and extent of tumor metastases in mice with transplanted, induced and spontaneous tumors. *Cancer 18:*985, 1965.
41. Wood, S., Jr. Experimental studies of the intravascular dissemination of ascitic V2 carcinoma cells in the rabbit, with special reference to fibrinogen and fibrinolytic agents. *Bull. Sw. Acad. Med. Sci. 20:*92, 1964.

PART III

42. Cook, E. S., Nutini, L. G. and Fardon, J. C. Resistance to transplanted and spontaneous isologous tumors in inbred strains of mice. *Acta Unio. Inter. Contr. Cancr.* 20:1541, 1964.
43. Ageenko, A. I. *Heterotransplantation of Malignant Neoplasms.* Moscow, 1960.
44. Clemmsen, J. On transplantation of tumor cells to normal and preirradiated heterologous organisms. *Am. J. Cancer 29:*313, 1937.
45. Clemmsen, J. *The influence of X-Radiation on the Development of Immunity to Heterologous Transplantation of Tumors.* Ejnar Munksgaard, Copenhagen and Oxford University Press, London, 1938.
46. Dagg, C. P., Karnofsky, D. A. and Roddy, J. Growth of transplantable human tumors in chick embryo and hatched chick. *Cancer Res. 16:*589, 1956.
47. Greene, H. S. N. Heterologous transplantation of human and other mammalian tumors. *Science 88:*357, 1938.
48. Greene, H. S. N. Heterologous transplantation of the Brown-Pearce tumor. *Cancer Res. 9:*728, 1949.
49. Greene, H. S. N. The heterologous transplantation of human melanomas. *Yale J. Biol. Med. 22:*611, 1950.
50. Greene, H. S. N. The transplantation of tumors to the brains of heterologous species. *Cancer Res. 11:*529, 1951.
51. Greene, H. S. N. The significance of the heterologous transplantability of human cancer. *Cancer 5:*24, 1952.
52. Greene, H. S. N. The transplantation of human brain tumors to the brains of laboratory animals. *Cancer Res. 13:*422, 1953.
53. Greene, H. S. N. The heterologous transplantation of the V_2 rabbit carcinoma. *Cancer Res. 13:*610, 1953.
54. Greene, H. S. N. Heterotransplantation of tumors. *Ann. N. Y. Acad. Sci. 69:* 818, 1957.
55. Greene, H. S. N. and Harvey, E. K. The growth and metastasis of amelanotic melanomas in heterologous hosts. *Cancer Res. 26:*706, 1966.
56. Greene, H. S. N. and Lund, P. K. The heterologous transplantation of human cancers. *Cancer Res. 4:*352, 1944.
57. Handler, A. H. Growth of a mouse leukemia in golden hamsters. *Transpl. Bull. 3:*153, 1956.
58. Herbut, P. A. and Kraemer, W. H. Heterologous transplantation of human tumors. *Cancer Res. 16:*408, 1956.
59. Lushbaugh, C. C. and Steiner, P. E. Intraocular transplantation of malignant lymphomas of the mouse, dog, and man in heterologous species. *Cancer Res. 9:* 299, 1949.
60. Jones, E. G. Heterologous transplantation of human malignant ovarian tumor. *Am. J. Obst. and Gynec. 51:*893, 1946.
61. Novikov, D. K. Heterotransplantation of transplantable tumors after pretreatment of donors. *Vopr. Onkol.* (Moscow) *10:*47, 1964.
62. Southam, C. M. Immunologic tolerance to human cancer transplants in rats. *Cancer Res. 26:*2496, 1966.
63. Toolan, H. W. Successful subcutaneous growth and transplantation of human tumors in x-irradiated laboratory animals. *Proc. Soc. Exptl. Biol. and Med. 77:*572, 1951.
64. Toolan, H. W. Growth of human tumors in cortisone treated laboratory animals: The possibility of obtaining permanently transplantable human tumors. *Cancer Res. 13:*389, 1953.
65. Tovell, H. M. M., Blackwood, C., Mandl, I. and Taylor, H. C. Heterologous growth of ovarian cancer. *Am. J. Obst. & Gynec. 85:*74, 1963.

66. Toolan, H. W. Transplantable human tumor. *Ann. N. Y. Acad. Sci. 76:*733, 1958.
67. Toolan, H. W., Winkler-Haemmerli, G. and Korngold, L. Studies on transplantable human tumors. I. Freezing. *Transpl. Bull. 4:*160, 1957.
68. Eichwald, E. J. and Chang, H. Y. The significance of anterior chamber in tumor transplantation. II. The nature of tumor growth beyond the anterior chamber. *Cancer Res. 11:*811, 1951.
69. Adams, R. A. Cheek pouch of the Syrian hamster and immunity to heterotransplantation of a murine leukaemia. *Nature 197:*1021, 1963.
70. Adams, R. A. Heightened immunity and susceptibility toward cheek pouch heterografts of a mouse leukemia in Syrian hamsters. *Cancer Res. 23:*1834, 1963.
71. Adams, R. A. Special property of the cheek pouch in heightened susceptibility to heterografts of a mouse leukemia. *Cancer Res. 23:*1841, 1963.
72. Billingham, R. E., Ferrigan, L. W. and Silvers, W. K. Cheek pouch of the Syrian hamster and tissue transplantation immunity. *Science 132:*1488, 1960.
73. Goldenberg, D. M., Witte, S., Hindringer, B. and Hartmann, G. Experimental chemotherapy of a human adenocarcinoma in the cheek pouch of the golden hamster: The effect of actinomycin C. *Arzneimittelforschung 16:*808, 1966.
74. Cohen, S. N. Comparison of autologous, homologous and heterologous normal skin grafts in the hamster cheek pouch. *Proc. Soc. Exptl. Biol. & Med. 106:*677, 1961.
75. Cardinali, G., Cardinali, G. and Handler, A. H. Effect of colchicine on human tumours transplanted in cheek pouch of Syrian hamster. *Nature 203:*90, 1964.
76. Delorme, E. J., Goodwin, C. M., Gowing, N. F. C., Moreman, K. G. and Wylie, J. A. H. Observations upon the behavior of human tumour cells when inoculated into the hamster cheek pouch using the Sanders-Shubik cheek pouch system for direct observation. *Brit. J. Exper. Path. 46:*530, 1965.
77. Engelbart, K. and Gericke, D. Oncolysis by clostridia. V. Transplanted tumors of the hamster. *Cancer Res. 24:*239, 1964.
78. Fulton, G. P. and Jackson, R. G. Cinephotomicroscopy of normal blood circulation in the cheek pouch of the hamster. *Science 105:*361, 1947.
79. Hertz, R. Suppression of human choriocarcinoma maintained in hamster cheek-pouch by extracts and alkaloids of Vinca rosea. *Proc. Soc. Exptl. Biol. and Med. 105:*281, 1960.
80. Patterson, W. B. Human tumor transplants in hamsters. Their usefulness in the study and treatment of patients with cancer. *Acta. Unio. Internat. Contra Cancr. 16:*714, 1960.
81. Sanders, A. G. and Shubik, P. A transparent window for use in the Syrian hamster. *Israel J. Exp. Med. 11:*118, 1964.
82. Schulte, C., Olson, K. and Stein, A. Heterologous transplantation of human tumors. *J.A.M.A. 179:*63, 1962.
83. Sommers, S. C., Reeves, G. and Reeves, E. Immunologic and chemotherapeutic effects on human melanoma heterotransplants. *Proc. Soc. Exptl. Biol. and Med. 123:*740, 1966.
84. Yohn, D. S., Hammon, W. McD. and Atchison, R. W. Serial heterotransplantation of a human adenocarcinoma, H. Ad. No. 1, in the cheek pouch of non-conditioned adult hamsters. *Fed. Proc. 20:*37, 1961.
85. Yohn, D. S., Hammon, W. M., Atchison, R. W. and Casto, B. C. Serial heterotransplantation of human adenocarcinoma No. 1 in the cheek pouch of unconditioned adult Syrian hamsters. *Cancer Res. 22:*443, 1962.
86. Yohn, D. S., Hammon, W. M. and Atchison, R. W. Influence of implant site on the immunologic response of unconditioned Syrian hamsters to heterotransplantable human tumors. *Cancer Res. 25:*484, 1965.

PART III

87. Bashford, E. F., Murray, J. A. and Haaland, M. Resistance and susceptibility to inoculated cancer. *Third Scientific Report, Imperial Cancer Research Fund*, London, 1908, p. 359.
88. Brunschwig, A., Southam, C. M. and Levin, A. G. Host resistance to cancer. Clinical experiments by homotransplants, autotransplants and admixture of autologous leukocytes. *Ann. Surg. 162:*416, 1965.
89. Carter, R. L. and Gershon, R. K. Studies on homotransplantable lymphomas in hamsters. I. Histologic responses in lymphoid tissues and their relationship to metastasis. *Am. J. Path. 49:*637, 1966.
90. Carter, R. L. and Gershon, R. K. Studies on homotransplantable lymphomas in hamsters. *Am. J. Path. 50:*203, 1967.
91. Crabb, E. D. A transplantable 9, 10-dimethyl-1, 2-benzanthracene sarcoma of the hamster. *Cancer Res. 6:*627, 1946.
92. Firtner, J. G., *et al.* Transplantable tumors of the Syrian (golden) hamster. I. Tumors of the alimentary tract, endocrine glands and melanomas. II. Tumors of the hemapoietic tissues, genitourinary organs, mammary glands and sarcomas. *Cancer Res. 21:*161, 1961.
93. Gericke, D. and Engelbart, K. Use of a transplantable myxosarcoma of the golden hamster for chemotherapeutic examinations. *Europ. J. Cancer 3:*25, 1967.
94. Gershon, R. K. and Carter, R. L. Studies on homotransplantable lymphomas in hamsters. II. The specificity of the histologic responses in lymphoid tissues and their relationship to metastasis. *Amer. J. Path. 50:*137, 1967.
95. Handler, A. H., Adams, R. A. and Farber, S. Further studies on the growth of homologous and heterologous lymphoma and leukemia transplants in Syrian hamsters. *Acta Unio. Internat. Contra Cancr. 16:*1175, 1960.
96. Southam, C. M., Moore, A. E. and Rhoads, C. P. Homotransplantation of human cell lines. *Science 125:*158, 1957.
97. Klein, E. and Sjogren, H. O. Humoral and cellular factors in homograft and isograft immunity against sarcoma cells. *Cancer Res. 20:*452, 1960.
98. Nutini, L. G., Fardon, J. C., Prince, J. E. and Duarte, A. G. Induced resistance to isologous and spontaneous tumors in inbred strains of mice. *Acta. Unio. Internat. Contra Cancr. 16:*110, 1960.
99. Snell, G. D. Histocompatibility genes of the mouse. II. Production and analysis of isogenic resistant lines. *J. Nat. Cancer Inst. 21:*843, 1958.
100. Staats, J. Standardized nomenclature for inbred strains of mice. Third listing. *Cancer Res. 24:*147, 1964.
101. Kampschmidt, R. E. and Upchurch, H. F. Effect of bacterial contamination of the tumor on tumor-host relationships. *Cancer Res. 23:*756, 1963.
102. Gross, L. *Oncogenic Viruses.* Pergamon Press, New York, 1962.
103. Furth, J. A meeting of ways in cancer research: Thoughts on the evolution and nature of neoplasms. *Cancer Res. 19:*241, 1959.
104. Hirsch, H. M. Some aspects of the problem of immunity against transplanted and spontaneous tumors. *Bact. Rev. 26:*336, 1962.
105. Holland, J. F. and Heidelberger, C. Human cancer the primary target—Guest editorial. *Cancer Res. 20:*975, 1960.
106. Stern, K. Host factors in neoplastic disease: A review of current concepts and trends in cancer research. *Hebrew Med. J. 1&2:*1, 1962.
107. Smithers, D. W. Cancer: An attack on cytologism. *Lancet 1:*493, 1962.
108. Hoag, W. G. Spontaneous cancer in mice. *Ann. N. Y. Acad. Sci. 108:*805, 1963.
109. Holland, J. F. Chemotherapy and chemopraxis of cancer. *Cancer Res. 21:*1086, 1961.

110. Scholler, J., Philips, F. S., Sternberg, S. S. and Bittner, J. J. A comparative study of chemotherapeutic agents in spontaneous mammary adenocarcinomas of mice and in transplants of recent origin. *Cancer 9:*240, 1956.

111. Scholler, J., Bittner, J. J. and Philips, F. S. Chemotherapeutic studies with transplants of spontaneous mammary tumors of mice growing in various hosts. *Cancer Res. 17:*605, 1957.

112. Scholiar, J. and Bittner, J. J. Further studies of chemotherapeutic agents in spontaneous mammary adenocarcinomas of mice and in transplants of recent origin. *Cancer Res. 18:*464, 1958.

113. Medawar, P. B. The immunology of transplantation. *Harvey Lecture Series 52:* 114, 1956-57.

114. Battista, A., Bloom, W., Loffman, M. and Feigin, I. Autotransplantation of anaplastic astrocytoma into the subcutaneous tissue of man. *Neurology 11:*977, 1961.

115. Bloom, W., Carstairs, K., Crompton, M. and McKissock, W. Autologous glioma transplantation. *Lancet 1:*77, 1960.

116. Grace, J., Perese, D., Metzgar, R., Sasabe, T. and Holdridge, B. Tumor autograft responses in patients with glioblastoma multiforme. *J. Neurosurg. 18:*159, 1961.

117. Mitts, M. G. and Walker, A. E. Autotransplantation of gliomas. *J. of Neuropath. and Exper. Neurol. 23:*324, 1964.

118. Nodler, S. H. and Moore, G. E. Autotransplantation of human cancer. *J.A.M.A. 188:*438, 1964.

119. Southam, C. M. and Brunschwig, A. Quantitative studies of autotransplantation of human cancer. Preliminary report. *Cancer 14:*971, 1961.

120. Southam, C. M., Brunschwig, A. and Dixon, Q. Autologous and homologous transplantation of human cancer. In: *Biological Interactions of Normal and Neoplastic Growth—A Contribution to the Host-Tumor Problem:* Henry Ford Hospital International Symposium, Brennan, M. J. and Simpson, W. L., Eds. Boston, Little, Brown and Company, 1962, pp. 723-738.

121. Sullivan, R. D. and Miller, E. Use of human cancer autotransplants in evaluation of chemotherapeutic agents. *Proc. Am. Assn. Cancer Res. 3:*154, 1960.

122. Vaitkevicius, V. K., Sugimoto, M., Reed, M. L. and Brennan, M. J. Effect of acute tissue injury on transplantability of autologous human cancer. *Cancer 18:*665, 1965.

123. Vaitkevicius, V. K., Sugimoto, M., Reed, M. L. and Brennan, M. J. Autologous transplantation of enzymatically prepared and freeze-preserved human tumors. *Cancer 17:*666, 1964.

124. Bittner, J. J. Spontaneous lung cancer in inbred stock mice and their hybrids. *Acta Unio. Internat. Contra Cancr. 5:*30, 1940.

125. Cloudman, A. M. *Spontaneous Neoplasms in Mice in Biology of the Laboratory Mouse,* Chapter 4. Snell, G. D., Ed. Dover, N. Y., 1941.

126. Dunn, T. B. Morphology and histogenesis of mammary tumors. In Mammary Tumors in Mice. *Publication 22, A.A.A.S.,* Moulton, F. A., Ed. Washington, 1945, p. 1.

127. Haddow, A. The influence of carcinogenic compounds and related substances on the rate of growth of spontaneous tumours of the mouse. *J. Path. & Bact. 47:* 567, 1938.

128. Lavrin, D. H., Blair, P. B. and Weiss, D. W. Immunology of spontaneous mammary carcinomas in mice. IV. Association of the mammary tumor virus with the immunogenicity of C3H nodules and tumors. *Cancer Res. 26:*929, 1966.

129. Lippincott, S. W., *et al.* A review of some spontaneous neoplasms in mice. *J. Nat. Cancer Inst. 3:*199, 1942.

PART III

130. Martin, D. S. Experimental design for chemotherapeutic cure of spontaneous mammary mouse carcinoma. *Proc. Am. Assn. Cancer Res. 3:*248, 1961.
131. Murphy, J. B. and Sturm, E. The effect of a growth-retarding factor from normal tissues on spontaneous cancer of mice. *J. Exper. Med. 60:*305, 1934.
132. Pullinger, D. B. and Iversen, S. Mammary tumour incidence in relation to age and number of litters in C3H$_f$ and RIII$_f$ mice. *Brit. J. Cancer 14:*267, 1960.
133. Scholler, J. Practical and theoretical considerations in the use of induced and spontaneous mammary tumors in cancer chemotherapy. *Ann. N. Y. Acad. Sci. 76:* 855, 1958.
134. Squartini, F. Responsiveness and progression of mammary tumors in high-cancer-strain mice. *J. Nat. Cancer Inst. 28:*911, 1962.
135. Strong, L. C. Extensive breeding as an adjunct to mammary gland carcinoma susceptibility in mice. *Proc. Soc. Exptl. Biol. and Med. 53:*257, 1943.
136. Taylor, A. and McKenna, G. F. A new mouse strain susceptible to mammary cancer. *Texas Rep. Biol. Med. 19:*706, 1961.
137. Woglom, W. H. The regression of spontaneous mammary carcinoma in the mouse. *J. Cancer Res. 7:*379, 1942.

Genetic and Molecular Biology Approaches to Cancer

Comparatively few studies have been done on the genetic and molecular approaches to cancer, and the available evidence strongly indicates that neither approach is likely to result in a practical cure or control of cancer within 50 to 100 years.

The genetic studies done thus far have shown quite convincingly that certain kinds of animal cancers involve genetic predisposition. This phenomenon is separate from that of compatibility of transplanted cancers (Chapter 14). Certain highly inbred strains of mice are much more likely to develop certain kinds of cancers than are other kinds of mice (1). There is also good evidence that some highly inbred strains of domestic animals are more susceptible to some cancers than are other members of the same species (2). Therefore, when considered as a biologic phenomenon, genetic predisposition to cancer appears to be a fact for some species. However, in terms of human cancer, the picture is quite different. Despite many studies, no one has ever convincingly demonstrated any special hereditary predisposition to the usual cancers in man. There have been a few cases of so-called cancer families, but statistical theory predicts that, in a large number of families, some will show a clustering of any situation under consideration, purely by chance.

In some groups of people, a particular kind of cancer sometimes appears to be much more common than in mankind generally. However, when careful studies have been done on these groups, the studies have brought to light a common environmental factor, such as food, prolonged exposure to local heat, parasites, or carcinogenic chemicals, that is the cause of the increased incidence of cancer.

There is no evidence that might suggest that any particular segment of the population has a markedly different susceptibility to cancer than mankind generally. In effect, there is no evidence that a condition of cancer proneness in part of the population might be responsible for most cancers in man. (There are a few cases of unusual cancers showing hereditary patterns, but they are quite rare.)

There is another way to approach the cancer problem genetically. Might it be possible to breed a condition of cancer resistance into people? In theory, this might be done, but it seems highly impractical. In order to breed special characteristics into or out of domestic animals, many generations of breeding are required. In mice, brother-sister matings for at least 20 generations are needed before a strain is considered reasonably well-defined genetically. In larger domestic animals, the number of generations needed to bring out or repress certain characteristics may be less than 20, but is almost always more than 5. Furthermore, the genetic characteristics that are the objects of most breeding endeavors in animals are generally obvious to the breeder before the animal reaches breeding age, so that he may select his breeding stock accordingly. However, susceptibility to cancer in man could not be known until long after the usual reproductive period. This may not be an insuperable obstacle but it is certainly a formidable one.

In addition, we do not yet have any idea which gene or combination of genes might be involved in cancer susceptibility in man. If a large group of human beings agreed to allow scientists and geneticists to arrange their marriages in an attempt to breed resistance to cancer into their descendants, we would still have to wait 10 to 20 generations before any substantial results could be seen. It is hard to believe that that many generations of people would follow such a protocol. Furthermore, we want a cure or control for cancer developed much sooner than 250 to 500 years from now.

Another possibility to consider is whether advanced scientific techniques may make it possible to change the genetic makeup of living people so as to render them less susceptible to cancer. We know of agents that can change the genetic code in some individual cells. These agents include high energy radiation and some chemicals. However, the changes affect only a few cells in the body, they are quite unpredictable, and the only relationship they seem to have to cancer is that of increasing its incidence. In order to change the genetic makeup of a living person's cells to instill a resistance to cancer, it would be necessary to change the genetic code in each of the billions of cells comprising the body, and to do it uniformly. Even if we knew which chromosomes were to be changed, and we do not, it should be clear that any approach of this nature is too impractical to deserve serious consideration.

If the geneticists and the other scientists studying DNA, RNA and the genetic code believe there are other ways in which they can translate their findings into a practical solution of the cancer problem, they have not made these ideas known. If, indeed, any scientists believe that there may be such a way they ought to describe it clearly so that we may judge its likelihood of success in a reasonable number of generations. Until the proponents of increased emphasis on the genetic approach to cancer research can explain how they intend to apply the information they hope to obtain to the problem of human cancer, it would be most unwise to devote any larger proportion of our meager financial resources to this area of research.

The molecular-biology approach to cancer presents additional problems. Molecular biology is a new field, and the scientists working in it do not yet know its extent or its limitations. As we know, there is always a tendency to exaggerate the potential value of any new scientific field. The theory underlying the statements made for the relationship of molecular biology to cancer seems attractive. It suggests that, if we know how organic molecules interact, we can find ways to identify and correct abnormalities in reactions of cells which, in the final analysis, are collections of organic molecules. Unfortunately, things are not that simple. The complexities of the reactions within a cell are great. It could take molecular biologists hundreds of years to analyze and define all the different reactions occurring at the molecular level. Whether at that time a relationship to cancer would emerge is far from certain.

There is another point that casts considerable doubt on the practical value of the molecular approach. This approach, concentrated as it is on events taking place inside a particular cell, virtually ignores the interrelationships and interaction between cells, tissues and organs in a living individual. In cell culture, for example, mammalian cells take on quite different attributes than they have in the living body.

Furthermore, the fundamental concepts of molecular biology have recently been challenged, on the basis of discrepancies between the theory and the reports of scientific observations. Commoner (3) has stated that "the entire conceptual basis of the molecular approach to biological questions must be revised: far from being a unique attribute of the inanimate DNA molecules in a cell's chromosomes repro- duction and heredity are properties of the whole intact cell."

Commoner also states that the meaning of the data and concepts of current molecular biology "has often been seriously distorted by an ill-considered effort to force them to answer questions to which such data cannot respond." Under these circumstances, it hardly seems prudent to rely on the molecular-biology approach for practical help in solving the cancer problem during the next few generations.

It is important to distinguish between molecular and cellular biology. The latter could provide us with useful clues to cancer in a reasonable time.

References

1. Taylor, A. and McKenna, G. F. A new mouse strain susceptible to mammary can- cer. *Texas Rep. Biol. Med. 19:*706, 1961.
2. Doyle, R., Garb, S., Davis, L. E., Meyer, D. K. and Clayton, F. Domesticated farm animals in medical research. In press. *Ann. N. Y. Acad. Sci.*
3. Bernhard, R. Crisis in biology. *Scientific Res. 1:*33, 1966.

SOME RESEARCH APPROACHES THAT DESERVE GREATER EMPHASIS

The following twelve chapters are devoted to a discussion of some of the research approaches to cancer that seem to be appropriate and hopeful components of a total national program. Some of them are being followed by a few scattered investigators and others by significant numbers of scientists, but none is currently being tackled on a scale that corresponds to its potential value and importance. Every approach we shall discuss deserves, in my opinion, a great increase in research effort. Some of the ideas and concepts put forward are my own, but they are based on the findings of other researchers. Some of the approaches discussed have been suggested by other cancer investigators, and appear to have been overlooked or inadequately pursued; one of the promising suggestions included here was made over 50 years ago, but has since been neglected.

One may wonder whether research leads developed many years ago and then discarded are worthy of further effort. Should one assume that these leads were not followed because they proved unfruitful? The history of medical research provides some guidance. Some of the most important medical discoveries were based on leads that had been developed and then temporarily forgotten for decades. The sulfonamides were found to have medical value when Domagk tested some chemicals which had been lying on a shelf for many decades. One of these chemicals happened to be prontosil, the forerunner of all the sulfonamide drugs.

The story of penicillin is equally constructive. In 1928, Fleming reported his discovery of penicillin and correctly predicted its possible value in the treatment of infections. Other scientists did not consider Fleming's discovery to be particularly significant, however, and looked upon it as a laboratory curiosity. They were convinced, in 1928, that no such thing as an antibiotic would be practical—that only antisera could affect the course of infectious diseases. Fleming himself believed that penicillin could be used to treat infections but, working alone, he could not obtain sufficient penicillin to perform the necessary studies. He was not a biochemist, and did not have the money to hire a biochemist to help him, and thus, for 12 years, penicillin remained a laboratory curiosity. Then, the outbreak of World War II spurred British authorities to assign several groups of scientists to search for better ways of treating the infected wounds that had killed so many British soldiers in World War I. The team of Chain and Florey came across Fleming's old reports and recognized their significance. Thus, with the necessary support and assistance, penicillin, a discovery which had been virtually ignored for 12 years, was quickly developed into a lifesaving medication.

The projects suggested here are only a few of those that could be selected as initial components of a major national program. They can be carried out as semi-independent parts of the total. For the over-all program to be successful, it is not necessary that all, or even a majority, of the component projects be successful. If a single one of the projects suggested is successful, the entire program would be a major success, and hundreds of thousands of lives would be saved each year.

CHAPTER 16

Improving Surgical Approaches to Cancer

At least 90 per cent of all cancer cures that have been effected in the past have resulted from surgical intervention. Over a million people have been saved by prompt and effective surgery and many millions more have had their lives prolonged and made more comfortable by surgical procedures. Even a relatively small percentage of increase in the effectiveness of operations for cancer would mean the saving of thousands of lives.

Since surgery constitutes the major area of cancer therapy today in terms of proven effectiveness, we might reasonably expect a continuing high level of support for research into the surgical approaches to cancer. However, the level of support for surgical research has been grossly inadequate. Many questions—practical questions which mean life or death to the patient—remain matters of controversy and disagreement among eminent surgeons. Studies which could give us the answers to these questions are well within our capabilities, but funds have not been available to pay for them.

Surgeons would like to know whether, in some kinds of cancer, a radical or a conservative operation would give the patient the best chance for survival. They would like to know whether anti-cancer drugs given before or after surgery are helpful or harmful to the patient. Another vital question is whether some surgical procedures, such as cautery, can increase cure rates.

Let us consider each of the problems that the surgeons face, and see how they could be resolved if a properly designed and supported national program were in existence.

In the case of some common types of cancer, particularly breast cancer, eminent surgeons disagree on the best surgical approach. On the one hand, there is the obvious desire to remove every bit of tissue that might harbor some cancer cells. Surgeons who follow this approach will do a radical mastectomy and remove large amounts of normal tissue, including muscle and lymph nodes. On the other hand, some surgeons believe that it is better to do a limited operation, a simple mastectomy, if the regional lymph nodes seem normal (1-11,

96). Their reasoning is that the regional lymph nodes are important body defenses, which filter out cancer cells, and which may also produce antibodies that keep the cancer, even at distant sites, in check—a point of view that is vigorously refuted by the experts who advocate radical mastectomy (97, 98). Thus far, there is no experimental evidence to indicate definitely which approach is better for the patient with breast cancer. Studies to settle this and related questions have been well within our technologic abilities for over a decade, but they have not been done because of inadequate financial support. Fortunately, the need for answers to this type of question has finally been recognized, and a special task force, appointed by the National Cancer Institute, has been given the mission of solving this problem (12). But similar questions in relation to the best surgical approach to other types of cancers are not yet being answered.

Surgeons have also been concerned with the problem of implantation of cancer cells in the incision. Rather frequently, after surgical removal of a cancer, regrowths occur in the area that was cut or handled, even when the surgeon was quite sure that he had not contaminated the operative area with cancer cells. Many surgeons have thought that such growth of cancers at the incision site indicate some unrecognized lapse of technique on their part. Yet, other factors may be involved. Long before most cancers in man are large enough to be diagnosed they are disseminating millions of cancer cells into the blood stream and lymph. Almost all these disseminated cells die, but a few may lodge and continue to grow *in an area that has been traumatized* (13, 101-106); the site of an incision would be such an area. Therefore, the question arises: Do the wound implants occur because the surgeon accidentally contaminates the area with cancer cells, or do they occur because cancer cells already in the circulation find the incision area to be fertile soil? The answer is of great practical importance. If it can be shown that implantation is largely the result of direct contamination of the operative area by the surgical procedure, it might be advisable to revise the procedures—with frequent changes of instruments, drapes, and so forth—even at the expense of prolonging the operation. On the other hand, if implantation primarily results from the other mechanism, such revisions of the surgical procedure would do little or no good; by prolonging an already lengthy operation, they may, in fact, increase operative mortality.

Fisher, Fisher and Feduska (101) state:

124

There are many clinical observations that surgery, chemotherapy, and even irradiation (all forms of trauma) may augment metastases. Such modalities may change host-tumor relationships allowing for unexpected neoplastic growth. In this regard it must be noted that surgeons have long practiced self-incrimination for local recurrences of tumor following an "adequate" operation when actually these recurrences may have been the result of a biological phenomenon beyond his control, i.e., circulating tumor cells lodging at a site of trauma.

Two procedures have been suggested for dealing with this problem. One is the irrigation of the operative area with solutions of anti-cancer drugs—a procedure recommended by some authorities (14-20). Would this be generally advisable? If it is an advisable procedure, what sort of solution should be used for the irrigation? Although some suggestions based on experimental evidence have been made, there is still a need for studies which will be clear and convincing to the surgeon who must make the final decision on the procedures to follow in a particular patient.

Nora and Preston (21) have pointed out:

Cancerocidal drugs used as irrigants for wounds seem logical as a method of reducing locally recurrent cancer after a resection for cancer. Published data on this subject is contradictory and at the present time these drugs cannot be recommended.

The subject is one of vital importance to patients and surgeons (22-32), but there is no answer yet.

The second suggested procedure involves the choice of suture material. It has been shown that when ordinary suture materials are used cancer tends to regrow around the sutures, but when iodized suture materials are used, such regrowth of the cancer does not occur (33-37). If further research confirms this finding, it would probably be worthwhile to use iodized suture materials in all operations for cancer.

The possible effects of wound irrigation with anti-cancer compounds and of the use of iodized suture materials are not necessarily related to the mechanism whereby implantation occurs at the incision lines. The mechanism could be direct contamination through the surgical procedure; or it could be that blood or lymph-borne cancer cells are finding a vulnerable area near the incision. Irrigation and the use of iodized suture materials could be effective in either case.

The regrowth of cancer along a suture line need not represent contamination by the needle. It could come about because the injury to the tissues pierced by the needle made them more vulnerable to blood-borne cancer cells.

This question can readily be answered by fairly simple experiments, as described below, and the answer would be very important to the surgeons operating on cancer patients.

Surgeons would also like to know whether it is helpful to a patient to receive any of the currently available anti-cancer drugs before, or shortly after, operation. We do know that these drugs are not curative when used in patients whose disease has progressed beyond the scope of surgery, but is it possible that if they were given just before surgery, they could prevent seeding of the cancers to distant sites during operative manipulation? Is it also possible that, if given soon after surgery when the total mass of cancer cells is small, anti-cancer drugs could significantly increase survival rates (38-55)?

The answers to these questions are not yet known (107, 108). It might seem, at first, that surgeons ought to give anti-cancer drugs before and after surgery anyway, in the hope that they would help the patient. Unfortunately, the drugs available today have some undesirable effects, too. They are all quite toxic and could increase postoperative death rates. Of equal concern is the fact that such drugs lower host resistance. Thus, they could lead to an increase in the growth of any remaining cancer metastases (56-58), and possibly could convert a surgical cure into a failure.

Obviously, surgeons cannot be expected to utilize an agent that could have such untoward effects, unless there is good evidence that the chances of helping the patient are greater than the chances of doing harm. Wolberg, Johnson and Curreri (58) have stated:

> One must be aware that the drugs used for adjunctive chemotherapy can produce complications by themselves and it is, therefore, hard to justify their use unless tumors appear to have a good chance of being affected at drug doses which can be tolerated in the postoperative period. This is particularly true because surgery alone may be curative. In every instance, the potential benefits must be carefully weighed against the potential harm of such chemotherapy.

Knock (59) has clearly summarized the problem and the hope for the future as follows:

This promise of early postoperative adjuvant chemotherapy of cancer is tempered by the knowledge that toxic anti-cancer drugs not active against the patient's own tumor can undermine wound healing, depress bone marrow, depress host resistance, and enhance tumor growth. Such needless injury inflicted on the cancer patient by use of toxic anti-cancer drugs presents both disturbing scientific and disturbing ethical implications.

The real hope for cancer control lies, however, in giving drugs matched to the chemical requirements of the patient's own tumor when such tumor is minimal, usually within 48 hours of tumor biopsy and operation.

Attempts to evaluate the effects of anti-cancer drugs on a particular patient's cancer are being made, but on a much smaller scale than this potentially valuable approach deserves. Several investigators have developed methods of studying tumor behavior in isolated perfused organs (60-67). The results to date are encouraging but are only preliminary and not yet applicable to most patients with cancer.

The possible usefulness of adjuvant immunotherapy has also been a matter of interest and concern to surgeons. Many of the problems applicable to adjuvant chemotherapy apply also to adjuvant immunotherapy (see Chapter 23).

The possible role of heat in the treatment of cancer has interested some outstanding surgeons. In certain advanced cancer cases, sharp dissection is out of the question; as a palliative procedure, electrocautery is sometimes used to remove part of the tumor. Byrne reported good results with this technique more than 75 years ago (68). Surprisingly, some heat-treated cancers have regressed entirely and many of the patients—apparently cured—have lived for many years in excellent health. This phenomenon was reported more than 60 years ago by Lomer (69); since then others (70-74) have had unexpectedly good results from local cautery of presumably incurable cancers. Some cases reported by Strauss and his associates (75-80) are particularly striking. Several investitgators have reported that heat potentiates the beneficial effects of radiation (73, 74, 81).

Crile has concluded (82):

The results of studies reported in the first 30 years of the century have been confirmed by our own observations, and suggest the following conclusions:

1. Some cancers, in both man and animals, are more susceptible to destruction by heat than are the tissues they grow in.

2. Heat acts synergistically with radiation in controlling the growth of many cancers.

3. The mechanism by which heat kills cells is poorly understood and deserves further study.

4. The uses of heat as an adjunct to the treatment of human cancers should be explored.

Some interesting studies of animal cancers have increased our understanding of the effects of heat on cancer cells (83-94). A classic study of Murphy and Sturm (88) in 1919 suggested that the heat affects the host response rather than the cancer itself. These investigators removed spontaneous cancers from mice. Each mouse was then exposed to dry heat between 55° and 63° C for five minutes, and then fragments of its own cancer were re-implanted into each mouse. Thus, the host, not the cancer was exposed to heat. In control animals, the cancers were removed and re-implanted on a similar time schedule, but without exposing the hosts to heat. In the control animals, 96 per cent of the animals developed a recurrence of their cancer, whereas in the heat-treated group, only 41 per cent developed a recurrence of cancer—a striking difference. Furthermore, since Murphy and Sturm used spontaneous cancers, their results probably have greater basic significance than studies on transplantable cancers. Of course, it may be impractical to utilize whole-body heating in man, but localized heat might invoke a response similar to that obtained in animals.

The studies of Popovic and Masironi (90-93) suggest that more than heat alone may be involved. They found that when the body of an animal was cooled, but the cancer kept at a normal temperature, the cancer regressed (90, 91); perhaps the use of differential heating could be adapted to treatment of cancer in man.

Localized heating of human cancers is practical only for those in accessible locations (95). It may be impossible to heat metastases in the brain, lung and other locations. There is a possibility, however, that heating of all the cancer cells in the body may not be necessary to control or cure the disease. One possibility is that heating the cancer may produce a subtle change in the antigenic nature of one or more of the constituents of the cancer, and that the modified antigen would provoke a greater than usual host response that also affects the unaltered antigen. This sort of occurrence has been described in other antigenic systems (*see* Chapter 23). It is also possible that heat applied to normal tissues that have been in close contact with cancer cells in some way increases their defenses against the cancer, and that some of these defending cells—i.e., lymphocytes—can migrate and successfully attack cancer cells at distant sites. Or, finally, the actual mechanism may be one that has not yet been suggested. Even though we do not yet have a clear understanding of the mechanism whereby heat affects the host-cancer relationship, there is convincing evidence from many sources that it does affect that relationship, and usually in a manner favorable to the host. Accordingly, it seems desirable to develop the use of heat into a practical therapeutic tool that our surgeons can use to help their patients. Undoubtedly, heat will eventually prove to have limitations in its therapeutic effectiveness, but this is true of all treatments. Once the limitations are clearly defined, it should be possible for surgeons to make better use of this kind of therapy.

We have considered a few of the areas of cancer research that are of particular interest in relation to surgery. There are others, but those described should suffice to show that important practical questions, the answers to which would help surgeons plan the best treatment for cancer patients, are still unanswered. The answers to most of these questions could have been found by techniques and procedures that have been within our national capabilities for decades. If one or more of these approaches would increase the cure rate of our current surgical procedures by even 10 per cent, that would mean a saving of 10,000 to 15,000 lives per year. The chances are that prompt and thorough exploration of these areas would improve surgical cure rates by much more than 10 per cent. Surely, this would be an important gain, well worth the modest cost.

Let us now turn to a consideration of the ways in which some of these questions facing surgeons can be answered. The quality of the evidence needed has to be such that it will convince surgeons of the value of using or omitting a particular procedure on their patients. It is doubtful that many surgeons would be convinced by evidence obtained solely on transplantable cancers in small animals (*see also* Chapter 14), nor is it by any means certain that evidence obtained solely on spontaneous cancers in rodents would be convincing. It seems likely that studies on spontaneous cancers in larger animals would be needed, before any extensive trials could be attempted in man.

Crile (86) has stated:

Finally, as an experimental method for dealing with actual tumors, which is very hard to do in small animals, I would strongly urge those of you who are interested in this to go to your local veterinary society and address them, give them the problem, and they will make arrangements with their individual clients to have dogs with incurable cancer, of which there are fantastic numbers, brought to you with the understanding that these dogs will be returned to their owners if you can help them. This has given us a wide experience in a spectrum of tumors very similar to those in human beings.

In principle, Crile echoes the belief of many outstanding surgeons that more studies ought to be done on spontaneous cancers in domestic animals. Under present conditions, his suggestion is probably the most feasible one, but surely a more effective and efficient way of arranging such studies can be found (*see* Chapter 29).

In relation to the specific areas of direct concern to surgeons, coordinated efforts by the surgeons and veterinarians ought to be developed and supported by adequate funds. One possible arrangement that seems practical and appropriate follows.

A group of distinguished surgeons, preferably a group elected by their colleagues, such as the officers of the American College of Surgeons, should be given the responsibility of identifying those problems relating to cancer surgery that deserve prompt solution. If the number of such problems is large, priorities can be assigned. A task force of surgeons should be assigned to each problem and given adequate financial support and authority to sub-contract with other groups. In all likelihood, these task forces would then make arrangements to combine with veterinary schools and clinics in planning for studies aimed at solving the problem.

Veterinary surgeons are well versed in the same surgical principles as those followed by surgeons on human patients. A useful arrangement might be to assign a young surgeon, who has just finished his residency, as a research fellow to a veterinary school or clinic. The veterinarians and the research fellow would carry out a project developed by the task force and make frequent reports to it. Each project should be done in triplicate, at three different locations, so that the results would be convincing. The details, as to species of animal and type of cancer to be used, may be left to the task force to work out jointly with the veterinarians. For some questions, experiments on a single species may be sufficient to provide the answers; for others, the surgeons may wish to have confirmatory results on two or more animal species before using the procedure in man.

After the animal studies have provided the necessary initial information, the task force would proceed to trials in specially selected human patients. It would probably be advisable to have the same task force follow the problem through from beginning to end.

In some situations, a surgical task force might decide that there are no satisfactory animal models, and start with studies on human cancer patients after careful consideration of the risks and potential gains to the individual patient.

The experimental procedures would vary in complexity. One study, designed to elucidate the mechanism of cancer recurrence in the operative wound, could be done quite simply. Domestic animals with spontaneous cancers would be anesthetized, and operated on at a site distant from the cancer, with incisions and manipulations of tissue equivalent to those involved in cancer surgery. The site of this operation should be far enough from the cancer to rule out any possibility of direct contamination with malignant cells during surgery. For example, if the cancer is in the abdominal cavity, the first operation could be done on a limb. Then, about 24 hours later, a second operation would be done, this one on the cancer itself—removing it with the same techniques and precautions used for humans. After the operations, the animals would be cared for optimally and observed frequently. If, in a series of animals, cancers develop in the first operative site (distant from the original cancer site) at a frequency comparable to that observed in the second operative site (the primary cancer), one could logically assume that the mechanism by which cancer develops in incisions is probably via blood and lymph spread, and not via direct contamination of the operative site during surgery. On the other hand, if cancer develops frequently in the second operative area but not the first, one could logically assume that the mechanism is probably direct contamination of the operative site.

Some of the research procedures for finding answers to other questions would probably be more complex. But, in all likelihood, several of the problems discussed in this chapter could be largely solved within three years of the start of a properly financed and supported program. Some of the other problems—those dependent on measurement of patient survival times after surgery—could take five to ten years. However, in virtually every case, a definitive answer—whether one way or another—would be of direct value to the surgeon and his patients. Surely, practical problems like these deserve prompt and adequate efforts at solution.

PART IV

References

1. Crile, G. Jr. Do ultraradical operations for cancer do more harm than good? *Surg., Gyn., and Obst. 100:*755, 1955.
2. Crile, G. Jr. Cancer of the breast: The surgeon's dilemma. *Cleveland Clin. Quart. 23:*179, 1956.
3. Crile, G. Jr. The present status of surgery in the treatment of cancer. *Postgrad. Med. 20:*118, 1956.
4. Crile, G. Jr. The case for conservatism in operations for cancer. *Surg. Clin. N. Amer. 38:*1215, 1958.
5. Crile, G. Jr. Results of simplified treatment of breast cancer. *Nat. Cancer Inst. Monograph 15:*125, 1964.
6. Crile, G. Jr. Results of simplified treatment of breast cancer. *Surg., Gyn., Obst. 118:*517, 1964.
7. Crile, G. Jr. Rationale of simple mastectomy without radiation for clinical stage 1 cancer of the breast. *Surg., Gyn., Obst. 120:*975, 1965.
8. Crile, G. Jr. Treatment of breast cancer by local excision. *Am. J. Surg. 109:*400, 1965.
9. Crile, G. Jr. Treatment of cancer of the breast. *Brit. J. Clin. Pract. 19:*193, 1965.
10. Crile, G. Jr. Simplified treatment of cancer of the breast. *Postgrad. Med. 37:*421, 1965.
11. Kaae, S. and Johanson, H. Breast cancer, a comparison of the results of simple mastectomy with postoperative roentgen irradiation by the McWhirter method with those of extended radical mastectomy. *Acta Radiol.* (supp.) *188:*155, 1959.
12. National Advisory Cancer Council, *Progress Against Cancer,* 1966, U. S. Dep't. of Health, Education, and Welfare, Washington, p. 45.
13. Fisher, B., Fisher, C. R., and Feduska, N. Trauma and the localization of tumor cells. *Cancer 20:*23, 1967.
14. Gibson, G. R. and Stephens, F. O. Experimental use of cetrimide in the prevention of wound implantation with cancer cells. *Lancet 1:*678, 1966.
15. McDonald, G. O., Edmonson, J. L., and Cole, W. H. Prevention of implantation of cancer cells in the wound by irrigation with anticancer agents. *Am. J. Surg. 101:*16, 1961.
16. McDonald, G. O., Gines, S. M. and Cole, W. H. Wound irrigation in cancer surgery. *A.M.A. Arch. Surg. 80:*920, 1960.
17. Smith, R. R. and Gehan, E. A. Effect of formaldehyde wound wash on development of local wound recurrences. *J. Nat. Cancer Inst. 23:*1339, 1959.
18. Venick, J. and Hoppe, E. T. The value of iodine compounds in the experimental treatment of wounds inoculated with cancer cells. *Surgery 59:*278, 1966.
19. Vernick, J. J., Magell, J., and Hoppe, E. T. Alkylating agents and indophor compounds for the prevention of local recurrence of cancer. *Surg. Forum 15:*336, 1964.
20. Gubareff, N., and Suntzeff, V. Preliminary report on application of iodine in prevention of surgical dissemination of viable malignant cells. *J. Surg. Res. 2:*144, 1962.
21. Nora, P. F. and Preston, F. W. Chemotherapy as an adjunct to surgery in the treatment of cancer. *Surg. Clin. N. Amer. 43:*39, 1963.
22. Ackerman, L. V., and Wheat, M. W., Jr. The implantation of cancer—An avoidable surgical risk? *Surgery 37:*341, 1955.
23. Beahrs, O. H., Phillips, J. W., and Dockerty, M. B. Implantation of tumor cells as a factor in recurrence of carcinoma of the rectosigmoid. *Cancer 8:*831, 1955.

24. Borehan, P. F. Surgical spread of cancer in urology. *Brit. J. Urol. 28:*163, 1952.
25. Cohn, I., Floyd, C. E., and Atik, M. Control of tumor implantation during operations on the colon. *Ann. Surg. 157:*825, 1963.
26. Cole, W. H. Recurrence in carcinoma of the colon and proximal rectum following resection for carcinoma. *A.M.A. Arch. Surg. 65:*264, 1952.
27. Goligher, J. C., Dukes, C. E. and Bussey, H. J. R. Local recurrence after spincter-saving excisions for carcinoma of the rectum and rectosigmoid. *Brit. J. Surg. 39:* 199, 1951.
28. Gottfried, G., Molomut, N., and Skaredoff, L. Effect of repeated surgical wounding on the growth rate of tumor graft. *Ann. Surg. 153:*138, 1961.
29. Smith, R. R., Thomas, L. B. and Hilberg, A. W. Cancer cell contamination of operative wounds. *Cancer 11:*53, 1958.
30. Sonneland, J. Accidental seeding of cancer in the operative area. *Northwest Med. 58:*1687, 1959.
31. Southwick, H. W., Harridge, W. H., and Cole, W. H. Recurrence at the suture line following resection for carcinoma of the colon. *Am. J. Surg. 103:*86, 1962.
32. Vaitkevicius, V. K., Sugimoto, M., Reed, M. L., and Brennan, M. J. Effect of acute tissue injury on transplantability of autologous human cancer. *Cancer 18:*665, 1965.
33. Cohn, I., Corly, R. G. and Floyd, C. E. Iodized sutures for control of tumor implantation in colon anastomosis. *Surg., Gynec. and Obst. 116:*366, 1963.
34. DiVincenti, F. C., and Cohn, I. The role of suture material on tumor implantation. *J.A.M.A. 191:*107, 1965.
35. Haverback, C. Z. and Smith, R. R. Transplantation of tumor by suture thread and its prevention. *Cancer 12:*1029, 1959.
36. Herter, F. P. and Sbuelz, B. Inhibition of tumor growth by iodized catgut. *J. of Surg. Res. 6:*393, 1966.
37. Keller, J. W., Kelley, H. G. and Kinsey, D. L. Efficiency of iodized suture in prevention of suture transferral of malignant tumors. *Cancer 19:*549, 1966.
38. Chirigos, M. A., Colsky, J., Humphreys, S. R., Glynn, J. P. and Goldin, A. Evaluation of surgery and chemotherapy in the treatment of mouse mammary adenocarcinoma 755. *Cancer Chemotherapy Reports* No. 22, 49, 1962.
39. Cole, D. R., Rousselot, L. M., Slattery, J. R., Tan, Y. L. and Gonzalez, E. M. Intraluminal cancer chemotherapy adjuvant to pulmonary resection. *J. Surg. Res. 5:*105, 1965.
40. Cruz, E. P., McDonald, G. O. and Cole, W. H. Prophylactic treatment of cancer; the use of chemotherapeutic agents to prevent tumor metastasis. *Surgery 40:* 291, 1956.
41. Knock, F. E. Coordinated surgical-chemical therapy of cancer. *J.A.M.A. 186:* 558, 1963.
42. Martin, D. S. An appraisal of chemotherapy as an adjunct to surgery for cancer. *Amer. J. Surg. 97:*685, 1959.
43. Martin, D. S. and Fugmann, R. A. Clinical implications of the interrelationship of tumor size and chemotherapeutic response. *Ann. Surg. 151:*97, 1960.
44. Martin, D. S., Fugmann, R. A. and Hayworth, P. Surgery, cancer chemotherapy, host defenses, and tumor size. *J. Nat. Cancer Inst. 29:*817, 1962.
45. McKibbin, B., Gazet, J. C. and Hoppe, E. T. Experimental use of anticancer compounds in the control of intraperitoneal malignant disease. *Surg. Forum 14:*131, 1963.
46. Moore, G. E. and Kondo, T. Study of adjuvant cancer chemotherapy by model experiments. *Surgery 44:*199, 1958.

PART IV

47. Moore, G. E. (Chairman) Present status of investigations in surgical adjuvant chemotherapy. Conference on experimental and clinical cancer themotherapy. *Nat. Cancer Inst. Monograph No. 3,* p. 107, 1960.
48. Moore, G. E., Ross, C. A. and Stiver, R. B. Chemotherapy as an adjuvant to surgery. *Am. J. Surg. 105:*591, 1963.
49. Mrazek, R., Economou, S., McDonald, G. O., Slaughter, D. and Cole, W. Prophylactic and adjuvant use of nitrogen mustard in the surgical treatment of cancer. *Ann. Surg. 150:*745, 1959.
50. Rousselot, L. M., Cole, D. R., Slattery, J., Grossi, C. E. and Gonzalez, E. M. Intraluminal chemotherapy adjuvant to surgery for cancer of the colo-rectum. *Ann. Surg. 162:*407, 1965.
51. Shapiro, D. M. and Fugmann, R. A. A role for chemotherapy as an adjunct to surgery. *Cancer Res. 17:*1098, 1957.
52. Sutow, W. W. Chemotherapy in childhood cancer (except leukemia) *Cancer 18:* 1585, 1965.
53. Tokuyama, H., Tukouka, J., Mizota, S., Satou, H., Tsunematsu, T. and Yamada, T. Critical considerations on the treatment of cancer: Effect of the administration of anticancer agents before, during, or after surgical operation. *Gann 54:*71, 1963.
54. Vernick, J. J., Oates, G. D., Magell, J., Fried, C. The use of anticancer agents for control of tumor growth in the peritoneal cavity after seeding with an experimental tumor. *J. Surg. Res. 4:*559, 1964.
55. Frei, E. III A commentary. Selected considerations regarding chemotherapy as adjuvant in cancer treatment. *Cancer Chemother. Rep. 50:*1, 1966.
56. Cole, W. H., Mrazek, R. G., Economou, S. G., McDonald, G. O., Slaughter, D. P. and Strehl, F. W. Adjuvant chemotherapy. *Cancer 18:*1529, 1965.
57. Kondo, T. and Ichihashi, H. Induction of metastases by treatment with carcinostatic agents. II. Depression of host resistance and antibody production. *Gann 55:*403, 1964.
58. Wolberg, W. H., Johnson, R. O. and Curreri, A. R. A reappraisal of surgical adjuvant cancer chemotherapy. *Surg., Gyn. and Obst. 120:*299, 1965.
59. Knock, F. E. Improved adjuvant chemotherapy for cancer. *Surg., Gyn. and Obst. 122:*991, 1966.
60. Folkman, J., Cole, P. and Zimmerman, S. Tumor behavior in isolated perfused organs: *In vitro* growth and metastases of biopsy material in rabbit thyroid and canine intestinal segment. *Ann. of Surg. 164:*491, 1966.
61. Folkman, J., Cole, P. and Zimmerman, S. Tumor behavior in isolated perfused organs: *In vitro* growth and metastases of biopsy material in rabbit thyroid and canine intestinal segment. *Ann. Surg. 164:*491, 1966.
62. Folkman, J., Long, D. M. and Becker, F. F. Tumor growth in organ culture. *Surg. Forum 13:*81, 1962.
63. Folkman, J., Long, D. M. and Becker, F. F. Growth and metastasis of tumor in organ culture. *Cancer 16:*453, 1963.
64. Furth, J. Studies of disease in organ culture: Summary, correlation and speculation. Symposium on organ culture, *National Cancer Inst. Monograph #11,* March, 1963, p. 250.
65. Knock, F. E. Sensitivity tests for cancer chemotherapy. *Arch. Surg. 91:*376, 1965.
66. Long, J. A. and Lyons, W. R. Small perfusion apparatus for study of surviving, isolated organs. *J. Lab. Clin. Med. 44:*614, 1954.
67. Richardson, G. S. and Ulfelder, H. Experiences with a simplified method of small organ perfusion. *Surgery 48:*237, 1960.
68. Byrne, A. Digest of 20 years' experience in the treatment of cancer of the uterus by galvanocautery. *Boston Med. & Surg. J. 121:*435, 1889.

69. Lomer, R. Zur Frage der Heilbarkeit des Carcinoms. *Zeitschr. f. Geburtsch. and Gyn. 50:*305, 1903.
70. Chrobak, R. Zur Behandlung des inoperablen Uterus-Karzinoms. *Wien. Klin. Woch. 18:*964, 1905.
71. Doyen, E. Traitement local des cancers accessibles par l'action de la chaleur au dessus de 55°. *Rev. de thérap. méd.-chir., Par. 77:*577, 1910.
72. Kiek, E. Zur Behandlung der bösartigen Geschwülste. *Zblatt. f. Chir. 551:*266, 1928.
73. Müller, C. Die Krebskrankheit und ihre Behandlung mit Röntgenstrahlen und hochfrequenter Elektrizität, resp. Diathermie. *Strahlentherapie 2:*170, 1913.
74. Wassink, W. F. The curative treatment of carcinoma recti by means of electrocoagulation and radium. *Arch. Chir. Neerl. 8:*313, 1956.
75. Strauss, A. A. Surgical diathermy of carcinoma of the rectum and its clinical end results. *Arch. Phys. Therap. 14:*212, 1933.
76. Strauss, A. A., Strauss, S. F., Crawford, R. A. and Strauss, H. A. Surgical diathermy of carcinoma of the rectum, its clinical end results. *J.A.M.A. 104:*1480, 1935.
77. Strauss, A. A., Strauss, S. F., and Strauss, H. A. New method and end results in treatment of carcinoma of the stomach and rectum by surgical diathermy (electrical coagulation). *South. Surg. 5:*348, 1936.
78. Strauss, A. A., Saphir, O., and Oppel, M. Development of absolute immunity in experimental animals and relative immunity in human beings due to necroses of malignant tumors. *Schweiz med. Wchnschr. 86:*606, 1956.
79. Strauss, A. A., Oppelm, M. and Saphir, O. Electrocoagulation of malignant tumors. *Am. J. Surg. 104:*37, 1962.
80. Strauss, A. A. Immunologic resistance to carcinoma produced by electrocoagulation. *Surg., Gyn. and Obst. 121:*989, 1965.
81. Prime, F. and Rohdenburg, G. L. Effect of combined radiation and heat on neoplasms. *Arch. Surg. 2:*116, 1921.
82. Crile, G., Jr. Heat as an adjunct to the treatment of cancer. *Cleveland Clin. Quart. 28:*75, 1961.
83. Ardenne, M. V. Spontanremission von Tumoren nach Hyperthermie. Ein Rückkopplungsvorgang? *Naturwissenchaften. 52:*645, 1965.
84. Crile, G., Jr. Heat as an adjunct to the treatment of cancer; Experimental studies. *Cleveland Clin. Quart. 28:*75, 1961.
85. Crile, G., Jr. Selective destruction of cancers after exposure to heat. *Ann. Surg. 156:*404, 1962.
86. Crile, G., Jr. (comment) in: Shingleton, W. W., Bryan, F. A., Jr., O'Quinn, W. L. and Krueger, L. C. Selective heating and cooling of tissue in cancer chemotherapy. *Ann. Surg. 156:*408, 1962.
87. Harris, J. J., Jones, W. C. and Woolley, G. W. The effect of temperature on tumor growth. *Proc. Am. Assoc. for Cancer Res. 3:*326, 1962.
88. Murphy, J. B. and Sturm, E. Effect of stimulation (heat) of the lymphocytes on rate of growth of spontaneous tumors in mice. *J. Exp. Med. 29:*31, 1919.
89. Shingleton, W. W., Bryan, F. A., Jr., O'Quinn, W. L. and Krueger, L. C. Selective heating and cooling of tissue in cancer chemotherapy. *Ann. Surg. 156:*408, 1962.
90. Popovic, V. and Masironi, R. Disappearance of euthermic tumors after 10-hour generalized hypothermia. *Life Sci. 4:*533, 1965.
91. Popovic, V. P. and Masironi, R. Disappearance of normothermic tumors in shallow (30°C) hypothermia. *Cancer Res. 26:*863, 1966.
92. Popovic, V. and Masironi, R. Effect of generalized hypothermia on normothermic tumors. *Am. J. Physiol. 211:*462, 1966.

93. Popovic, V. and Masironi, R. Enhancement of 5-fluorouracil action on normothermic tumors by generalized hypothermia. *Cancer Res. 26:*2353, 1966.
94. Westermark, N. Effect of heat upon rat-tumors. *Skand. Arch. F. Physiol. 52:* 257, 1927.
95. Woodhall, B., Pickrell, K. L., Georgiade, N. G., Mahaley, M. S. and Dukes, H. T. Effect of hyperthermia upon cancer chemotherapy: Application to external cancers of head and face structures. *Ann. Surg. 151:*750, 1960.
96. Crile, G., Jr. The smaller the cancer, the bigger the operation? *J.A.M.A. 199:* 736, 1967.
97. Haagenson, C. D. and Miller, E. Is radical mastectomy the optimal surgical procedure for early breast carcinoma? *J.A.M.A. 199:*739, 1967.
98. Urban, J. A. What is the rationale for an extended radical procedure in early cases? *J.A.M.A. 199:*742, 1967.
99. Rubin, P. Carcinoma of the breast. General introduction. *J.A.M.A. 199:*742, 1967.
100. Rubin, P. Comment: Controlled clinical trials. *J.A.M.A. 199:*745, 1967.
101. Fisher, B., Fisher, E. R. and Feduska, N. Trauma and the localization of tumor cells. *Cancer 20:*23, 1967.
102. Agostino, D. and Cliffton, E. E. Trauma as a cause of localization of blood-borne metastases: Preventive effect of heparin and fibrinolysin. *Ann. Surg. 161:*97, 1965.
103. Alexander, J. W. and Altemeier, W. K. Susceptibility of injured tissues to hematogenous metastases: An experimental study. *Ann. Surg. 159:*933, 1964.
104. Jewell, W. R. and Romsdahl, M. M. Recurrent malignant disease in operative wounds not due to surgical implantation from the resected tumor. *Surgery 58:* 806, 1965.
105. Jones, F. S. and Rous, P. On the cause of the localization of secondary tumors at points of injury. *J. Exper. Med. 20:*404, 1914.
106. Raichev, R. and Andreev, V. The problem of injury and the development of matastases. *Khirurgija* (Sofia) *13:*1045, 1960. In *Excepta Med. Amst. Sect.* XVI, 10, 298.
107. Decker, D. G., et al. Adjuvant therapy for advanced ovarian malignancy. *Am. J. Obstet. & Gyn. 97:*171, 1967.
108. Moore, G. E. Chemotherapy in stage 1 breast cancer. *J.A.M.A. 199:*744, 1967.

Improving the Effectiveness of Radiotherapy

Radiotherapy, although less effective in the treatment of cancer than surgery, has cured thousands of patients and provided temporary relief and prolongation of life to many millions more. Still, there are reasons to believe that radiotherapy could be used much more effectively if we knew how it actually affects cancer. Unfortunately, some research leads which were developed as far back as 30 and 40 years ago have not been adequately followed up. There is a reasonable chance that properly planned and supported research in radiotherapy could lead to a cure of a much higher percentage of patients, and increase the life expectancy of many others who cannot as yet be cured.

The mechanism by which radiation cures some cancer patients and helps others is not clear. The source of radiation may be an x-ray machine or a radioactive element such as radium, radon or cobalt. Thus far, we have little evidence that the source of the radiation makes a great deal of difference in the way radiation affects cancers, but the possibility that this is so cannot be ruled out. It is generally believed that the main anti-cancer effect of radiation results from a direct killing of vulnerable cells by the ray (1). The vulnerability of particular cells to radiation appears to depend on several factors. Many radiologists believe that rate of division is the major factor—that rapidly dividing cells are more vulnerable to radiation. Thus, Bacq and Alexander (2) state:

> The use of ionizing radiations in cancer therapy is not due to any inherent differences in response of normal and malignant cells, but depends on the greater sensitivity of dividing cells.

This, of course, points to a major limitation to the expanded use of radiotherapy. If the effect of radiation does indeed depend entirely, or largely, on the greater sensitivity of dividing cells, then rapidly dividing *normal* cells are quite vulnerable. As was pointed out in Chapter 5, some normal cells which are essential to life, including those in the bone marrow and those lining the gastrointestinal tract, multiply more rapidly than most cancer cells. Therefore, if the entire body is irradiated, any procedure that selectively kills the more rapidly multiplying cells is likely to kill the patient before destroying all cancer cells. To avoid this, radiologists beam the radiation at discrete areas of cancer, avoiding exposure of the remainder of the patient's body. Thus, radiation is useful primarily in cancers that are radiosensitive and that are not widely disseminated; it is much less useful in the treatment of metastases throughout the internal organs and, unfortunately, these are the cancers for which better treatment is most needed.

There is, however, significant experimental evidence, as well as clinical evidence, that the beneficial effects of radiation on cancer may be based on other mechanisms besides cell division. Friedman (3) points out that:

A number of phenomena were observed which suggested that there are different ways whereby irradiation affects cancer and tissue.

He goes on to say (4):

We who look at irradiated tumors through a microscope and observe crude histologic changes, find that mitosis, or the absence of it, is only of partial consequence in the irradiation destruction of a tumor. . . .

One of the most radiosensitive of all tissues is lipoid histiocytosis; a single dose of 250r. is lethal for half these tumors. One sees no mitosis there whatever. . . .

Many radiosensitive lesions [cancers] have occasional or no mitosis, while some tumors with many mitotic figures are highly resistant.

Other clinical observers have suggested the possibility of an abscopal effect (5, 6), which is one that occurs at a site distant from the site of irradiation.

The effectiveness of radiation therapy is markedly influenced by the oxygen tension in the area directly surrounding the particular cell being bombarded by rays. The higher the oxygen tension, the greater the effect. This oxygen effect applies to all cells, normal and cancerous. Patt states (7):

In general, the radiation dose required to induce a degree of change in the absence or near absence of oxygen comparable to that produced in air is increased by a factor of about three. It is important to stress that the oxygen effect increases very sharply from levels around zero to about 10 per cent oxygen, and then plateaus at levels approaching the physiological or normal ambient tension.

This oxygen effect seems to be one reason for the failure of radiation to cure many cancers. The interiors of cancers are essentially anoxic (*see* Chapter 5). This is a consequence of the abnormal vasculature (8). However, the normal body cells are well supplied with oxygen, so that the oxygen effect tends to make radiation less toxic to cancer cells, but more toxic to normal cells, including those of bone marrow and gastrointestinal tract. Bacq and Alexander have described the importance of the oxygen effect (9). They have suggested methods for counteracting it, including the use of vasodilators (10)—which seems impractical in view of the physiology of the circulation (*see* Chapter 20)—and the use of a compression chamber (10) which has also been suggested by Moses (11). However, there have been no controlled studies to indicate whether or not a compression chamber might be helpful.

It is possible, and even likely, that the oxygen effect may help explain one aspect of clinical radiotherapy of cancer. It has long been known that radiotherapy is much more effective when given in divided doses over a period of several weeks than when given as a single dose. It may be that, when divided doses are given, the outer layers of cancer cells, which are well supplied with oxygen, are killed, but not the inner layers. The death of the outer layers may stimulate blood vessels to proliferate deeper into the cancer mass, bringing in more oxygen, and therefore making the next layer more sensitive to radiation. This has been likened to a "peeling-off" effect (12). On the other hand, the greater effectiveness of divided doses may be related to an entirely different effect of radiation—improvement of immunologic defenses.

In some popular descriptions of radiotherapy of cancer, the process is likened to the shooting of a gun. The rays are compared to bullets, and the cancer cells to targets. According to such a theory, better aim and greater intensity of fire should increase the effectiveness of radiotherapy. Clinical experiences suggest that this concept is oversimplified and misleading. For example, increasing the dose of radiation beyond a certain level may worsen the patient's chances instead of improving them. Garcia (13) reported on two large groups of patients with carcinoma of the cervix. There were about 500 patients in each group. One group, in which patients received 3,000r of radiation in 30 days, had a 6 per cent recurrence rate of their cancers. The group that received more radiation—4,000r units—had an 18 per cent recurrence rate, three times as high.

Furthermore, patients receiving preoperative radiotherapy may have a higher mortality rate than those who do not (14), although some authors have reported that *small amounts* of preoperative irradiation are helpful to patients (15). Thus, the picture is far from clear.

When the Atomic Energy Commission was requesting large sums of money from Congress for its nuclear reaction program, it emphasized the potential peaceful uses of atomic energy, stressing in particular that more powerful sources of radiation would produce a much higher cure rate of cancers. In general, this expectation has not been met. While it is true that a relatively few patients have received more benefit from cobalt radiation than they would have received from regular x-ray machines, most patients who would benefit from radiotherapy do not, apparently, need the extra energy of the cobalt source. Our existing sources of radiation provide more than enough energy, and increasing their size and energy output does not appear to be necessary. Instead, we need to take a closer look at the mechanisms which are responsible for the effects of radiation therapy on cancer, to see whether we are omitting or neglecting some approaches that could lead to a marked increase in the cure rate.

A recurrent theme in radiation research is the suggestion that radiation in some manner increases host resistance to the cancer. One way of achieving this would be to alter the antigenicity of the cancer. More than half a century ago, Lepper (16) and Wedd, Morson, and Russ (17) reported that the injection of irradiated cancers into animals produced an immunity to those cancers. There were, of course, flaws in their studies (such as the use of non-inbred animals with transplantable cancers), but their observations still deserve consideration. A decade later, Wood and Prigosan (18) were not able to produce immunity by inoculating irradiated tumor tissue, but this may have been due to the dose of radiation they used. Large doses kill cancer cells, and alter their antigenicity drastically, while smaller doses attenuate the activity of cancer cells and may alter their antigenicity to a more appropriate degree. About 25 years ago, Goldfeder (19) suggested that further research be done on radiation-attenuated cancer implants.

There is also evidence that suggests that small doses of x-rays may stimulate host resistance in a nonspecific manner. Nakahara and Murphy (20) studied this phenomenon on mice with transplanted cancers. In 1919, Nakahara (21) reported changes in the lymphoid organs after small doses of x-rays, and, a few years later, Murphy, Maisin, and Sturm (22) reported that x-rays induced local resistance to spontaneous mouse cancer. They state:

> It is evident from our experiments that as far as mouse cancer is concerned, the beneficial result from x-ray therapy is due to the reaction in the normal tissues induced by the rays, not to any direct effect on the cancer cells.

It seems likely that Murphy and his colleagues were incorrect in the second part of their conclusion, and that x-rays have some direct effects on cancer cells. Nevertheless, their observations of effects on the normal tissues, stimulating them to repel the cancer cells, seem quite valid and deserving of further study.

The British investigators Russ, Chambers, Scott and Mottram came to similar conclusions (23, 24). They suggested (23) that there are at least three effects of x-rays in relation to cancer. First, there is a direct effect on the cancer cells. Second, large doses of radiation *reduce* host immunity and favor growth of the tumor. Third, small doses of radiation *increase* host immunity and help control the cancer. They go on to suggest that the radiologist, by giving a primary cancer a killing dose of radiation, may be indirectly encouraging growth of metastases by lowering host resistance. In France, Rubens (25) also reached this conclusion, and suggested that the effectiveness of radiotherapy is due as much to the lymphoid connective tissue reactions the rays provoke as to the destructive effects they may produce on cancer cells.

These important studies (21-25) were all done more than 40 years ago, and yet we still do not have a clear-cut description of the mechanism of action of radiation on cancer cells, nor have we developed practical ways to utilize such information to increase the effectiveness of radiotherapy.

More than 25 years ago, Russ and Scott (26) showed that x-rays could affect cancer growth when the cancer itself was not irradiated.

In recent years, there has been a renewal of interest in the question the effects of radiation on cancer and on the host bearing the cancer. Vermund (27) and Strenstrom, Vermund *et al.* (28) have suggested that an important aspect of radiation therapy involves the effect on the tumor bed—the host tissues in which the cancers grow. Silk, Hawtrey and MacIntosh (29) have shown that there are indirect effects of irradiation of cancers. Mitchell (30), working with spontaneous mouse cancers, showed that irradiated cancer cells can affect recurrences of these cancers. Haddow and Alexander (31) have developed an immunologic method of increasing the vulnerability of sarcomas to x-rays. Kaplan (32) has pointed out the importance of host nutritional factors in the effectiveness of radiotherapy. He indicates that little work is being done in this area, and that much more should be done.

One of the most vital questions to be answered concerns the effect of radiation on metastases as well as on the primary cancer. Oich, Eck and Smith (33) did a study of this important subject in 1959; so did Kallenbach and Gregl (34) in 1962.

Several studies have been done on combinations of radiation and other therapy (35, 36).

Other studies over the past fifty years (37-42) have opened areas for additional research in radiotherapy of cancer. For example, Mitchell and Mitchell (44) have uncovered an important aspect of radiotherapy. In a recent article they reported that Miss R. D. Saunders, a scientist at a radiotherapeutic center in a hospital in England, noted that patients whose radiation treatment for lip cancer started on Monday seemed to have a better outcome than those whose treatment started on Thursday. Mitchell and Mitchell reviewed the hospital records and found a highly significant difference in recurrence rates. Since no treatments were given on Saturday or Sunday, the spacing of the two rest days appears to be the critical factor. The sequence 5-0-0-2 resulted in a recurrence rate only one-third of the recurrence rate with sequence 2-0-0-5. In the subgroup consisting of patients under 70 years of age, the 5-0-0-2 sequence produced a recurrence rate of only one-ninth that of the 2-0-0-5 sequence. In every other respect, both groups of patients were alike. The authors believe that the difference in response is related to host factors.

Where do we stand today in radiation treatment of cancer? Empirically, radiotherapists have discovered that radiation can cure some cancers and affect others. Yet more than fifty years after the discovery that x-rays can affect cancer, we still do not understand how this happens. To a major extent, this deficiency is a result of completely inadequate support for research on radiation effects on cancer. If we knew more about this vital field, the chances are good that the efficiency of radiotherapy could be improved, with a consequent saving of many more lives.

Let us now consider what should be done and how. Since we need to know all the ways in which radiation affects the host-cancer relationship, some of the specific questions that ought to be answered are:

1. Does radiation therapy alter the antigenicity of cancer cells in a way that enables the host to produce more and better antibodies to the cancer cells?

   a. If so, would it be advisable to remove a cancer or part of it, irradiate it, and then implant it into the same patient?

   b. What dose range and schedule would be most efficient?

2. Does radiation therapy improve host defenses in a nonspecific stimulatory manner?

   a. Does radiation have to hit the cancer cell to affect it?

   b. What dose range and schedule would be most efficient?

3. Does radiation therapy have an important effect on the host blood vessels that proliferate to the cancer? (*see* Chapter 19).

4. Can we find better ways of selecting patients most likely to benefit from radiotherapy?

5. To what extent does host nutritional status affect the cure rate of radiation therapy?

   a. Is general host nutrition the main factor?

   b. Are there specific nutritional factors, such as particular amino acids or vitamins, that can improve the cure rate of radiation therapy?

   c. Are there any nutritional factors that might lower the cure rate of radiation therapy?

6. Does radiation affect metastases in the same way that it affects the primary cancer?

7. Can combinations of radiotherapy, chemotherapy and immunotherapy give better results than any of these alone?

The research approaches to these problems will require the coordinated efforts of scientists in several fields. It has become increasingly clear that the selection of the proper experimental model is of great importance. The use of transplanted rodent cancers can hardly be considered satisfactory, unless the results are confirmed with spontaneous cancers. The general objections to the use of transplantable cancers have been discussed in Chapter 14. Kaplan (43) has pointed out the need for more studies on the effects of radiotherapy on cancers in the original host. He states:

. . . I think we should all be aware of the pitfalls of working with transplantable tumors. I think there is much to be learned from them, but basically the transplant and its host are foreign bodies to one another, even if they come from the same strain.

I think there is need for much more work with tumors, either induced or spontaneous, arising in the original host.

In radiotherapy studies, there are also some drawbacks to the use of small animals, simply because of their size. Radiation has a certain degree of spread; in order to irradiate a mouse cancer and not the entire animal, special shielding procedures, often including anesthesia, are needed, and these might influence the results. Furthermore, the relationship of absorption of radiation energy to body size may introduce major errors. For these reasons, it seems imperative to do studies on animals whose size at least approximates that of man. As a satisfactory size range, we might accept initially ⅕ to 5 times the mass of an adult human being, or 30 to 750 lbs. This would include most dogs, swine, and some cattle. With increasing experience, this range might be narrowed or broadened.

To carry out these studies, task forces including radiotherapists, pathologists and veterinarians should be given the missions, and the facilities and support to carry them out. Within the veterinary medical profession, there are now specialties corresponding to many of those in human medicine. Thus, there are veterinary radiologists and veterinary pathologists. Although their numbers are small, they should be able to provide invaluable assistance in designing and carrying out these missions.

We have had the technical facilities to work on most of these vital studies for more than 20 years, and we should have had the answers to many of the questions about radiotherapy for cancer years ago. Any further delay would be inexcusable.

References

1. Bacq, Z. M. and Alexander, P. *Fundamentals of Radiobiology.* Academic Press, N. Y., 1955.
2. *Ibid.,* p. 202.
3. Friedman, M. Patterns of tumor regression and cell death. In *Research in Radiology,* Kaplan, H. S., Ed. Publication 571, Nat. Acad. Sci., Washington, 1958, p. 9.
4. *Ibid.,* p. 10, 11.

5. Chamberlain, R. H. 3. Possible role of abscopal effects (Lorenz and Hollcroft): Status of sensitizers; Status of combined radiation and chemotherapy. In: *Research in Radiology*, Kaplan, H. S., Ed. Publication 571, Nat. Acad. Sci., Washington, 1958, p. 109.
6. *Ibid.*, p. 113.
7. Patt, H. M. 2. Oxygen effect and modification by oxygen binding agents; theoretical basis of Gray's proposal for use of high O_2 in therapy. In: *Research in Radiology*, Kaplan, H. S., Ed. Publication 571, Nat. Acad. Sci., Washington, 1958, p. 51.
8. *Ibid.*, p. 53.
9. Bacq, Z. M. and Alexander, P., *op. cit.*, pp. 209, 216.
10. *Ibid.*, p. 217.
11. Moses, L. E. 4. Comments on the design of a clinical high oxygen experiment. In: *Research in Radiology*, Kaplan, H. S., Ed. Publication 571, Nat. Acad. Sci., Washington, 1958, p. 67.
12. Kohn, H. I. In: *Research in Radiology*, Kaplan, H. S., Ed. Publication 571, Nat. Acad. Sci., Washington, 1958, p. 60.
13. Garcia, M. In: *Research in Radiology*, Kaplan, H. S., Ed. Publication 571, Nat. Acad. Sci., Washington, 1958, p. 48.
14. Tildon, T. T. and Hughes, R. K. Complications from preoperative irradiation therapy for lung cancer. *Ann. Thor. Surg. 3:*307, 1967.
15. Hoye, R. C. and Smith, R. R. The effectiveness of small amounts of preoperative irradiation in preventing the growth of tumor cells disseminated at surgery. *Cancer 14:*284, 1961.
16. Lepper, E. H. The immunity to rat sarcoma produced by grafts of sarcoma which have been irradiated by radium. *Arch. Middlesex Hosp. 33:*89, 1914.
17. Wedd, B. H., Morson, A. C., and Russ, S. On the immunity conferred upon mice by radium-irradiated mouse carcinoma. *J. Path. and Bact. 18:*566, 1914.
18. Wood, F. C. and Prigosan, R. E. No immunity produced by inoculating irradiated tumor tissue. *J. Cancer Res. 9:*287, 1925.
19. Goldfeder, A. Relation between radiation effects and cell viability as indicated by induced resistance to transplanted tumors. *Radiology 39:*426, 1942.
20. Nakahara, W. and Murphy, J. B. Studies of x-ray effects. VII. Effect of small doses of x-rays of low penetration on the resistance of mice to transplanted cancer. *J. Exp. Med. 33:*429, 1921.
21. Nakahara, W. Studies on x-ray effects. III. Changes in the lymphoid organs after small doses of x-rays. *J. Exp. Med. 29:*83, 1919.
22. Murphy, J. B., Maisin, J. and Sturm, E. Local resistance to spontaneous mouse cancer induced by x-rays. *J. Exp. Med. 38:*645, 1923.
23. Russ, S., Chambers, H., Scott, G. M. and Mottram, J. C. Experimental studies with small doses of x-rays. *Lancet 1:*692, 1919.
24. Russ, S., Chambers, H., and Scott, G. M. On the local and generalized action of radium and x-rays on tumour growth. *Proc. Roy. Soc. London.* Series B. *92:*125, 1921.
25. Rubens, D. H. Radiumthérapie et défense de l'organisme contre le cancer épithélial. *J. Méd. Franc. 10:*128, 1921.
26. Russ, S. and Scott, G. M. The effect of x-rays upon tumour growth when the tumour itself was not irradiated. *Brit. J. Radiol. 13:*267, 1940.
27. Vermund, H. The significance of the tumor bed reactions in the radiation treatment of malignant tumors. *Am. J. Roentgenol. 82:*678, 1959.
28. Strenstrom, K. W., Vermund, H., Mosser, D. G. and Marvin, J. F. Effects of roentgen irradiation on the tumor bed. *Radiation Res. 2:*180, 1955.

PART IV

29. Silk, M. H., Hawtrey, A. O. and MacIntosh, I. J. C. Indirect effects during x-irradiation of malignant tumors. *Cancer Res. 18:*1257, 1958.
30. Mitchell, J. R. Effects of irradiated tumor cells on spontaneous mammary tumor recurrences in C3H mice. *Growth 26:*47, 1962.
31. Haddow, A. and Alexander, P. An immunological method of increasing the sensitivity of primary sarcomas to local irradiation with x-rays. *Lancet 1:*452, 1964.
32. Kaplan, H. S. Factors in the host and tumor bed. 1. Role of nutrition, vascular bed and stroma. In: *Research in Radiology,* Kaplan, H. S., Ed. Publication 571, Nat. Acad. Sci., Washington, 1958, p. 43.
33. Oich, P. D., Eck, R. V. and Smith, R. R. An experimental study of the effect of external radiation on a "primary" tumor and its distant metastases. *Cancer 12:* 23, 1959.
34. Kallenbach, H. and Gregl, A. Über die Veränderung der Metastasenhäufigkeit nach Röntgenganzbestrahlung im Tier-experimentellen Modellversuch. *Med. Klin. 57:* 1621, 1962.
35. Koldovsky, P. and Lengerova, A. A combination of specific antitumour therapy and x-ray irradiation. *Folia Biol.* (Prague) *6:*441, 1960.
36. Vermund, H., Hodgett, J. and Ansfield, F. J. Effects of combined roentgen irradiation and chemotherapy on transplanted tumors in mice. *Amer. J. Roentgenol. Rad. Ther. and Nuc. Med. 85:*559, 1961.
37. Murphy, J. B. and Morton, J. J. The effect of Roentgen rays on the rate of growth of spontaneous tumors in mice. *J. Exp. Med. 22:*800, 1915.
38. Wood, F. C. and Prime, F. D. Lethal dose of roentgen-rays for cancer cells. *J.A.M.A. 74:*308, 1920.
39. Clemmesen, J. *Influence of X-radiation on the Development of Immunity to Heterologous Transplantation of Tumors.* London, Oxford U. Press, 1938.
40. Cohen, L. Immunity and resistance in clinical cancer. *South African Med. J. 30:* 161, 1956.
41. Ludovici, P. P., Pock, R. A., Christian, R. T., Riley, G. M. and Miller, N. F. Detection of characteristic differences in the irradiation sensitivity of four human cell strains. *Rad. Res. 14:*141, 1961.
42. Summers, W. C. A model of tumor growth in irradiated hosts. *Nature 205:*414, 1965.
43. Kaplan, H. S. *Research in Radiology.* Publication 571, Nat. Acad. Sci., Washington, 1958, p. 50.
44. Mitchell, J. S. and Mitchell, L. M. Fractionation in radiotherapy of cancer of the lip. *Acta Radiologica 6:*299, 1967.

Plant Materials as Sources of Anti-Cancer Medications

In the earliest days of cancer research, attention was focussed mainly on plant materials. Then, as the value of synthetic chemicals in other areas of medicine became apparent, the emphasis shifted to synthetic chemicals. Since 1960, however, there has been a gradual increase in the number of studies being done on the use of plant materials for anti-cancer effects.

There are sound reasons for giving a considerable degree of attention to plant materials in general; in addition, it may prove helpful to invest an extra degree of effort in studies on a special class of plant materials, the differential growth inhibitors.

Let us first consider the historic relationship of plant materials in general to human medicine. Virtually all of the earliest effective medications were of plant origin. Long ago men, who by modern standards would be considered primitive, recognized the therapeutic value of many of the plants that we still use today as sources of potent drugs. We have, of course, purified the plant extracts; in some cases the active ingredients have been synthesized and modifications made. Nevertheless, the basic discoveries that led to the current use of most of these drugs must be credited to these men. Some of the still important medications of plant origin are:

The digitalis glycosides, such as digitoxin, ouabain and lanatoside that are used for the treatment of heart failure.

The belladonna alkaloids—atropine and homatropine.

The opium alkaloids—morphine and codeine.

The cinchona alkaloids—quinine and quinidine.

The salicylates—including methyl salicylate (oil of Wintergreen) and aspirin, which is a synthetic derivative. (The term salicylates comes from the botanical name Salix, meaning willow—an original source.)

Colchicine, a material found in the meadow saffron.

The Rauwolfia alkaloids, including reserpine.

It is of interest that some of the drugs of plant origin cannot be synthesized as yet in the laboratory, even though the purified drugs have been available for decades and their chemical structure is definitely known. The digitalis glycosides fall into this classification.

It is pertinent to ask why scientifically unsophisticated men were able to discover such important plant medications for various diseases, but not for cancer. Apparently, these men were able to observe and reason from a rather direct and immediate effect of a plant material on a symptom. For example, if the headache of a person went away within an hour or two after he had chewed willow bark, a cause-effect relationship was suggested; if other members of the group observed the same thing, the utility of willow bark would become part of the folk-lore of the group. This type of direct observation probably was not effective in cases of cancer. The disease was usually internal, and its effects were gradual and insidious. If a primitive man with cancer did eat parts of a plant that had anti-cancer effects, he would have to keep eating it for weeks or months to determine whether he was improving. Even if such a thing happened, which seems unlikely, there would be no way of relating the effects of the plant to cancer, rather than to a wide variety of internal disturbances. Accordingly, the fact that primitive men who found so many useful medications did not, to our knowledge, find a treatment for cancer cannot be used as an indication of the rarity or lack of anti-cancer materials in plants. It is entirely possible that we may find scores of anti-cancer drugs in plants (just as we have found hundreds of digitalis glycosides), provided our techniques of searching are sound.

In the past few years, two plant materials have been found that are useful in the treatment of human cancer and related diseases. The materials, vinblastine and vincristine, are derived from the common periwinkle (Vinca rosea). Vinblastine can produce cures in some cases of choriocarcinoma in women (1). It is also effective in Hodgkin's disease, which has certain features similar to cancer, and can provide temporary help in some leukemias (2, 3). Recently, Scott and Voight (4) reported that vinblastine has an unusually good effect on cases of Kaposi's sarcoma, a form of cancer that differs in some respects from most cancers and is quite rare in the United States. Although vinblastine has not been used long enough in these cases to allow us to use the term "cure," the results thus far suggest that cures may be produced. Thus far, *all* of the three patients treated by Scott and Voight appear to be free of the sarcoma and in good health, including the first patient who was treated five years before the authors' report. Vincristine is known to be helpful in some leukemias of children and possibly in some solid cancers, although our information about its usefulness in these cases is incomplete. The mechanism of action of these two alkaloids is unclear. They block mitosis in metaphase, as does colchicine. However, some authorities believe that the anti-cancer effects may result from a different action than that on mitosis. In any event, the discovery that a common garden plant has anti-cancer properties and is useful in treating human cancers is a hopeful sign, and suggests that a wider and more intensive search of plant materials might turn up more, and more effective, anti-cancer agents.

A number of investigators (5-51, 72-80, 95-103) have tested plant extracts for effects against experimental cancers in animals; and a few such tests have been made on cancers in man (94, 105). Some active principles have been purified (81-93). A rather high proportion of the materials tested seem to have a significant effect. A group of researchers at the University of Texas (13-24) have been doing outstanding work on the effects of plant extracts on cancer in animals. In one study, they tested extracts of 498 plants on a transplantable mammary carcinoma grown in inbred mice (20). Extracts of 25 plants inhibited tumor growth significantly: this constitutes 5 per cent of the plants tested. However, the follow-up tests on spontaneous mouse tumors have been proceeding slowly, and results are not yet known. In a later report (22) it was stated that in the total program of testing a single type of crude extract from 1,500 plants approximately 4.5 per cent of the extracts inhibited growth of the transplanted tumor by 40 per cent or more. The authors of the report state: "The leads which have developed indicate an area which should receive much more attention." Thus far, however, this area has not received a fraction of the attention it deserves.

There are about one million known plant species, and an attempt to test each one for anti-cancer activities would involve a task much greater than our national resources in personnel and space could handle at this time, even under a national goal program. If there were a way to narrow down the kinds of plants to be tested, a desired material might be found much sooner. In the past, plants selected for such tests were often chosen because they were known to contain toxic principles. Sometimes the toxic nature of the plant was revealed by the sickness or death of animals eating it; at other times through the use of the plant by primitive tribes in making arrow poisons and other poisons. The reasoning has been that since the plant is toxic to mammals, perhaps a small dose could be relied upon to produce some change in the host that would be short of the effects

149

of toxicity. This method has been quite successful in finding medications for other diseases; accordingly, there is good reason to test such plants for possible anti-cancer effects. Unfortunately, the number of plants known to be toxic to animals or suitable for making poisons is quite small, and would not provide enough different species for a comprehensive program. Furthermore, all plants selected in this fashion would almost inevitably cause serious toxic side reactions.

An additional group of plants should be tested, and perhaps the method for selecting such plants could be based on the ecologic patterns of the plants. It has been known for many years that some plants secrete growth inhibitors that interfere with the growth of competing plants. Since 1832 (52), this has been a matter of interest to botanists, although it has only been in the last few decades that any really intensive research has been done in the area, and the field of study is still in its early stages. The aspect of the growth inhibitors that may be of interest in cancer research is their selectivity. They do not interfere with all growing cells—only with some. Most of the growth inhibitors are selective in terms of the species they affect. For example, it has been reported that the black walnut tree (53-57) secretes into the soil an inhibitor that prevents apple trees, tomatoes and certain additional plants from growing nearby, while several other plants, such as peach, pear, and wheat, are reported to be unaffected. Furthermore, the growth inhibitors affect certain parts of the competing plant, but not others. Some inhibitors stunt root growth, others affect stems or leaves (58-60), others prevent germination of seeds.

Only a handful of plant growth inhibitors have been tested for their effects on animal cells, but the results have been encouraging. Protoanemonin, a material produced by *Anemone pulsatilla* inhibits rapidly multiplying cells of plant and animal origin, but not resting cells. It does not, to the best of our knowledge, have a differential effect on animal cells of diverse origins, but the studies on this material have not been extensive enough for definite conclusions to be drawn.

One plant growth inhibitor, parasorbic acid (sometimes called hexenolactone), which is found in substantial amounts in the ripe berries of the mountain ash (Sorbus aucuparius) and also in other plants, appears to have an interesting differential effect on animal cells. Several authors (61-63) have reported that it inhibits animal cells of fibroblast origin; yet in the same concentrations it apparently does not affect cells of epithelial origin. Years ago, it was reported that parasorbic acid produced complete cures of the Jensen sarcoma in rats (61, 64). One wonders what effect this material might have in other sarcomas, particularly in man, but I have not been able to find any reports of such studies. It may well be that parasorbic acid has been tested by several investigators who found it unsuitable or too toxic, and could not report the results, since editors of scientific journals have usually discouraged reports of essentially negative data. However, the key point is that a material known to be a differential plant growth inhibitor (65-69) has been shown to have a differential effect on some animal cells, and, in addition, has been reported to be effective in curing at least one type of animal cancer.

There have been a few other scattered reports of plant growth inhibitors retarding the growth of cancers but there is not enough information available to determine whether or not these particular inhibitors deserve further study. On the other hand, since so few plant growth inhibitors have been tested for effects on animal cells, including cancers, the few positive reports constitute an encouraging proportion of the total.

Certainly, there seems to be adequate reason to test all the currently known plant growth inhibitors on cancers (and many of these have been tested). However, this would not be sufficient. In a rather extensive review of the botanical literature (58), I found less than 20 plant growth inhibitors of known chemical composition, and less than 40 plants that were reported to produce inhibitors of unknown composition. This is not an indication of a scarcity of plant growth inhibitors, but an indication of markedly inadequate support for studies on the inhibitors. One may find evidence of plant growth inhibitors in almost any garden. For example, I observed that young ragweeds seemed to produce an inhibitor which affected corn markedly. Another observer has noted that ragweed also inhibits radishes (70), and the experiment he performed indicated that the mechanism was production of a growth inhibitor rather than any competition for nutrients.

There are certain ecologic growth patterns of plants that give good clues to the existence of differential growth inhibitors. These patterns could enable us to pick out the plants most likely to secrete such inhibitors. Then, studies could be concentrated on the extracts of such plants. In ecologic terms, the "single stand" consists of a substantial grouping of plants of the same species that grow together, excluding all other competing multicellular plants from the area. There may be other factors, besides the production of differential growth inhibitors, to account for some of the single stands, but the chances are that, if most plants that are found to grow in single stands in the wild state were investigated, a substantial proportion would be found to secrete differential growth inhibitors.

A second type of ecological pattern that may indicate the presence of growth inhibitors is the "fairy ring" (59, 71). In this pattern, a plant is surrounded by a ring of other plants, each at a substantial distance from the first and from each other. (Sometimes, there is an additional ring, a substantial distance from the first ring.) This pattern may be due to secretion of an homologous growth inhibitor, which affects plants of the same species, keeping them from growing too close to each other. Such patterns may be seen in desert plants, and also in some forest and meadow plants.

Studies of plant communities may also provide leads to plants that secrete differential growth inhibitors. If, for example, it is found that plant A is widely distributed, but is hardly ever found growing close to plant B, even when the habitat seems suitable, there is a good chance that plant B is producing an inhibitor.

There are enough clues to the differential growth inhibitors to make it possible for trained botanists, selecting species to be used in a coordinated study, to choose a much larger proportion of plants with differential growth inhibitors than could be selected on the basis of chance or availability.

The mechanics of studying plant growth inhibitors on cancers should, ideally, involve the coordinated efforts of scientists of several different disciplines. Botanists and plant ecologists should be given the primary responsibility for selecting the plants to be studied. Sometimes, the natural stands of these plants would be large enough to supply all the material needed for testing. In other situations, it might be necessary to grow additional plants in greenhouses or prepared fields.

The extraction of the plant fractions to be used for testing should probably be the responsibility of biochemists and pharmaceutical chemists. The testing of the extracts in animals with cancer could be done by M.D.'s, D.V.M.'s, and Ph.D.'s in Pharmacology, with the help of research assistants and technicians.

A suggested testing procedure would involve the use of extracts which, starting with a crude material containing many ingredients, are made purer and purer. It would be impractical to first separate and purify all the compounds in a plant, and then test each purified material, because there are thousands of compounds in each plant, and the time and effort needed to isolate each one would be excessive. Unfortunately, we do not have any idea of the chemical structure of the anti-cancer drugs being sought, so that we cannot try to isolate a particular compound or group of compounds. However, the method of proceeding from crude to more purified extracts enables us to narrow the search. Also, in the event that a particular purification process destroys the active material, that fact would be readily apparent, since the more purified extract would be less effective than its cruder predecessor.

In performing the tests, it is vital that the schedule of administration of the plant materials be such that an active cancer growth inhibitor, which may be rapidly excreted by a mouse, will not be falsely excreted by mice to be missed by the screen. Accordingly, the usual method of screening anti-cancer drugs in mice has a basic disadvantage, in that it allows a potentially useful drug that is fairly rapidly excreted by mice to be missed by the screen. Accordingly, the usual type of screening procedure would probably be inadequate for testing for growth inhibitors; a procedure that provides for longer exposure of the mouse to the test drug would be needed.

References

1. Hertz, R., Lipsett, M. B. and Moy, R. H. Effect of vincaleukoblastine on metastatic choriocarcinoma and related trophobastic tumors in women. *Cancer Res. 20:*1050, 1960.
2. Johnson, I. S., Wright, H. F., Svoboda, G. H. and Vlantis, J. Anti-tumor principles derived from *Vinca rosea* Linn. I. Vincaleukoblastine and Leurosine. *Cancer Res. 20:*1016, 1960.
3. Whitelaw, D. M. and Teasdale, J. M. Vincaleukoblastine in the treatment of malignant disease. *Canad. Med. Assoc. J. 85:*584, 1961.
4. Scott, W. P. and Voigt, J. A. Kaposi's sarcoma: Management with vinblastine. *Cancer 19:*557, 1966.
5. Belkin, M. Effect of podophyllin on transplanted mouse tumors. *J. Pharmacol. & Exper. Therapy 93:*18, 1948.
6. Hartwell, J. L., Johnson, J. M., Fitzgerald, D. B. and Belkin, M. Siliciolin, a new compound isolated from Juniperus silicicola. *J. Am. Chem. Soc. 74:*4470, 1952.
7. Belkin, M. and Fitzgerald, D. B. Tumor-damaging capacity of plant materials. I. Plants used as cathartics. *J. Nat. Cancer Inst. 13:*139, 1952.
8. Belkin, M., Fitzgerald, D. B. and Felix, M. D. Tumor-damaging capacity of plant materials. II. Plants used as diuretics. *J. Nat. Cancer Inst. 31:*741, 1952.
9. Belkin, M. and Fitzgerald, D. B. Tumor-damaging capacity of plant materials. III. Plants used as pesticides. *J. Nat. Cancer Inst. 13:*889, 1953.
10. Fitzgerald, D. B., Belkin, M., Felix, M. D. and Carroll, M. K. Tumor-damaging capacity of plant materials. IV. Conifers. *J. Nat. Cancer Inst. 13:*895, 1953.
11. Belkin, M. and Fitzgerald, D. B. Tumor-damaging capacity of plant materials. V. Miscellaneous plants. *J. Nat. Cancer Inst. 14:*607, 1953.

12. Fitzgerald, D. B., Belkin, M., Felix, M. D., Carroll, M. K., Hartwell, J. L. and Leiter, J. Distribution of tumor-damaging lignans among conifers. *J. Nat. Cancer Inst. 18:*83, 1957.

13. Taylor, A., Carmichael, N., McKenna, G. F. and Burlage, H. M. Inhibition of the growth of egg cultivated tumor tissue by extracts of *Cooperia pedunculata* herb. *Proc. Soc. Exptl. Biol. & Med. 77:*841, 1951.

14. Taylor, A., McKenna, G. F. and Burlage, H. M. Cancer chemotherapy experiments with plant extracts. *Texas Rep. Biol. & Med. 10:*1062, 1952.

15. McKenna, G. F., Taylor, A. and Burlage, H. M. Chemotherapy experiments with plant extracts and transplantable tumors. *Texas Rep. Biol. & Med. 12:*500, 1954.

16. Taylor, A., McKenna, G. F. and Burlage, H. M. Anticancer activity of plant extracts. *Texas Rep. Biol. & Med. 14:*538, 1956.

17. McKenna, G. F., Taylor, A. and Carmichael, N. Cancer chemotherapy with plant extracts. *Texas Rep. Biol. & Med. 16:*203, 1958.

18. Dalal, U. C., Taylor, A. and McKenna, G. F. The effect of plant extracts on egg cultivated tumor tissue. *Texas Rep. Biol. & Med. 16:*439, 1958.

19. McKenna, G. F., Taylor, A. and Gibson, B. S. Further studies of plant extracts in cancer chemotherapy. *Texas Rep. Biol. & Med. 17:*123, 1959.

20. McKenna, G. F., Taylor, A. and Gibson, B. S. Extracts of plants and cancer chemotherapy. *Texas Rep. Biol. & Med. 18:*233, 1960.

21. McKenna, G. F., Taylor, A. and Albers, C. C. Essential oils, plant extracts and chemicals from plants in cancer chemotherapy. *Texas Rep. Biol. & Med. 19:*321, 1961.

22. McKenna, G. F. and Taylor, A. Screening plant extracts for anticancer activity. *Texas Rep. Biol. & Med. 20:*214, 1962.

23. McKenna, G. F. and Taylor, A. The effect of feeding *Chelidonium majus L.* on the incidence of mammary tumors in mice. *Texas Rep. Biol. & Med. 20:*64, 1962.

24. Taylor, A. and Taylor, N. C. Protective effect of Symphytum officiale on mice bearing spontaneous and transplant tumors. *Proc. Exptl. Biol. & Med. 114:*772, 1963.

25. Hardinge, M. G., Courville, D. A., Hardinge, M., Fujikawa, B. and Harvey, R. Action of plant extracts on transplanted mouse tumors screening data. I. *Cancer Res. 21:*573, 1961.

26. Bekker, E. E., Rodinova, E. G., Iangulova, I. V., Petrova, M. A., Koroleva, V. G., Maevskii, M. M., Romanenko, E. A., Urazova, A. P., Bondareva, A. S., Mazaeva, V. G., Timoschechkina, M. E. and Mol'kob, I. N. Antitumor properties of extracts from the mycelia of various fungi. *Antibiotiki* (Moscow) *6:*488, 1961.

27. Cain, B. F. Tumour inhibitors from plant sources. Part I. *J. Chem. Soc. 509:* 2599, 1961.

28. Hauptlab, J. W. and Schering, A. G. The effect of live and killed yeasts on tumours of mice. *Naturwissenschaften 48:*576, 1961.

29. Carraz, P. G. and Oddoux, L. Recherche d'activité antitumorale chez les myceliums d'homobasidies en culture. *Thérapie 17:*22, 1962.

30. Mayhew, W. G. and Roe, E. M. F. Mode of inhibitory action of tragacanth powder on the growth of the Landschutz ascites tumour. *Brit. J. Cancer 16:*163, 1962.

31. Lewisohn, R., Leuchtenberger, C., Leuchtenberger, R. and Laszlo, D. Effect of intravenous injections on yeast extract on spontaneous breast adenocarcinomas in mice. *Proc. Soc. Exptl. Biol. & Med. 43:*558, 1940.

32. Lewisohn, R., Leuchtenberger, C., Leuchtenberger, R., Laszlo, D. and Bloch, K. Action of yeast extract on transplanted and spontaneous malignant tumors in mice. *Cancer Res. 1:*799, 1941.

33. Mordarski, M. Oncostatic properties of actinomycetes. II. *In vivo* studies. *Arch. Immun. Ter. Dosw. 8:*305, 1960.
34. Nakanishi, K., Tada, M., Yamada, Y. and Ohashi, M. Isolation of lampterol, an antitumour substance from Lampteromyces japonicus. *Nature 197:*292, 1963.
35. Navashin, S. M., Fomina, J. P. and Koroleva, V. G. A study of the antitumour action of actinoxanthine and polymycin in cultures of human cancer cells. *Antibiotiki* (Moscow) *6:*912, 1961.
36. Pelner, L. and Rhoades, M. G. Host-tumor antagonism. XVII. Experimental treatment of breast cancer in dogs with an hydrolysate of certain plant seeds (oncolysin). *J. Am. Geriatrics Soc. 9:*136, 1961.
37. Pugh, L. H., Lechevalier, H. A. and Solotorovsky, M. Antitumour activity of a substance produced by a strain of Helminthosporium. *Antibiotics & Chemotherapy 12:*310, 1962.
38. Schultz, R. D. and Norman, D. Cytocidal activity of plant auxin analogues against the Ehrlich ascites carcinoma. *Nature 206:*276, 1965.
39. Vester, F. and Mai, W. Zur Kenntnis der Inhaltsstoffe von Viscum album. I. *Zschr. Physiol. Chem. 322:*273, 1960.
40. Selawry, O. S. and Vester, F. Study of the fractions of *Viscum album.* II. Tumor inhibiting fractions. *Zschr. Physiol. Chem. 324:*262, 1961.
41. Selawry, O. S., Vester, F., Mai, W. and Schwartz, M. R. Zur Kenntnis der Inhaltsstoffe von Viscum album. II. Tumorhemmende Inhaltsstoffe. *Zschr. Physiol. Chem. 324:*262, 1961.
42. Vester, F. and Nienhaus, J. Cancerostatische Protein-komponenten aus Viscum album. *Experientia 21:*197, 1965.
43. Shohat, B., Gitter, S. and Lavie, D. Antitumor activity of cucurbitacins: Metabolic aspects. *Cancer Chemotherapy Rep. 23:*19, 1962.
44. Sokoloff, B., Funaoka, K., Fujisawa, M., Saelhof, C. C., Taniguchi, E., Bird, L. and Miller, C. An oncostatic factor present in the bark of Hippophae rhamnoides. *Growth 25:*401, 1961.
45. Sokoloff, B., Saelhof, C. C., Fujisawa, M., Funaoka, K. and Miller, C. A critical study on the oncostatic factor present in Caltha palustris. *Growth 26:*71, 1962.
46. Sokoloff, B., Saelhof, C. C., McConnell, B., Taniguchi, E. and Funaoka, K. An oncostatic factor present in Euphorbia amygdaloides. *Growth 26:*77, 1962.
47. Tanaka, T., Fukuoka, F. and Nakahara, W. Mechanism of antitumor action of some plant polysaccharides. *Gann, 56:*529, 1965.
48. Tanimura, A. Studies on the anti-tumour component in the seeds of Coix lacrymajobi L. var. Ma-yuen Stapf. II. The structure of coixenolide. *Chem. Pharm. Bull.* (Tokyo) *9:*47, 1961.
49. Ukita, T. and Tanimura, A. Studies on the anti-tumour component in the seeds of Coix lacrymajobi L. var. ma-yuen stapf. I. Isolation and anti-tumour activity of coixenolide. *Chem. Pharm. Bull.* (Tokyo) *9:*43, 1961.
50. Vargha, L., Toldy, L., Feher, O., Horvath, T., Kasztreiner, E., Kuszmann, J. and Landvae, S. New sugar derivatives with cytostatic activity. *Acta Physiol. Acad. Sci. Hung. 19:*305, 1961.
51. Abbott, B. J., Leiter, J., Hartwell, J. L., Perdue, R. E., Jr., and Schepartz, S. A. Screening data from the Cancer Chemotherapy National Service Center Screening Laboratories. XXXII. Plant extracts. *Cancer Res. 26:*391, 1966.
52. DeCandolle, M. A. *Physiologie Vegetale.* T. *3:*1474, 1832.
53. Cook, M. T. Wilting caused by walnut trees. *Phytopathology 11:*346, 1921.
54. Massey, A. B. Antogonism of the walnuts *(Juglans nigra L.* and *Juglans cinerea L.)* in certain plant associations. *Phytopathology 15:*773, 1925.

55. Schneiderhan, F. J. The black walnut *(Juglans nigra L.)* as a cause of the death of apple trees. *Phytopathology 17:*529, 1927.
56. Davis, R. F. The toxic principle of *Juglans nigra* as identified with synthetic juglone and its toxic effects on tomato and alfalfa plants. *Am. J. Bot. 15:*620, 1928.
57. Brooks, M. G. Effect of black walnut trees and their products on other vegetation. West Virginia Univ., *Agr. Exp. Sta., Bull. 347:*1, 1951.
58. Garb, S. Differential growth-inhibitors produced by plants. *Botanical Rev. 27:* 422, 1961.
59. Cooper, W. S. and Stoesz, A. D. The subterranean organs of *Helianthus scaberrimus. Bull. Torrey Bot. Club 58:*67, 1931.
60. Erickson, R. O. and Rosen, G. W. Cytological effects of protoanemonin on the root tip of *Zea mays. Am. J. Bot. 36:*317, 1949.
61. Heaton, T. B. The effect of inhibition of connective tissue growth by means of substances present in tissue extracts. *J. Path. Bact. 32:*565, 1929.
62. Medawar, P. B. A factor inhibiting the growth of mesenchyme. *Quart. J. Exp. Physiol. 27:*147, 1937.
63. Royle, J. G. Some effects of hexenolactone on tissue cultures. *Growth 9:*275, 1945.
64. Medawar, P. B., Robinson, L. and Robinson, R. A synthetic differential growth inhibitor. *Nature 151:*195, 1943.
65. Hauschka, T., Toennies, G. and Swain, A. P. The mechanism of growth inhibition of hexenolactone. *Science 101:*383, 1945.
66. Hauschka, T. Effects of the growth-inhibitor, hexenolactone, on flatworms. I. Absence of axial gradient pattern in the tissue-differential response. II. Chemical mechanism of tissue damage. *Growth 10:*193, 1946.
67. Briggs, R. Effects of the growth inhibitor, hexenolactone, on frog embryos. I. Effects on diploid embryos. II. Differential effects on haploid and diploid embryos. *Growth 10:*45, 1946.
68. Cornman, I. Alteration of mitosis by coumarin and parasorbic acid. *Am. J. Bot. 33:*217, 1946.
69. Cornman, I. The responses of onion and lily mitosis to coumarin and parasorbic acid. *J. Exp. Biol. 23:*292, 1947.
70. Personal communication.
71. Curtis, J. T. and Cottam, G. Antibiotic and autotoxic effects in prairie sunflower. *Bull. Torrey Bot. Club 77:*187, 1950.
72. Anon. Plants supply promising antitumor agents. *Chem. & Eng. News 44:*64, 1966.
73. Batrak, G. E., Popova, E. V. and Furs, I. T. New Medicinal Agents of a Vegetable Origin. *Trud. Ukranian Acad. Med. Sci. Publ.,* Kiev, 1959.
74. Bianchi, E., Caldwell, M. E. and Cole, J. R. Deoxypodophyllotoxin; an antitumor agent from *Bursera microphylla* A. Gray (Burseraceae). *Abstracts, 4th International Symposium on The Chem. of Natural Products* (IUPAC), Stockholm, 1966, pp. 47-48.
75. Cole, J. R. and Buchalter, L. Isolation of a potential antitumor fraction from *Rumex hymenosepalus. J. Pharm. Sci. 54:*1376, 1965.
76. Galbraith, W., Jones, R. L. and Roe, E. Tumour inhibition by tragacanth powder. *Brit. Empire Cancer Campaign, 38th Ann. Rep., 1960* (Pt. 2): 45.
77. Galbraith, W., Mayhew, E. and Roe, E. M. F. Mode of inhibitory action of tragacanth powder on the growth of the Landschutz ascites tumour. *Brit. J. Cancer 16:*163, 1962.

78. Hartwell, J. L. Plant remedies for cancer. *Cancer Chemotherapy Rep.* 7:19, 1960.
79. Hovy, J. W. H. Cytostatic properties of *Opunta maxima* (E., Abstract). *Biochem. Pharmacol.* 8:71, 1961.
80. Konopa, J., Jereczek-Morawska, E., Matuszkiewicz, A. and Nazarewicz, T. Antitumor substances from Bryonia alba L. (Preliminary Report) *Neoplasma 3:*335, 1965.
81. Kupchan, S. M., Aynehchi, Y., McPhail, A. T. and Sim, G. A. The isolation and structural investigation of two novel cytotoxic sesquiterpenoid dilactones from *Elephantopus elatus* (Compositae). *Abstracts, 4th Inter. Symposium on The Chemistry of Natural Products* (IUPAC). Stockholm, p. 62, 1966.
82. Kupchan, S. M., Aynehchi, Y., Cassidy, J. M., McPhail, A. T., Sim, G. A., Schnoes, H. K. and Burlingame, A. L. The isolation and structural elucidation of two novel sesquiterpenoid tumor inhibitors from *Elephantopus elatus*. *J. Am. Chem. Soc.* 88:3674, 1966.
83. Kupchan, S. M., Barboutis, S. J., Knox, J. R. and Lau Cam, C. A. Tumor inhibitors. XIII. Beta-solamarine: Tumor inhibitor isolated from *Solanum dulcamara*. *Science 150:*1827, 1965.
84. Kupchan, S. M., Bright, A. and Macko, E. Tumor inhibitors. II. Alkaloids of *Ervatamia dichotoma*. Isolation, crystallization, and pharmacological properties of coronaridine. *J. Pharm. Sci.* 52:598, 1963.
85. Kupchan, S. M., Cassady, J. M., Bailey, J. and Knox, J. R. Tumor inhibitors. XII. Gaillardin, a new cytotoxic sesquiterpene lactone from *Gaillardia pulchella*. *J. Pharm. Sci. 54:*1703, 1965.
86. Kupchan, S. M. and Doskotch, R. W. Tumor inhibitors. I. Aristolochic acid, the active principle of Aristolochia indica. *J. Med. Pharmaceut. Chem. 5:*657, 1962.
87. Kupchan, S. M., Doskotch, R. W., Bollinger, P., McPhail, A. T., Sim, G. A. and Renauld, S. Tumor inhibitors. XIV. The isolation and structural elucidation of a novel steroidal tumor inhibitor from Acnistus arborescens. *J. Am. Chem. Soc. 87:* 5805, 1965.
88. Kupchan, S. M., Doskotch, R. W. and Vanevenhoven, P. W. Tumor inhibitors. III. Monocrotaline, the active principle of *Crotalaria spectabilis*. *J. Pharm. Sci. 53:* 343, 1964.
89. Kupchan, S. M., Hemingway, R. J. and Doskotch, R. W. Tumor inhibitors. IV. Apocannoside and cymarin, the cytotoxic principles of *Apocynum cannabinum* L. *J. Med. Chem. 7:*803, 1964.
90. Kupchan, S. M., Hemingway, J. C. and Knox, J. R. Tumor inhibitors. VII. Podophyllotoxin, the active principle of *Juniperus virginiana*. *J. Pharm. Sci. 54:*659, 1965.
91. Kupchan, S. M., Knox, J. R. and Kelsey, J. E. Tumor inhibitors. V. Calotropin, a cytotoxic principle isolated from *Asclepias curassavica* L. *Science 146:*1685, 1964.
92. Kupchan, S. M., Knox, J. R. and Udayamurthy, M. S. Tumor inhibitors. VIII. Eupatorin, new cytotoxic flavone from *Eupatorium semiserratum*. *J. Pharm. Sci. 54:*929, 1965.
93. Kupchan, S. M., Patel, A. C. and Fujita, E. Tumor inhibitors. VI. Cissampareine, new cytotoxic alkaloid from *Cissampelos pareira*. Cytotoxicity of bisbenzylisoquinoline alkaloids. *J. Pharm. Sci. 54:*580, 1965.
94. Nabeya, K. and Iijima, Y. Clinical experience in use of anti-cancerous drug W.T.T.C. (E., Abstract) *Gann 51 (Suppl.):*61, 1960.
95. Pelc, J., Sobotka, J., Tobiska, J., and Kapoun, K. Antitumor substances from Euphorbia amygdaloides. Experiments with Walker rat tumour. *Neoplasma 5:* 140, 1958.

96. Petrova, M. F., Pukhalskaya, E. Ch. and Menshikov, G. P. A factor isolated from Hippophae ramnoides, inhibiting the growth of transplanted animal tumours. *Bull. Eksp. Biol. Med.* (Moscow) *2:*102, 1959.
97. Pukhalskaya, E. Ch., Petrova, M. F. and Massagetov, P. S. An antitumor factor in the bark of Hippophae rhamnoides. *Bull. Eksp. Biol. Med.* (Moscow) *6:*57, 1957.
98. Svoboda, G. H., Poore, G. A., Simpson, P. J. and Boder, G. B. Alkaloids of *Acronychia baueri* Schott. I. Isolation of the alkaloids and a study of the antitumor and other biological properties of acronycine. *J. Pharm. Sci.* *55:*758, 1966.
99. Tobiska, J., Pelc, J., Sobotka, J. and Kapoun, K. Antitumor substances found in Euphorbia amygdaloides. I. Experiments with Crocker tumour. *Neoplasma 4:* 125, 1957.
100. Tochkov, A., Ivanⁿ , V., Sobeva, V., Gantcheva, Tz., Rangelova, St. and Toneva, B. Antibacterial, antiviral, antitoxic and cytopathogenic properties of protoanemonin and anemonin. *Antibiotiki* (Moscow) *10:*918, 1961.
101. Tochkov, A. and Rangelova, St. Biological activity of Ranunculaceae. *Trud. Nauch. Inst. Epid. and Mikr.* (Sophia) *6:*41, 1959.
102. Tochkov, A. and Sobeva, V. Microbiological and cytopathological aspects of the activity of Ranunculaceae. *Mikrob. Zhur.* *22:*24, 1960.
103. Ulubelen, A., Caldwell, M. E. and Cole, J. R. Isolation of an antitumor proteinaceous substance from *Gutierrezia sarothrae* (Compositae). *J. Pharm. Sci. 54:* 1214, 1965.
104. Ulubelen, A. and Cole, J. R. Preliminary phytochemical investigation of *Maytenus trichotomus* (Celastraceae). *J. Pharm. Sci. 54:*1763, 1965.
105. Fellmer, C. and Fellmer, K. E. Maintenance therapy with a Viscum album preparation, "Iscador", following irradiation of genital carcinomas. *Krebsarzt. 21:* 174, 1966.

The Blood Supply to Cancer

In 1959, a group of medical students at Albany Medical College, working under the author's supervision, carried out a study of cancers transplanted to the hamster cheek pouch. Small pieces of cancers from patients who had been operated on were implanted under the mucous membrane of the cheek pouch of anesthetized hamsters (*see* Chapter 14). The rapid development of a blood supply to the tumor was impressive. The cheek pouch, like other mucous membranes, is pink and has many capillaries, but normally no large vessels can be seen. After the fragment of cancer had been implanted, however, some remarkable changes occurred. An extensive network of small blood vessels developed to the cancer, and a small artery was apparent within six days, leading from a large artery of the host to the cancer. The newly evident vessel began at a site quite distant from the cancer. Within another week, while the cancer grew to the size of a pea, the small artery increased in size until it was as large as the hamster's internal carotid artery, one of the largest in the body. Simple irritation of the hamster cheek pouch did not produce anything similar in blood vessel response. Virtually all the hamsters with implanted cancers developed these large arteries supplying the tumors, and the origin of the arteries was always quite a distance from the cancer. Thus, they were not arteries inside the cancer or arteries produced directly by the cancer cells. They were arteries that the host produced, and that supplied blood to the growing cancer, apparently enabling it to grow and endanger the host.

A search of the literature revealed that similar observations have been made by several investigators. An early researcher, Goldman, stated in 1907 (1):

> We find that in the growing tumour extensive new formation of blood vessels happens. This is most apparent in the zone of proliferation. . . .
>
> I mentioned that the impetus which gives rise to the proliferation of blood vessels emanates from the invading cell.

An important question is what Goldman had in mind when he used the term "impetus." Later investigators became more specific in their use of terms.

In 1908, Russell (2) in Great Britain pointed out that in a transplantable cancer: . . . there is a rich development of new blood-vessels from the capillaries of the host.

In 1939, Ide, Baker and Warren (3) reported some studies, performed at the University of Rochester School of Medicine, in which they had used a transparent ear chamber in a rabbit. They implanted a cancer, called the Brown-Pearce epithelioma (named after the discoverers), into the rabbits' ears and observed the development of blood vessels. For comparison, they also implanted small pieces of normal tissue under some of the chambers. They observed that the tumor transplants induced new blood vessel formation by the third to eighth day, and that the proliferation was maintained. They state:

> In the deep chamber no observable change took place in the size of the tumor fragment until the vessels began to proliferate; immediately thereafter one could detect expansion.

By contrast, the implanted normal tissues provoked a slight and short-lived blood vessel proliferation. Ide, Baker and Warren point out:

> Control tissue transplants were observed under the same conditions and illustrated the profound lack of ability of normal tissues to stimulate blood vessel growth quickly enough to maintain growth in this type of acute experiment in contrast to the rapid growth of vessels called forth by the tumor transplant.

They add that:

> By contrast, the rapid blood vessel growth toward and into the tumor transplant is very striking. . . .

Some of the conclusions of these investigators are of particular interest:

> Tumor growth is grossly visible within twenty-four hours following the beginning of visible blood vessel growth.

> If blood vessel growth is not observed, the transplant fails to take as shown by subsequent biopsy.

Finally, of the greatest significance to future research:

Since the rapidly growing tumor tissue is able to initiate in an unprepared site an adequate blood supply which is characteristic in pattern and not observed in the controls and the repair sites, it is probable that the tumor may be elaborating a vessel growth stimulating substance.

In 1945, Algire and his colleagues at the National Cancer Institute (4) performed a series of ingenious experiments, using transparent chambers sutured into skin flaps of mice. In some mice, the tissue under the chamber was cut into, to produce a small wound. In these mice with inflammation but no cancer, Algire first found dilation of the adjacent normal vessels; then, on the fifth or sixth day, proliferation of new capillaries, which lasted until about the ninth day. Some of the new capillaries became larger and turned into arterioles and venules (the smallest arteries and veins, not usually visible to the unaided eye). By the twelfth day, the vascularity reached approximately the level of the surrounding connective tissue, and no significant further vascularization took place.

In another group of mice, bits of normal mouse tissue were transplanted under the transparent chamber. On the fourth or fifth day after this procedure, new capillaries appeared, with a peak reached on the eleventh day. By the sixteenth day, the volume of blood vessels in the area had dropped to about the level of the surrounding connective tissue.

We should note that when new blood vessels were formed, either as a result of healing of injury or the transplantation of normal tissue, the total volume of blood vessels in the test area stabilized at about the volume of blood vessels in the surrounding connective tissue.

Next, Algire and his colleagues transplanted some fragments of mouse cancer under the transparent chamber. New capillary sprouts were seen by the third day following. By the fifth day, many widely dilated and newly proliferated capillaries were seen, and in Algire's words:

Growth of the tumor (cancer) became evident with the accomplishment of this initial vascularization.

By the fifth day the volume of blood vessels in the cancer area approximated that of the surrounding connective tissue. By the seventh day, it was about double that of the surrounding connective tissue. In Figure 19-1, these data from Algire's paper (4) are summarized. The effect of the cancer implanation differed from the effects

161

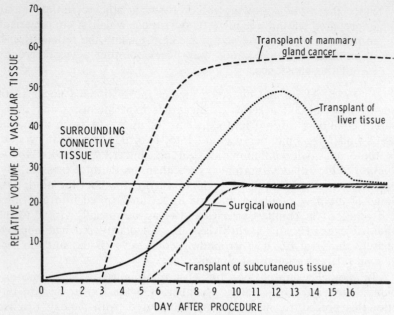

Figure 19–1. The effect of some procedures on tne relative volume of blood vessels, under a transparent chamber in mice, compared to the volume of blood vessels in the surrounding connective tissue (adapted from Algire et al., Ref. 4)

of the other procedures in several ways. The cancer induced blood vessel proliferation much sooner; the rate was much higher; and the blood vessel volume never returned to that of the surrounding normal connective tissues.

Algire also observed that the new capillary sprouts to the cancer came not only from capillaries that originally supplied the tissues around the area, but ". . . even from vessels in a nerve trunk at some distance from the tumor." This careful observation may be of crucial importance, since it has been confirmed by others, and since it may provide a useful clue to the effects of cancer on host vascularization.

Let us consider some of the comments which Algire and his colleagues, more than 20 years ago, made about the significance of their studies. They state:

> The results presented indicate 1) that the rapid growth of tumor transplants is dependent upon the development of a rich vascular supply, and 2) that an outstanding characteristic of the tumor cell

is its capacity to elicit continuously the growth of new capillary endothelium from the host. A fundamental problem arising from these considerations is that of the nature of the factors responsible for the stimulation of vascular proliferation. It seems worth emphasizing that tumor tissue elicited capillary growth as early as 3 days after implication, whereas 6 days elapsed prior to the beginning of capillary proliferation in a wound site. This fact suggests that, if the capillary proliferation is a response to a specific substance, this substance, as produced by the tumor cells, is more rapidly effective than is that from traumatized tissues.

Algire and his colleagues then go on to a most important suggestion:

It is entirely possible that the change in the tumor cell that enables it to evoke capillary proliferation is the only change necessary to give the tumor cell its increased autonomy of growth relative to the normal cell from which it arose. In other words, it seems quite possible that the primary difference between the malignant cell and the normal cell from which it arose may be that the malignant cell is able to provoke a continued vascular proliferation.

Thus, we can see that this group of investigators considered the ability of the cancer cell to provoke the host to supply it with blood vessels to be an important, perhaps the major, difference between cancer and normal cells. Although Algire and his colleagues continued their work on the blood vessels of cancer for several more years (5-13), I have not found any evidence that they tried to find out *how* the cancer provoked the host blood vessel response.

In 1956, Algire, in collaboration with Merwin, also of the National Cancer Institute, reported on some extensions of Algire's original work (12). They used the transparent chamber technique to study the effects of normal tissue implants and implants of mammary adenocarcinoma C3HBA. They observed:

No sprouts grew from host vessels adjacent to grafts of normal tissue, whereas a rich network of sprouts grew from vessels adjacent to grafts of tumor tissue.

(They note that there are a few other kinds of tumor that do not seem to induce the proliferation of host vessels, at first. But one of these tumors, a lymphoma, does induce blood vessel proliferation after it reaches a certain thickness.)

They concluded that:

The host vessels adjacent to grafts of tumor tissue produced, in each case, a rich network of vessels which provided almost all the vessels for the tumor graft. These findings confirm previous reports in the literature that grafts of tumor tissue may stimulate host vessels more than do grafts of normal tissue.

A study by Waters and Green (14), carried out at the University of North Carolina and Indiana University around 1958, also points to the importance of the blood vessels to the cancer. These researchers used transplantable ovarian granulosa-cell cancers in mice. They stated:

It appeared that the capillary bed of the connective tissue surrounding these neoplasms was being stimulated toward proliferation. This resulted in a dense bed of vessels available to the neoplasm. . . .

This observation indicated that the tumor in some unknown fashion, was inducing a proliferation of capillaries. It leads one to speculate that a substance from the tumor was diffusing into the surrounding connective tissue to produce an effect upon its vasculature.

They went on to suggest:

The circulatory pattern of neoplasms appears to be a fertile field for investigation. There is no small possibility that more knowledge in this sphere could be applied therapeutically, since checking this acquisition of a blood supply might restrict tumor growth.

In 1964, Goodall, Sanders and Shubik, a group of investigators at the Chicago Medical School, adapted the transparent tissue chamber to study the growth of blood vessels to tumors in the hamster cheek pouch (15). They, too, noted that new blood vessels developed rather rapidly.

The usual time for the establishment of new functional capillaries was between 3 and 6 days for each tumor.

Several different types of tumors were used, and the new capillaries that grew in followed patterns that varied with the type of tumor. The authors stated:

The host apparently contributes the vascular tissue, but the tumor determines its morphology. . . .

Warren and Shubick (16) in 1966 studied transplants of melanomas, pigmented skin cancer, in the hamster cheek pouch. They found that by the second day there was dilatation of the capillary bed, and by the third day a blood-vessel pathway through the tumor was visible. They stated:

Whereas previously growth of the tumor mass was not great, a phase of rapid growth now ensues.

Let us consider the significance of all these studies and observations. For more than half a century, scientists in several leading institutions have been impressed with the ability of cancers to stimulate the proliferation of host blood vessels to the cancer more effectively, much more promptly, and over a more prolonged period of time than occurs following trauma or implantation of normal tissues. It has been observed (3, 4) that the ability of an implanted tumor to grow rapidly seems to follow upon, and be dependent on, the proliferation of the host blood vessels. A leading expert in this area of research, Algire, suggested that the markedly enhanced ability to induce host blood vessel proliferation may be the major characteristic differentiating cancer cells from nonmalignant cells. Above all, we should note that several investigators (3, 4, 14) have come to the conclusion that cancers secrete some agent into the surrounding tissue, and that this agent in turn stimulates the proliferation of host blood vessels. The suggestion by Waters and Green (14) that further research into the nature of this agent may produce important leads to therapy seems to be a sound one.

If we can determine the chemical nature of the agent that stimulates production of blood vessels by cancers, it may be possible to design an effective antidote. The details of such a procedure are too complex to be considered here. The science of pharmacology, however, has progressed so far that it is often possible to design and synthesize an antidote to a particular chemical agent. For example, dimercaprol was designed specifically as an antidote to lewisite, a toxic war gas, and has been found a useful antidote to other toxic materials as well (17, 18). Pralidoxime was designed as an antidote to anticholinesterase chemicals, such as certain insecticides, and has proven to be lifesaving in some cases (19-21).

Antidotes or blocking agents have also been designed and synthesized to oppose the actions of several materials that occur naturally in the body, such as acetylcholine, epinephrine and histamine. Thus, there seems to be a good chance that pharmacologists could design,

165

and chemists synthesize, an antidote to the blood vessel stimulating material secreted by cancers, *provided* it could be isolated and identified.

The first and most difficult step is the isolation of the active material. Once this has been done, chemists will probably be able to identify its chemical structure in a reasonable period of time. The chances are that the blood vessel stimulating factor is rapidly destroyed in the body; if the factor were absorbed into the blood stream, its effects would extend far beyond the tumor. Accordingly, the usual types of extracts made from tumors may show no activity, since the active material could have been destroyed in the process of making the extract. This sort of problem has recurred again and again in medicine. It was the cause of the long delay in producing insulin, even though most scientists felt sure that insulin existed and had even named it before its actual discovery. Nevertheless, scientists have solved these difficult problems in the past, and an appropriate team, with adequate support, should have a good chance of solving this one.

A team consisting of several expert biochemists could be given the responsibility for making the various tumor extracts and fractions thereof, and a group of other scientists the responsibility of testing the responses of blood vessels to the extracts. The test animal could be hamster, mouse or rabbit, initially, although preparations found to be active ought to be tested in several species. The fractions produced by the biochemists would be injected into the appropriate test site in the experimental animal, using a modification of one of the transparent chamber preparations described by earlier investigators (3, 4, 11, 13, 15, 16). For controls, the biochemists would prepare extracts of normal tissues in the same manner. Should one of the cancer extracts show a markedly greater effect than extracts of normal tissues in causing host blood vessel proliferation, that extract would be further fractionated until a relatively pure material, ready for chemical analysis, is obtained. It may turn out that injections of a liquid preparation of extracts have too brief an effect. In that case, the extract could be absorbed by some inert solid material, made into a pellet, and implanted in such a way as to permit slow diffusion into the test area. Of course, it would then be necessary to perform an additional control study to find out whether the presumed inert material is really inert.

One may argue against this proposal because, in a sense, it is an all-or-none type of experiment. That is, if positive results are obtained, its value would be clear. But if all results are negative—if the biochemists are unable to prepare a tumor extract possessing the sought-for response—the effort would be entirely wasted. In case of a negative outcome, we would not know whether the reason is that the cancer does not produce a diffusible blood vessel growth-stimulating factor, or that the biochemists do not yet have the necessary techniques to prepare an active extract of such a factor. Nevertheless, the potential value of a discovery of such a factor produced by cancers seems so great, in terms of finding a possible treatment for the disease, that this approach deserves a vigorous, prompt and continuing effort. If such a blood vessel growth-stimulating factor is found, the discovery might also be of value in planning the treatment of diseases that are characterized by lack of adequate blood supply to an area.

References

1. Goodmann, E. The growth of malignant disease in man and the lower animals, with special reference to the vascular system. *Lancet 2:*1236, 1907.
2. Russell, B. R. G. The nature of resistance to the inoculator of cancer. *Scientific Rep. Imperial Cancer Res. Fund. 3:*341, 1908.
3. Ide, A. G., Baker, N. H. and Warren, S. L. Vascularization of the Brown-Pearce rabbit epithelioma transplant as seen in the transparent ear chamber. *Am. J. Roentgenol. Radiotherap. 42:*891, 1939.
4. Algire, G. H. and Chalkley, H. W. Vascular reactions of normal and malignant tissues in vivo. I. Vascular reactions of mice to wounds and to normal and neoplastic transplants. *J. Nat. Cancer Inst. 6:*73, 1945-1946.
5. Algire, G. H., Legallais, F. Y. and Park, H. D. Vascular reactions of normal and malignant tissue in vivo. II. The vascular reaction of normal and neoplastic tissues of mice to a bacterial polysaccharide from Serratia marcescens (Bacillus prodigiosus) culture filtrates. *J. Nat. Cancer Inst. 8:*53, 1947.
6. Algire, G. H., Chalkley, H. W. and Earle, W. R. Vascular reactions of normal and malignant tissues in vivo. III. Vascular reactions of mice to fibroblasts treated in vitro with methylcholanthrene. *J. Nat. Cancer Inst. 11:*555, 1951.
7. Algire, G. H. and Legallais, F. Y. Vascular reactions of normal and malignant tissues in vivo. IV. The effect of peripheral hypotension on transplanted tumors. *J. Nat. Cancer Inst. 12:*399, 1951.
8. Algire, G. H., Legallais, F. Y. and Anderson, B. F. Vascular reactions of normal and malignant tissues in vivo. V. The role of hypotension in the action of a bacterial polysaccharide on tumors. *J. Nat. Cancer Inst. 12:*1279, 1952.
9. Algire, G. H., Lagallais, F. Y. and Anderson, B. F. Vascular reactions of normal and malignant tissues in vivo. VI. The role of hypotension in the action of components of podophyllin on transplanted sarcomas. *J. Nat. Cancer Inst. 14:*879, 1954.
10. Algire, G. H. Vascular reactions of normal and malignant tissues in vivo. VII. Observations on vascular reactions in destruction of tumor homografts. *J. Nat. Cancer Inst. 15:*483, 1954.

11. Algire, G. H. and Merwin, R. M. Vascular patterns in tissues and grafts within transparent chambers in mice. *Angiology 6:*311, 1955.
12. Merwin, R. M. and Algire, G. H. The role of graft and host vessels in the vascularization of grafts of normal and neoplastic tissue. *J. Nat. Cancer Inst. 17:*23, 1956.
13. Algire, G. H. and Legallais, F. Y. Recent developments in the transparent-chamber technique as adapted to the mouse. *J. Nat. Cancer Inst. 10:*225, 1949.
14. Waters, H. G. and Green, J. A. The vascular system to two transplantable mouse granulosa-cell tumors. *Cancer Res. 19:*326, 1959.
15. Goodall, C. M., Sanders, A. G. and Shubik, P. Studies of vascular patterns in living tumors with a transparent chamber inserted in hamster cheek pouch. *J. Nat. Cancer Inst. 35:*497, 1965.
16. Warren, B. A. and Shubik, P. The growth of the blood supply to melanoma transplants in the hamster cheek pouch. *Lab. Invest. 15:*464, 1966.
17. Sulzberger, M. D. and Baer, R. L. Development and use of BAL: A review with particular reference to arsenical dermatitis. *J.A.M.A. 133:*293, 1947.
18. Stocken, L. A. and Thompson, R. H. S. Reactions of British Anti-Lewisite with arsenic and other metals. *Physiol. Rev. 29:*168, 1949.
19. Davies, D. R. and Green, A. L. The kinetics of reactivation, by oximes, of cholinesterase inhibited by organo-phosphorus compounds. *Biochem. J. 63:*529, 1956.
20. Green, A. L. and Smith, H. J. The reactivation of cholinesterase inhibited with organophosphorus compounds. Part 1. Reactivation by 2-oxaldoximes. *Biochem. J. 68:*28, 1958.
21. Grob, D. and Johns, R. J. Use of oximes in treatment of intoxication by anticholinesterase compounds in normal subjects. *Am. J. Med. 24:*497, 1958.

A Suggestion for Improvement of Cancer Chemotherapy—Overlooked for Over 50 Years

In Chapter 19, we considered the ability of cancers to induce proliferation of host blood vessels, and directed our attention to those vessels that were outside the cancer itself and that brought blood to the cancer. In this chapter, we will consider a different group of blood vessels, those that are inside the cancer.

These blood vessels differ in several important respects from the blood vessels that are found in nonmalignant growths or in most normal tissues. First, the volume of blood vessels inside cancers is usually much higher than the volume of blood vessels inside normal tissues (1, 2). Second, the blood vessels within the cancer are sinusoids, that is, vessels with a much larger internal diameter than capillaries, but with a wall consisting of only a single layer of cells (1, 3, 4). Third, these sinusoids are tortuous in shape, winding around each other, doubling back on their courses, and joining with one another (3), so that the blood flow through them is irregular, inefficient, and slow (4, 5). It is essential that we keep in mind the distinction between the *amount* of blood in a cancer (which is much higher than normal) and the *rate* at which blood flows into and through the cancer (which is much lower than normal). Fourth, the sinusoids do not differentiate into arterioles and venules (1), and do not have any contractile smooth muscle around them. As a result, the sinusoids do not respond to vasoconstrictor drugs which cause normal blood vessels to constrict (6).

With these points in mind, let us go back to 1913 and the studies of Walker and Whittingham (6) in the research department of the Royal Cancer Hospital in Glasgow, Scotland. These two scientists were evaluating reports by earlier investigators that certain toxic materials injected into mice with cancer caused necrosis (death) of most of the cancer; the mechanism that had been suggested was a selective action of the toxic materials on certain unknown abnormal enzymes believed to be present in cancer cells. The earlier investi-

169

gators, Wassermann (7) and Neuberg, Caspari and Löhe (8), had reported that, when they injected their materials, most of the blood vessels in the animals' bodies constricted and blanched, but the blood vessels in the cancers did just the opposite—they dilated. These observations suggested to Walker and Whittingham that the effects of the materials tested might have been on blood vessels rather than on enzymes, and they proceeded to design an experiment to clarify the point. In 1912, they did not have the variety of vasoconstrictor drugs that are available today, and they worked with two agents: Ernutin, a preparation of ergot, and a pituitary extract. They used mice with transplanted cancers, and injected one of the drugs either intravenously or subcutaneously. They observed that the entire body of the mouse blanched, except for the cancer, which did not blanch. They reasoned from this that, since the blood vessels in the rest of the animal's body constricted and those in the cancer did not, a greater amount of blood than usual flowed through the cancer while the vasoconstrictor drugs were exerting their effects. This was a logical conclusion, since the blood in the animal at a given moment is incompressible; if the regular vessels constrict, the blood pressure would rise and cause a passive dilation of the cancer sinusoids.

Then, Walker and Whittingham made a suggestion for the future when anti-cancer drugs might become available. They said:

> It seems possible that something might be done towards producing an effect on cancer cells by injecting substances which will tend to kill the cells, in combination with something which will contract the blood vessels of the body, such as pituitary extract and Ernutin. The passive dilatation of the vessels in the tumour should collect the toxic substance there, though, of course, it will be diffused over the whole body to a less extent.

In other words, Walker and Whittingham suggested that anti-cancer drugs be given together with vasoconstrictors, so that the constriction of the normal vessels and secondary passive dilatation of the vessels in the cancer would shunt more of the anti-cancer drug to the cancer and less to the normal tissues. Despite a careful search and inquiries from experts in the field of cancer chemotherapy, I have not been able to find any evidence that the suggestion of Walker and Whittingham has ever been tested in animals or in human patients. Yet, in the intervening years, other studies have been reported (4, 9, 10, 11) that tend to support strongly the findings and the suggestion of Walker and Whittingham.

170

In 1959, the Russian scientist, Natadze (9), found that a vaso-constrictor (epinephrine) increased blood flow through both trans-plantable and spontaneous cancers.

In 1962, Urbach (4), working at Temple University School of Medicine in Philadelphia found that human skin cancers have blood vessels with the same structural and functional abnormalities as the experimental tumors of mice. Urbach made two vital points.

> The emphasis in this field has been on the development of more active and more specific chemical agents. But newer and better chemicals will not have much success if one cannot get them to the tumor cells.

And:

> It thus appears to me that only when methods are devised to cir-cumvent the anatomical road block, posed by the peculiar prop-erties of the tumor circulation, will the chemotherapy of cancer become truly effective.

In 1964, Abrams (10) reported on an ingenious diagnostic study, which he had done at Stanford University School of Medicine. He had a patient with symptoms that suggested a cancer of the kidney, and was faced with the problem of making a definite diagnosis by x-ray. First, he performed a regular diagnostic radiologic procedure, which involved injecting a radio-opaque material into the artery sup-plying the kidney suspected of having the cancer. With complex machines, a series of x-rays was taken of the kidney at rapid rates (up to 2 per second). Since the radio-opaque material in the blood ves-sels blocked the passage of x-rays, it produced on the x-ray film a shadow outline of the blood vessels in and around the kidney. Then, after allowing the patient to rest for 30 minutes, Abrams injected epinephrine (adrenalin), a potent vasoconstrictor, into the same artery, and 50 seconds later, repeated the injection of radio-opaque material and the taking of x-rays. The epinephrine caused constric-tion of the normal blood vessels, but not of those to and within the cancer. Therefore, the radio-opaque material went mainly into the cancer rather than into the kidney proper, and the x-rays showed a clear and dramatic outline of the blood vessels to the cancer and of the cancer itself. The cancer was subsequently removed surgically.

Thus, Abrams demonstrated that in man the blood vessels supply-ing a cancer respond differently from normal blood vessels to epi-nephrine, a vasoconstrictor. In effect, he showed that the findings of

Walker and Whittingham on mice more than 50 years earlier were applicable to man.

One of Abrams' conclusions is of particular significance:

> In inoperable patients, selective chemotherapeutic perfusion of the tumour may be accomplished by pharmacological blockage of adjacent normal vessels.

In 1965, Goodall, Sanders and Shubik (11) at the Chicago Medical School, studying cancers grown in the hamster cheek pouch, were unable to find any evidence that the blood vessels in the cancers were able to constrict. Although these observations were considered preliminary, they are of interest since they fit the pattern described by others.

It is important to consider the extent to which blood flow per minute through cancers is less than blood flow per minute through normal tissues. An outstanding study of this problem was done by Gullino and Grantham (5) in 1961, at the National Cancer Institute. They worked with mice and rats and found that the blood flow through a gram of cancer tissue was much smaller than the blood flow through a gram of normal parent tissue. Gullino and Grantham state:

> If the blood flow of hepatomas (liver cancers) in rats and mice follows the same laws which regulate the general circulation, it can be expected that a substance injected into the host will circulate roughly 20 times through the liver before passing once through the hepatoma. In view of these facts, the effectiveness of certain chemotherapeutic agents may have to be re-evaluated because the dose received by the tumor per unit of time may be very small.

Some apparently contradictory results have come from a later study of Gullino and Grantham (12). They reported in 1962 that, in their special experimental preparation, epinephrine *reduced* blood flow through the cancer. The most likely reason for this is the special nature of the preparation used by Gullino and Grantham. They allowed a transplanted tumor to destroy a host organ (usually an ovary) completely, and noted that the original vessels of the organ then supplied blood to the cancer. Thus, they apparently measured the response of the normal blood vessels that were taken over by the cancer. We cannot be sure that this is the entire story, however. As things stand, most researchers who have studied the problem (6-10) report that drugs that constrict normal blood vessels do not constrict blood vessels inside cancers. Cater, Adair and Grove (13) found that the effects of injected epinephrine on tumor blood flow depended on the dose and rate of administration. Kruuv, Inch and McCredie (14) reported that isoproterenol, a vasodilator, decreased tumor blood flow.

It seems important that the effects of vasoconstrictors on cancer blood flow be clarified; the drugs used should have a minimal direct effect on the heart, and the experimental preparations should be reasonably close in nature to the types of cancer that occur in man. If the findings of the majority of earlier investigators are corroborated, we might eventually—by choosing the optimum dose of the most appropriate vasoconstrictor—be able to get a much larger proportion of blood containing an anti-cancer drug into the cancer per unit of time. If so, treatments that today merely relieve symptoms and prolong life for a few months may in some cases become curative. Accordingly, this avenue of research seems to be one that deserves prompt and extensive investigation.

Let us consider what steps ought to be taken. Two projects which could probably provide meaningful answers within a year or two could be carried on simultaneously. I will describe them in a somewhat simplified fashion.

1. An experiment could be done to measure how much of a drug actually gets into a cancer, since it is vital to know this. Any one of several drugs may be used as a marker. They need not be anti-cancer drugs; indeed, certain other drugs may be more suitable for this purpose, since at this stage of the study we need not consider what effect the drug will have. The marker drug should be one that can be given by vein, that is well distributed in the tissues, and that can readily be measured in tissues and serum by accurate, reproducible techniques. Some drugs that fit these qualifications are chlorpromazine, phenylbutazone, and sodium salicylate.

Experimental animals with cancer would be divided randomly into two groups. The animals of one group would receive a predetermined amount of the marker drug intravenously at a constant, predetermined rate. After a set amount of time had passed, the experimental animal would be sacrificed quickly and painlessly, and the cancer and several normal organs and tissues removed and quickly frozen. Then, by chemical assay, the concentration of the marker drug found in the cancer and in the normal organs and tissues would be measured. In the second group of animals, a vasoconstrictor drug would be given by injection just after the state of the administration

173

of the marker drug, and then a similar procedure would be followed. Findings in the two groups of experimental animals would then be compared. If the cancers in the animals receiving the vasoconstrictor drugs have a higher concentration of the marker drug, it would be reasonable to assume that an anti-cancer drug would also reach the cancer in higher concentrations when a vasoconstrictor is used. Several pilot studies would be needed to determine the most appropriate concentration and rate of administration of both the marker and vasoconstrictor drugs. To reduce the chances of error, the animals of the two groups would be tested alternately, that is, an animal from group A, one from group B, and so on.

The choice of an experimental animal for this study would depend largely on technical factors. A few scientists are able to give intravenous injections to mice with a high rate of success, but many cannot. Rats might be used, or hamsters. Rabbits would probably be an excellent choice because of their size.

2. In another project, the aim would be to find out whether a vasoconstrictor added to an anti-cancer drug would significantly improve the life duration of the subject. Since it does not appear to be practical at this time to try a controlled experiment with these drugs on human patients, it may be worthwhile to try such an experiment on large farm animals with spontaneous cancer. An excellent experimental animal would be the Hereford cow or steer with eyelid cancer (*see* Chapter 29). Animals with eyelid cancer of comparable extent would be selected randomly; every other animal would receive, intravenously, a standard anti-cancer drug believed to be fairly effective against such cancers. The other animals would receive the same drug, in the same manner, but with the addition of a vasoconstrictor that would raise the blood pressure about 50 mm of mercury, and keep it at that level while the anti-cancer drug is circulating. Evaluation of the response of the animals would then be made by a veterinarian who did not know which treatment each animal received. (If desired, a similar experiment could be run, with the use of intra-arterial rather than intravenous routes of injection.) Such a study could be completed much sooner, and at a much lower cost, than any comparable studies in man.

In summary, the possible role of selected vasoconstrictors in cancer chemotherapy, suggested by Walker and Wittingham (6) over 50 years ago, deserves exploration. As recently as 1966, Dr. Wittingham (15) indicated that he still considered this approach worthy of further study.

References

1. Algire, G. H. and Chalkley, H. W. Vascular reactions of normal and malignant tissues in vivo. I. Vascular reactions of mice to wounds and to normal and neoplastic transplants. *J. Nat. Cancer Inst. 6:*73, 1945-1946.
2. Ide, A. G., Baker, N. H. and Warren, S. L. Vascularization of the Brown-Pearce rabbit epithelioma transplant as seen in the transparent ear chamber. *Am. J. Roentgenol. Radiotherap. 42:*891, 1939.
3. Waters, H. G. and Greene, J. A. The vascular system of two transplantable mouse granulosa-cell tumors. *Cancer Res. 19:*326, 1959.
4. Urbach, F. Anatomy and pathophysiology of skin tumor capillaries. *Nat. Cancer Inst. Monograph 10:*539, 1963.
5. Gullino, P. M. and Grantham. F. H. Studies on the exchange of fluids between host and tumor. II. The blood flow of hepatomas and other tumors in rats and mice. *J. Nat. Cancer Inst. 27:*1465, 1961.
6. Walker, C. and Whittingham, H. The effect of general contraction of the peripheral blood-vessels upon mouse cancers. *Lancet 1:*1010, 1913.
7. Wassermann. *Beiträge zum Problem: Geschwülste von der Blutbahn aus therapeutisch zu beeinflussen. Deutsche Medicinische Wochenschrift.* Dec. 1911, cited by Walker and Whittingham (6).
8. Neuberg, Caspari and Lohe. *Weiteres über Heilversuche an Geschwulstkranken Tieren mittels tumeraffiner Substanzen.* Berliner Klinische Wochenschrift, July 1912, cited by Walker and Whittingham (6).
9. Natadze, T. G. Regulation of blood circulation in malignant tumors. *Vopr. Onkol.* (Moscow) *5:*14, 1959.
10. Abrams, H. L. Altered drug response of tumour vessels in man. *Nature 201:* 167, 1964.
11. Goodall, C. M., Sanders, A. G. and Shubik, P. Studies of vascular patterns in living tumors with a transparent chamber inserted in hamster cheek pouch. *J. Nat. Cancer Inst. 35:*497, 1965.
12. Gullino, P. M. and Grantham, F. H. Studies on the exchange of fluids between host and tumor. III. Regulation of blood flow in hepatomas and other rat tumors. *J. Nat. Cancer Inst. 28:*211, 1962.
13. Cater, D. B., Adair, H. M. and Grove, C. A. Effects of vasomotor drugs and "mediators" of the inflammatory reaction upon the oxygen tension of tumours and tumour blood-flow. *Brit. J. of Cancer 20:*504, 1966.
14. Kruuv, J. A., Inch, W. R. and McCredie, J. A. Blood flow and oxygenation of tumors in mice. II. Effects of vasodilator drugs. *Cancer 20:*60, 1967.
15. Whittingham, H. Personal communication, 1966.
16. Natadze, T. G. Functional peculiarity of blood circulation in tumours. In *VIII International Cancer Congress.* Moscow, Medgiz Publishing House, 1962, p. 233.

The Invasiveness of Cancer

A basic feature of cancer is its ability to invade neighboring tissues. This invasiveness distinguishes cancers from benign tumors, which are readily curable by simple surgical techniques. What it is that enables cancers to invade normal tissues is not clearly understood, but there seem to be several mechanisms involved. First, cancer cells appear to modify the properties of the matrix or ground substance in which normal cells lie. This matrix, which is normally a gel, usually presents a barrier to cell movement and infiltration, but cancer cells seem to be able to surmount this obstacle.

Second, cancer cells probably have some way of passing through layers of normal cells that are tightly cemented together by an intercellular substance. We are quite confident that cancer cells do this, because cut sections of cancerous areas show such penetration microscopically. Perhaps cancer cells secrete a substance that dissolves the intercellular cement between two normal cells, or perhaps the cancer cell kills a normal cell with a secreted toxin or enzyme, and then moves into the space formerly occupied by the normal cell.

Third, cancer cells apparently have the ability to flow or move in an ameboid manner. It is likely that these three mechanisms are interrelated, but evidence for such relationships is not yet clear. Let us, therefore, consider each of these mechanisms of invasion separately.

Ability to Penetrate Ground Substance

In normal tissues, the cells are embedded in a jelly-like mass which provides a degree of firmness and cohesion. This jelly-like material is, ordinarily, relatively impermeable.

Cameron (1), a consulting cancer surgeon, who has written the most comprehensive review on cancer invasiveness states:

> It is now firmly established that in any tissue the individuals cells, the collagen reticulin and elastic fibres, and the blood and lymph capillaries are firmly embedded in an amorphous viscous gel of ground substance. There are no free channels or tissue spaces as

such, and the whole cemented mass presents a uniform homogenous barrier to permeation and penetration.

The viscosity of the ground substance can vary, and certain enzymes are capable of changing it from the gel into the sol form. In the latter state, it is readily traversed by most materials, particulate as well as soluble. The ground substance is made up of a mixture of proteins and mucopolysaccharides. Its exact structure is complex and not fully understood, but it is known to contain hyaluronic acid, chondroitin, chondroitin sulfate, heparitin sulfate and keratosulphate (2).

It seems logical that in order for cancer cells to invade normal tissues they must have some mechanism that enables them to penetrate through the ground substance. There is some experimental evidence that this is actually the case.

In 1928, Duran-Reynals (3) first reported that certain extracts of normal organs had the capacity to increase the spread of vaccinia virus. A large number of studies followed; they showed that the spread of invasive organisms and of non-living particulate matter through living tissues and organs could be enhanced by extracts of certain normal cells and body fluids (4-15), bacteria (16-27), leeches (28, 29) and other biological materials. The agent that increased the spread through tissues was named "spreading factor" by Duran-Reynals, its discoverer. The potential importance of a spreading factor in cancer was recognized early, and a number of studies showed the presence of one or more spreading factors in several animal cancers (30-39). Spreading factors have been found in a variety of human cancers also (40-65). In addition, studies have been done on the effects of added spreading factors on cancer growth (66-77). Although the results of these studies have not been clear-cut or consistent, improvements in technique may provide important information.

Despite the initial promise of this approach in cancer research, it has apparently received comparatively little attention over the past 20 years, although the publication of Cameron's book (1) may be expected to increase interest in the area. It may be worthwhile to consider some of the reasons for the slow progress along this research route and consider ways to improve it.

One important obstacle seems to be a matter of semantics. Duran-Reynals in his fundamental early studies referred to "spreading factors"; some other investigators, about the same time, used the term "diffusing factors." It is important to note that the plural "spreading factors" was used by Duran-Reynals (78, 79), and that Fleming (80), and McClean and Hale (81) also used the plural "diffusing factors." In 1940, however, Chain and Duthie (82) reported on "Identity of hyaluronidase and spreading factor." They showed clearly that hyaluronidase, an enzyme which hydrolyzes the hyaluronic acid in the ground substance, was *a* spreading factor. They did not, however, demonstrate that it was the *only* spreading factor; indeed, some of their findings suggest that they were dealing with more than one spreading factor. They found, for example, that bacterial and snake venom solutions produced bigger spreads than might have been expected from the hyaluronidase content. This discrepancy was dismissed as the result of edema, but a more logical explanation is that other spreading factors besides hyaluronidase were present.

Nevertheless, many succeeding scientists assumed that hyaluronidase is *the* spreading factor or at least the most important spreading factor, and did their studies with hyaluronidase. Some studies with hyaluronidase did not reveal significant connections with cancer (83, 84). Furthermore, Kiriluk, Kremen and Glick (85), searching for hyaluronidase in human and animal tumors, concluded that the hyaluronidase found did not come from the cancer cells but from the bacteria within the tumor. Since almost all the animal studies were done on transplantable cancers, which carry large numbers of bacteria, Kiriluk *et al.* have raised a critical point. On the other hand, some of the studies that showed hyaluronidase or another spreading factor in cancers were done with precautions against bacterial contamination (33, 34). Yet, even if there were no increase in hyaluronidase in cancers, it would still be vital to find out whether there is an increase in other spreading factors. The evidence for the existence of more than one kind of spreading factor is impressive (86-90). Several studies have demonstrated the complexities involved in assessing the actions of hyaluronidase or other spreading factors (91-100).

We do not yet have incontrovertible evidence that spreading factors are important in the invasiveness of cancer. But observations on the clinical course of cancer strongly suggest that such factors may, indeed, be present. Cameron has used the term "hyaluronidases" in place of spreading factors. He has indicated (101), however, that "spreading factors" might be a better term in some contexts. He has summarized the possible role of hyaluronidase in cancer as follows:

> The possible role of hyaluronidase in the pathogenesis of tumours may be summarized and presented in the form of two alternative

CHAPTER 21

hypotheses. The first and more limited concept is supported by a good deal of circumstantial evidence and may be simply stated: 1) Tumour cells persistently secrete excess hyaluronidase which is directly responsible for malignant invasiveness and indirectly facilitates tumour growth by enhanced nutrition. The alternative hypothesis is more speculative and is merely an extension of the above to include responsibility for cellular proliferation. It may be stated: 2) The persistent secretion of excess hyaluronidase is the fundamental difference between the neoplastic and the normal cell and is directly responsible for all manifestations of cancer. If there is any truth in either hypothesis then it is obvious that the inhibition of tumour hyaluronidase would be of inestimable benefit to the cancer patient. Previous suggestions that hyaluronidase might play some part in malignant invasiveness have not been universally accepted because of an alleged lack of experimental proof that tumour cells actively produce hyaluronidase. This opinion is based on the inconclusive results obtained in the enzyme assay of tumour extracts.

There are, however, a number of indirect methods that indicate that cancer cells do produce hyaluronidase. In summarizing these observations, Cameron presents other impressive arguments to bolster the concept that hyaluronidases (or other spreading factors) are vital to cancer invasiveness, and he answers the objections and criticisms that have been raised to this concept (103).

Another situation that seems to have been partially responsible for the lessened support given to studies on spreading factors may have been a failure to realize that even quite small spreading factor concentrations could account for cancer invasiveness. Many of the early studies on spreading factors utilized the factors produced by bacteria, and tests and assays were designed to measure their potency. The invasiveness of bacteria, however, is several orders of magnitude greater than the invasiveness of cancer cells. In the pre-antibiotic period, it was not uncommon to see some streptococcal infections spread at the rate of several centimeters per day. Cancers spread much more slowly; accordingly, it is logical to expect cancer spreading factors to be much less potent than bacterial spreading factors. Williams (104) found that pseudoneoplasia occurred when the rate of infusion of hyaluronidase was as low as 3×10^{-8} mgm per minute. Commenting on this, Cameron states: (105)

If this figure bears any relationship to the rate of liberation in true neoplasia, then the hyaluronidase content of most tumours

179

must be very low indeed, and require extraordinary sensitive methods for its detection.

Cameron makes the important suggestion that the method of Bollet, Bonner and Nance (101) be used since it is a highly sensitive indicator of hyaluronidase. But the development of additional methods, suitable for demonstrating various kinds of spreading factors in low concentrations, should be given a high priority.

It would be helpful if, at the same time, studies were done on anti-spreading factors, and if any materials found to possess an anti-spreading factor action were tested in animals with cancer. In such tests, prolonged administration should be utilized, and in addition to the usual measurements of cancer growth rate and animal longevity, observations should be made of invasive capacity of the cancer. It is possible that an effective inhibitor of spreading factors that are elaborated by cancer might not significantly change the rate of tumor enlargement, or, by itself, the survival time. Yet, an arrangement that prevented invasion of normal tissues might make it possible for surgeons to remove completely cancers that might have been considered inoperable before because of their size and location. This could come about if a spreading factor inhibitor were able, for a period of time, to change an invading cancer into a non-invading benign growth.

Cameron (107) is quite optimistic about the possible value of an antidote to hyaluronidase (spreading factor). He states:

> If hyaluronidase secretion is the responsible mechanism (for invasion), then total inhibition of the enzyme would convert the most malignant growth to a relatively innocuous benign tumour, harmful only from pressure effects, amenable to simple local surgery, but in many situations requiring no further treatment. The extent of dissemination at the onset would not limit the value of such treatment; pre-existing secondary deposits would simply be converted to multiple encapsulated non-metastasizing benign tumours.

Ability to Penetrate Intercellular Cement

Virtually nothing is known about the ability of any organisms or cells to penetrate intercellular cement. Indeed, little is known about the basic composition or properties of intercellular cement. It would be worthwhile to support a series of studies designed to find out more about this material and its properties. Then, studies could be done to determine how cancer cells can penetrate this cement and how such penetration might be prevented.

Ameboid Motion

There is general agreement that cancer cells exhibit ameboid movement during some phases of their life cycle. Precise studies on this feature of cancer are lacking, however. We ought not assume that ameboid motion of cancer cells is nearly so rapid as the motion of parasitic and saprophytic ameba.

One possibility is that a drug that inhibits movement of the parasitic or saprophytic ameba might also inhibit the ameboid movement of cancer cells but would not act as an amebacide. If we were to find a drug that inhibits ameboid motion without killing the cells, it might have a good chance of being non-toxic to most normal cells. (Effects on leukocytes might pose problems.) Such a drug, given over a long period of time might provide a reasonably adequate control for cancer.

This is an approach to which general biologists, parasitologists and microbiologists could make major contributions.

The entire area of cancer invasiveness, of which a few facets have been presented, deserves intensive research.

References

1. Cameron, E. *Hyaluronidase and Cancer.* Pergamon Press, Oxford, 1966, p. 2.
2. *Ibid.*, p. 3.
3. Duran-Reynals, F. Exaltation de l'activité du virus vaccinal par les extraits des certains organes. *Comp. Rend. Soc. Biol.* (Paris) *99:*6, 1928.
4. Claude, A. and Duran-Reynals, F. On existence of factor increasing tissue permeability in organs other than testicle. *J. Exper. Med. 60:*457, 1934.
5. Christensen, J. F. Reynals permeability factors in urine. *Hospitalstid. 81:*572, 1938.
6. Madinaveitia, J. Comparison of diffusing factors from different sources and preparation of concentrates from bull testicle. *Biochem. J. 33:*347, 1939.
7. Duran-Reynals, F. General permeability-increasing effect of factor from mammalian testicle on blood capillaries. *Yale J. Biol. and Med. 11:*601, 1939.
8. Head, J. J. and Thomas, R. M. Spreading effect of testicle extract upon areas of acute inflammation produced by physical agents. *Yale J. Biol. and Med. 12:*69, 1939.
9. Fellowes, O. N. and Hudson, N. P. Duran-Reynals (spreading) factor in adult and fetal guinea-pig organs as it affects vaccinia virus. *Am. J. Hyg.,* Sect. B. *30:*11, 1939.
10. Greenberg, B. E. and Gargill, S. L. Relation of hyaluronidase in seminal fluid to fertility. *Human Fertil. 11:*1, 1946.
11. Eichenberger, E. Mucinolytic ferment in normal and pathological human sperm; contribution to problem of male sterility. *Gynaecologia 121:*288, 1946.
12. Kurzrok, R., Leonard, S. L. and Conrad, H. Hyaluronidase—Role in human infertility. *Am. J. Med. 1:*491, 1946.

13. Hechter, O. and Hadidian, Z. Hyaluronidase activity of spermatozoa. *Endocrinology 41:*204, 1947.
14. Anlyan, A. J. and Starr, A. Beta-glucuronidase activity of spinal and ventricular fluids in humans. *Cancer 5:*578, 1952.
15. Duran-Reynals, F. Further studies on influence of testicle extract upon effect of toxins, bacteria and viruses and on Schwartzman and Arthus phenomena. *J. Exper. Med. 58:*451, 1933.
16. Duran-Reynals, F. Studies on a certain spreading factor existing in bacteria and its significance for bacterial invasiveness. *J. Exp. Med. 58:*161, 1933.
17. Duran-Reynals, F. Extent of local dispersion of infectious agents as factor in resistance to infection. *J. Exper. Med. 61:*617, 1935.
18. McClean, D. A factor in culture filtrates of certain pathogenic bacteria which increases permeability of tissues. *J. Path. and Bact. 42:*477, 1936.
19. McClean, D. Capsulation of streptococci and its relation to diffusion factor (hyaluronidase). *J. Path. and Bact. 53:*13, 1941.
20. Evans, D. G. Protective properties of alpha antitoxin and antihyaluronidase occuring in Clostridium welchii type A antiserum. *J. Path. and Bact. 55:*427, 1943.
21. McClean, D. and Rogers, H. J. Detection of bacterial enzymes (hyaluronidase and lecithinase) in infected tissues. *Lancet 2:*434, 1944.
22. Crowley, N. Hyaluronidase production by hemolytic streptococci of human origin. *J. Path. and Bact. 56:*27, 1944.
23. Kass, E. H. and Seastone, C. V. Role of mucoid polysaccharide (hyaluronic acid) in virulence of Group A streptococci. *J. Exper. Med. 79:*319, 1944.
24. MacLennon, L. D. Hyaluronidases in infected wounds. *Lancet 2:*433, 1944.
25. Humphrey, J. H. Hyaluronidase production by pneumococci. *J. Path. and Bact. 56:*273, 1944.
26. Kass, E. H., Lichstein, H. C. and Warshren, B. A. Occurrence of hyaluronidase and lecithinase in relation to virulence in Clostridium welchii. *Proc. Soc. Exptl. Biol. and Med. 58:*172, 1945.
27. Schwabacher, H., Cunliffle, A. C., Williams, E. O. and Harper, G. J. Hyaluronidase production by staphlococci. *Brit. J. Exper. Path. 26:*124, 1945.
28. Claude, A. Spreading properties of leech extracts and formation of lymph. *J. Exper. Med. 66:*353, 1937.
29. Claude, A. Spreading properties and mucolytic activity of leech extracts. *Proc. Soc. Exptl. Biol. and Med. 43:*684, 1940.
30. Duran-Reynals, F. and Stewart, F. W. The action of tumor extracts on the spread of experimental vaccinia of the rabbit. *Am. J. Cancer 15:*2790, 1931.
31. Boyland, E. and McClean, F. A factor in malignant tissues which increases the permeability of the dermis. *J. Path. and Bact. 41:*533, 1935.
32. Okano, K., Kaku, T. and Hamada, S. The spreading factor in Yoshida sarcoma. *Gann 42:*260, 1951.
33. Balazs, E. A. and Von Euler, J. Hyaluronidase content of necrotic tumor and testis tissue. *Cancer Res. 12:*326, 1952.
34. Valle Jimeniz, A. Relacion entre el factor difusor y el crecimiento e invasion de los tumores transplantados. (Relationship between the diffusion factor and the growth and invasiveness of transplanted tumours.) *Rev. Esp. Oncologia 2:*1, 1953.
35. Biryukova, L. S. Hyaluronidase distribution in rabbits with tumours and after anti-tumour serum. *Bjull. Eksp. Biol. Med 50:*90, 1960.
36. Grossfeld, H. Production of hyaluronic acid by fibroblasts growing from explants of Walker tumor 256: production of hyaluronidase by the tumor cells. *J. Nat. Cancer Inst. 27:*543, 1961.

37. Carr, A. J. The activities of some glycosidases in experimental tumours. *Scot. Med. J. 7:*114, 1962.

38. Carr, A. J. The relation to invasion of glycosidases in mouse tumours. *J. Path. Bact. 89:*239, 1965.

39. Fishman, W. H. and DeLellis, R. Rapid method for localizing beta-glucuronidase in populations of human leucocytes and of mouse Ehrlich carcinoma cells. *Nature 212:*312, 1966.

40. McCutcheon, M. and Coman, D. R. Spreading factors in human carcinomas. *Cancer Res. 7:*379, 1947.

41. Fishman, W. H. and Anlyan, A. J. The presence of high beta-glucuronidase activity in cancer tissue. *J. Biol. Chem. 169:*449, 1947.

42. Fishman, W. H. and Anlyan, A. J. The comparison of the beta-glucuronidase activity of normal, tumor and lymph node tissues of surgical patients. *Science 106:*66, 1947.

43. Fishman, W. H., Anlyan, A. J. and Gordon, E. Beta-glucuronidase activity in human tissues; some correlations with processes of malignant growth and with the physiology of reproduction. *Cancer Res. 7:*808, 1947.

44. Baggi, G. and Borghi, U. Modificazione del fenomeno di diffusione nel cancerosi. (Changes in the spreading phenomenon in cancer patients.) *Boll. Soc. Med. Chir. Modena 52:*432, 1953.

45. Fishman, W. H., Baker, J. R. and Borges, P. R. F. Localization of β-glucuronidase in some human tumors. *Cancer 12:*240, 1959.

46. Fishman, W. H. and Bigelow, R. A comparative study of the morphology and glucuronidase activity in 44 gastrointestinal neoplasms. *J. Nat. Cancer Inst. 10:*1115, 1950.

47. Fishman, W. H., Borges, P. R. F. and Baker, J. R. Localization of beta-glucuronidase in certain tumors. *Proc. Am. A. Cancer Res. 2:*297, 1958.

48. Fishman, W. H., Markus, R. L., Page, O. C., Pfeiffer, P. H. and Homburger, F. Studies on effusions. I. Glucuronidase and lactic acid in neoplastic effusions of the pleura and peritoneum. *Am. J. M. Sc. 220:*55, 1950.

49. Harvey, S. R. and Panse, T. B. Oral cancer and beta-glucuronidase activity. *Indian J. Med. Res. 48:*692, 1960.

50. Kasdon, S. C., Fishman, W. H. and Homburger, F. Beta-glucuronidase studies in women. II. Cancer of the cervix uteri. *J.A.M.A. 144:*892, 1950.

51. Kasdon, S. C., Homburger, F., Yorshis, E. and Fishman, W. H. Beta-glucuronidase studies in women. VI. Premenopausal vaginal fluid values in relation to invasive cervical cancer. *Surg., Gynec. and Obst. 97:*579, 1953.

52. Lorincz, A., Novelli, J., McGoogan, L. S. and Odell, L. D. Beta-glucuronidase activity in human female genital cancer. *Am. J. Obst. and Gynec. 61:*527, 1951.

53. Monis, B., Banks, B. M. and Rutenburg, A. M. Beta-D-glucuronidase activity in malignant neoplasms of man: a histochemical study. *Cancer 13:*386, 1960.

54. Monis, B. and Rutenburg, A. M. Histochemical demonstration of beta-D-glucuronidase in malignant tumors. *J. Histochem. and Cytochem. 4:*498, 1956.

55. Odell, L. D., Burt, J. and Bethea, R. Beta-glucuronidase activity in human female genital cancer. *Cancer Res. 9:*362, 1949.

56. Odell, L. D., Priddle, H. D. and Burt, J. C. Activity of beta-glucuronidase in human female genital tissues and in vaginal secretion. *Am. J. Clin. Path. 20:*133, 1950.

57. Pico, C. and Baccellato, C. Beta-glucuronidase in the gastric juice of patients with malignant stomach neoplasms. *Ann. ital. chir. 33:*479, 1956; cited in *Chem. Abstr. 52:*20600 e, 1958.

PART IV

58. Pico, C. Changes of beta-glucuronidase in human gastric juice of patients with stomach carcinoma after gastric resection. *Rass. Ital. Gastroenterol. 3:*569, 1957; cited in *Chem. Abstr. 52:*1484, 1958.
59. Podilchak, M. D. and Petrus, V. S. O faktore pronitsaemosti v opukholyakh cheloveka. (The permeability factor in human tumours.) *Med. Zhur. 22:*35, 1952.
60. Rauramo, L. The significance of beta-glucuronidase content in the vaginal fluid of patients with cancer of the uterus. *Scandinav. J. Clin. and Lab. Invest. 11:*285, 1959.
61. Rauramo, L. The significance of tissue beta-glucuronidase content in patients with cancer of the uterus. *Scandinav. J. Clin. and Lab. Invest. 11:*290, 1959.
62. Rich, C. and Myers, W. P. L. Excretion of acid mucopoly-saccharides in the urine of patients with malignant neoplastic diseases. *J. Lab. Clin. Med. 54:*223, 1959.
63. Rozin, D. L. k voprosu o vzaimootnoshenii gialuronovoi kisloty s ekstraktami zlokachestvennykh opukholei cheloveka. (The relation between hyaluronic acid and extracts of human malignant tumours.) *Vopr. Onkol. 21:*97, 1952.
64. Whitaker, B. L. Plasma β-glucuronidase levels in breast cancer. *Brit. J. Cancer 14:* 471, 1960.
65. Bartalos, M. and Gyorkey, F. Beta-glucuronidases: Their significance and relation to cancer. *J. Amer. Geriatrics Soc. 11:*21, 1963.
66. Duran-Reynals, F. The effect of testicle extract and of normal serum on a transplantable epithelial tumor of the rabbit. *J. Exp. Med. 54:*493, 1931.
67. Sturm, E. and Duran-Reynals, F. Properties of causative agent of chicken tumor; effect of testicle extract on rate of growth of chicken tumor I. *J. Exper. Med. 56:* 711, 1932.
68. Duran-Reynals, F. and Claude, A. Further experiments on effect of testicle extract on agent of chicken tumor I. *Proc. Soc. Exptl. Biol. and Med. 32:*67, 1934.
69. Prime, F. and Haagansen, C. D. The effect of testicular extract on animal neoplasms. *Amer. J. Cancer 20:*630, 1934.
70. Tanzer, R. C. The effect of testicular extract on the growth of transplantable mouse tumors. *J. Exper. Med. 55:*455, 1932.
71. Seifter, J. and Warren, G. H. Effect of purified hyaluronidase on growth of Sarcoma 37 in mouse. *Proc. Soc. Exptl. Biol. and Med. 75:*796, 1950.
72. Koreneva-Zubkova, O. P. and Gragerova, R. B. Vliyanii testikulyavnogo ekstrakta na rost pereritoi kartsinouy krolika pri vnutrikozhnon vredenii. (The influence of testicular extract on the growth of transplanted carcinoma in the rabbit by intradermal injection.) *Med. Zhur. 20:*82, 1950.
73. Podilchak, M. D. Vliyanie stafilokokkovoi gialuronidazy na rost i techenie adenokartsinomy myshi. (The effect of staphylococcal hyaluronidase on the growth and course of adenocarcinoma of mice.) *Med. Zhur. 21:*51, 1951.
74. Luhrs, von W. and Willig, H. Über den Einfluss von Hyaluronidase und 2, 4, 6-Triethylenimino-1,3,5-Triazin (T.E.M.) auf das Wachstum des Jensen-Sarkoms der Ratte. (The effect of Hyaluronidase and of TEM on the Jensen Rat sarcoma.) *Dtch. Gesundh. Wes. 7:*1537, 1952.
75. Luhrs, von W. and Willig, H. Weitere tierexperimentelle Untersuchungen über den Einfluss von Hyaluronidase auf das bösartige Wachstum. (The influence of hyaluronidase upon malignant growth.) *Arch. Geschwulstforsch. 6:*183, 1953.
76. Russo, G. and Terranova, T. Influenza della ialuronidasi sul tumore di Walker. (The action of hyaluronidase on the Walker tumour.) *Boll. Soc. ital. Pat.* (Torino) *3:*52, 1953.
77. Fujita, K. and Iwase, S. Influence of mucin and hyaluronidase upon the growth of chicken sarcoma (with special regard to the histological observations). *Nagoya J. Med. Sci. 16:*298, 1954.

78. Duran-Reynals, F. Spreading factors and their significance: resistance of connective tissue and tissue permeability. *Ann. Inst. Pasteur. 57:*597, 1936.
79. Duran-Reynals, F. Tissue permeability and the spreading factors in infection: A contribution to the host: parasite problem. *Bact. Rev. 6:*197, 1942.
80. Fleming, D. S. Spreading factors and bacterial infection (role of hyaluronidase). *Am. J. Med. Sci. 211:*374, 1946.
81. McClean, D. and Hale, C. W. Diffusing factors; hyaluronidase activity of testicular extracts, bacterial culture filtrates and other agents that increase tissue permeability. *Biochem. J. 35:*159, 1941.
82. Chain, E. and Duthie, E. S. Identity of hyaluronidase and spreading factor. *Brit. J. Exper. Path. 21:*324, 1940.
83. Coman, D. R., McCutcheon, M. and Zeidman, I. Failure of hyaluronidase to increase the invasiveness of neoplasms. *Cancer Res. 7:*383, 1947.
84. Pirie, A. A hyaluronidase and a polysaccharide from tumors. *Brit. J. Exper. Path. 23:*277, 1942.
85. Kiriluk, L. B., Kremen, A. J. and Glick, D. Mucolytic enzyme systems. XII. Hyaluronidase in human and animal tumors, and further studies on the serum hyaluronidase inhibitor in human cancer. *J. Nat. Cancer Inst. 10:*993, 1950.
86. Hobby, G. L., Dawson, M. H., Meyer, T. and Chaffee, E. Relationship between spreading factor and hyaluronidase. *J. Exper. Med. 73:*109, 1941.
87. Meyer, K., Chaffee, E., Hobby, G. L. and Dawson, M. H. Hyaluronidases of bacterial and animal origin. *J. Exper. Med. 73:*309, 1941.
88. Cameron, E. Op. Cit., p. 5.
89. Coman, J. and Levvy, G. A. Comparison of different glycosidase activities in conditions of cancer. *Brit. J. Cancer 11:*487, 1957.
90. Benditt, E. P., Schiller, S., Mathews, M. B. and Dorfman, A. Evidence that hyaluronidase is not the factor in testicular extract causing increased vascular permeability. *Proc. Soc. Exptl. Biol. and Med. 77:*643, 1951.
91. Haas, E. Mechanism of invasion, antiinvasin I, enzyme in plasma (which destroys hyaluronidase). *J. Biol. Chem. 163:*63, 1946.
92. Haas, E. Antiinvasin II, An enzyme in plasma. *J. Biol. Chem. 163:*101, 1946.
93. Haas, E. Mechanism of invasion, proinvasin I, enzyme (which protects hyaluronidase) in pathogenic bacteria and in venoms. *J. Biol. Chem. 163:*89, 1946.
94. Hale, C. W. Diffusing factors; action of reducing agents on hyaluronic acid and other polysacchardies. *Biochem. J. 38:*362, 1944.
95. Hale, C. W. Diffusing factors; influence of environmental conditions on activity of hyaluronidase. *Biochem. J. 38:*368, 1944.
96. Hoffman, D. C., Parker, F., Jr. and Walker, T. T. Effect of testicle extract on Rous sarcoma. *Am. J. Path. 7:*523, 1931.
97. Lacassagne, A., Loiseleur, J. and Rudali, G. Action inverses l'hyaluronidase et d'un sérum antihyaluronidase sur l'évolution du carcinome mammaire chez la souris. (Inverse action of hyaluronidase and antihyaluronidase serum upon the development of mammary carcinoma of mice.) *Comp. Rend. Acad. Sci.* (Paris) *244:* 1587, 1957.
98. Mathews, M. B. and Dorfman, A. Inhibition of hyaluronidase. *Physiol. Rev. 35:* 381, 1955.
99. Pike, R. M. The production of hyaluronic acid and hyaluronidase by some strains of group A streptococci. *Ann. N. Y. Acad. Sci. 52:*1070, 1950.
100. Golde, A. Les mucopolysaccharides dans quelques sarcomes aviaires cultivés *in vitro*. (Mucopolysaccharides in fowl sarcomas cultivated *in vitro.) Comp. Rend. Soc. Biol.* (Paris) *150:*349, 1956.
101. Cameron, E. Personal communication.

PART IV

102. Cameron, E. *Op. cit.,* p. 63.
103. *Ibid.,* p. 19.
104. Williams, R. G. The effects of continuous local injection of hyaluronidase on skin and subcutaneous tissue in rats. *Anat. Rec. 122:*349, 1955.
105. Cameron, E. *Op. cit.,* p. 73.
106. Bollet, A. J., Bonner, W. M. and Nance, J. L. The presence of hyaluronidase in various mammalian tissues. *J. Biol. Chem. 238:*3522, 1963.
107. Cameron, E., *Op. cit.,* p. 135.
108. Meyer, K. The biological significance of hyaluronic acid and hyaluronidase. *Physiol. Rev. 27:*335, 1947.
109. Wied, G. L. and Sechelmann, F. J. K. Aktivitätsbestimmung der Beta-Glukuronidase in der Gynäkologie. *Zentralbl. Gynäk. 74:*2033, 1952.
110. Conchie, J. and Levvy, G. A. Localization of beta-glucuronidase in normal and cancer cells. *Nature 184:*1709, 1959.
111. Ozaki, M. Malignant tumours and the spreading factor. *Gann. 42:*97, 1951.
112. Ozaki, M. Malignant tumours and the spreading factor. *Kumamoto Med. J. 4:* 119, 1952.
113. Thomson, D. L. Spreading Factors (Hyaluronidase) Review. *McGill, Med. J. 13:* 51, 1944.
114. Aylward, F. X. Chemical nature of Reynals spreading factor from mammalian testicle. *Proc. Soc. Exptl. Biol. and Med. 36:*477, 1937.
115. Aylward, F. X. Physiologic properties of Reynals diffusion factor. *Proc. Soc. Exptl. Biol. and Med. 49:*342, 1942.
116. Claude, A. and Duran-Reynals, F. Chemical properties of purified spreading factor from testicle. *J. Exper. Med. 65:*661, 1937.
117. Bachtold, J. G. and Gebhardt, L. P. The determination of hyaluronidase activity as derived from its reaction kinetics. *J. Biol. Chem. 194:*635, 1952.
118. Easty, G. C. and Easty, D. M. An organ culture system for the examination of tumour invasion. *Nature 199:*1104, 1963.
119. Greenstein, J. P. Method of evaluating thymonucleodepolymerase activity in normal and tumor tissues. *J. Nat. Cancer Inst. 2:*357, 1942.
120. Grossfeld, H. Method for determination of permeability of animal cells *in vitro. Protoplasma 29:*272, 1938.
121. Humphrey, J. H. Diffusing factors: Kinetics of action of hyaluronidase from various sources upon hyaluronic acid with note upon anomalies encountered in estimation of N-acetyl glucosamine. *Biochem. J. 40:*435, 1946.
122. Leonard, S. L., Perlman, P. L. and Kurzrok, R. Turbidmetric method for determining hyaluronidase in tissue extracts. *Endocrinology 39:*261, 1946.
123. McClean, M. Methods of assay of hyaluronidase and their correlation with skin diffusing activity. *Biochem. J. 37:*169, 1943.
124. Swyer, G. I. M. and Emmens, C. W. A modified method for the viscometric assay of hyaluronidase. *Biochem. J. 41:*29, 1947.
125. Tolksdorf, S., McCready, M. H., McCullagh, D. R. and Schwenk, E. The turbidometric assay of hyaluronidase. *J. Lab. Clin. Med. 34:*74, 1949.
126. Bacharach, A. L., Chance, M. R. A. and Middleton, T. R. Biologic assay of diffusing factor. *Biochem. J. 34:*1464, 1940.
127. Madinaveitia, J. and Quibell, T. H. H. Diffusing factors; action of testicular extracts on viscosity of vitreous humor preparations (in relation to mucinase). *Biochem. J. 34:*625, 1940.
128. Madinaveitia, J. and Quibell, T. H. H. Diffusing factors; effect of salts on action of testicular extract on viscosity of vitreous humor preparations. *Biochem. J. 34:* 456, 1941.

129. Favilli, G. Effect of testicle extract on red blood cells *in vitro*. *J. Exper. Med. 54:*197, 1931.

130. Favilli, G. Influence of organ extracts on permeability to water of sea-urchin eggs. *J. Cell. and Comp. Physiol. 2:*1, 1932.

131. Favilli, G. Mucolytic effect of several diffusing agents, and of diazotized compound (azoprotein). *Nature 145:*866, 1940.

132. Favilli, G. and McClean, D. Influence of testicular extract upon fragility of red blood cells and upon dispersion of indian ink particles in dermis. *J. Path. and Bact. 38:*153, 1934.

133. Hechter, O. Hyaluronidase–mechanism of action in skin. *Science 104:*409, 1946.

134. Hechter, O. Spreading factors–importance of mechanical factors in action on skin. *J. Exper. Med. 85:*77, 1947.

135. Hechter, O. Mechanisms of spreading factor action. *Ann. N. Y. Acad. Sci. 52:* 1028, 1950.

136. Hirst, G. K. Effect of polysaccharide-splitting enzyme (from leech extract) on streptococcal infection. *J. Exper. Med. 73:*443, 1941.

137. Hoffman, D. C. Effect of testicular extract on filterable virus. *J. Exper. Med. 53:*43, 1931.

138. McClean, D. Influence of testicle preparation on dermal permeability and response to vaccine virus. *J. Path. and Bact. 33:*1045, 1930.

139. McClean, D. Further observations on testicular extract and its effect upon tissue permeability. *J. Path. and Bact. 34:*459, 1931.

140. McClean, D. Action of diffusion factors on tissue permeability. *Lancet 1:*797, 1941.

141. McClean, D. and Hale, C. W. Mucinase and tissue permeability. *Nature 145:* 867, 1940.

142. Pijoan, M. Action of testicle preparations on infective power of bacteria. *J. Exper. Med. 53:*37, 1931.

143. Rogers, H. J. Influence of hydrolysates of hyaluronate upon hyaluronidase production by micro-organisms. *Biochem. J. 40:*583, 1946.

144. Sannella, L. S. Effect of testicular extract on distribution and absorption of subcutaneous saline solution. *Yale J. Biol. and Med. 12:*433, 1940.

145. Tichomirov, D. M. Effect of enzymes from malignant tumors on elastic tissue *in vitro*. *Virchows Arch. F. Path. Anat. 292:*310, 1934.

146. Day, T. D. Connective tissue permeability and the mode of action of hyaluronidase. *Nature 160:*785, 1950.

147. Day, T. D. Mode of action of hyaluronidase. *British Empire Cancer Campaign 28th Annual Report,* p. 172, 1950.

148 Bergavist, S. Synergism between staphlococci and tubercle bacilli as manifestation of spreading factor. *Nord. Med. 33:*513, 1947.

149. Boyland, E., Wallace, D. M. and Williams, D. C. Enzyme activity in relation to cancer. Inhibition of urinary beta-glucuronidase of patients with cancer of the bladder by oral administration of 1:4 saccharolactone and related compounds. *Brit. J. Cancer 11:*578, 1957.

150. Bronfenbrenner, J. and Sulkin, S. E. Nature of deteterious effect of local application of staphlococcus bacteriophage (role of Reynals spreading factor). *J. Infect. Dis. 65:*64, 1939.

151. Dux, C., Guerin, M. and LaCour, F. Sur la presence de l'hyaluronidase dans les tumeurs humanines et expérimentales examinees par le test MCP. (On the presence of hyaluronidase in human and experimental tumors examined by the MCP test.) *Bull. Assoc. Franc. P. L'Etude Du Cancer 35:*427, 1948.

PART IV

152. Fishman, W. H. B-glucuronidase, method of preparation and purification. *J. Biol. Chem. 127:*367, 1939.
153. Fishman, W. H. Increase in B-glucuronidase activity of mammalian tissues induced by feeding glucuronidogenic substances. *J. Biol. Chem. 136:*229, 1940.
154. Fishman, W. H., Green, S., Homburger, F., Kasdon, S. C., Nieburgs, H. E., McInnis, G. and Pund, E. R. Beta-glucuronidase studies in women. VII. Premenopausal vaginal-fluid beta-glucuronidase values in relation to in situ cancer of the cervix. *Cancer 7:*729, 1954.
155. Gibertini, G. Osservazioni sul contento in fermenti muchinolitici (mesomucinasi) dei tumori. (Observations on the hyaluronidase content of tumours.) *Tumori 28:* 317, 1942.
156. Humphrey, J. H. Diffusing factors: Action of hyaluronidase preparations from various sources upon some substrates other than hyaluronic acid. *Biochem. J. 40:* 442, 1946.
157. Leighton, J. Contribution of tissue culture studies to an understanding of the biology of cancer: A review. *Cancer Res. 17:*929, 1957.
158. Madinaveitia, J. Diffusing factors; concentration of mucinase. *Biochem. J. 35:* 447, 1941.
159. Smoylovska, E. Y. Variations in permeability of normal and tumorous tissues in hypotonic solution. *Med. Zhur. 7:*881, 1937.
160. Gasic, G., Loebel, F. and Badinez, O. Cementing substances in metastasizing and non-metastasizing transplantable tumours in mice. *Nature 185:*864, 1960.
161. Gersh, I. and Catchpole, H. R. The organization of ground substance and basement membrane and its significance in tissue injury, disease and growth. *Am. J. Anat. 85:*457, 1949.
162. Ghose, T. The role of spreading factors (hyaluronidase) in metastasis. *Indian J. Med. Sci. 14:*190, 1960.
163. Simpson, W. L. Mucolytic enzymes and invasion by carcinomas. *Ann. N. Y. Acad. Sci. 52:*1125, 1950.
164. Maiskii, I. N., Kozlova, N. A. and Nilovskii, M. N. The production of an anti-hyaluronidase horse serum and its effect on metastasization of Brown-Pearce carcinoma in rabbits. *Byull, Eksper. Biol. I. Med. 50:*86, 1960. (Consultant's Bureau translation—*Bull. Exp. Biol. and Med. 50:*1178, 1960.)
165. Gopal-Ayengar, A. R. and Simpson, W. L. Hyaluronidase and the growth of malignant epithelial tumors. *Cancer Res. 7:*727, 1947.
166. Meyer, K. and Chaffee, E. Mucopolysaccharides of skin—indication for identity of spreading factor with hyaluronidase. *J. Biol. Chem. 138:*191, 1941.
167. Chain, E. and Duthie, E. S. Mucolytic enzyme (musinase) in extracts (identity with spreading factor). *Nature 144:*977, 1939.
168. Christensen, J. F. Kallikrein (circulatory hormone from pancreas) as Reynals factor. *Nature 142:*36, 1938.

Cancer Cell Secretions

For generations, physicians have suspected that cancer cells secrete one or more substances that affect the host. The clinical observation that cancer patients lose weight, even when the cancer is in a non-vital area and too small to metabolize much nutrient, suggested to doctors that the cancer changes host functions through some chemical that diffuses to areas distant from the cancer. This concept is in accord with our knowledge of the ways in which some pathogenic bacteria, including streptococci, *C. tetanus, C. diphtheriae,* and the gas gangrene group, affect the host. These bacteria produce toxins that diffuse into the host and affect the functioning of tissues and organs that are free of the invading bacteria. The toxins of several bacteria have been isolated and purified.

There is now impressive, and virtually conclusive, evidence that cancer cells, too, produce chemicals that modify host functions. Several types of effects on the host have been reported. We do not yet know whether there are a multitude of cancer cell secretions (or toxins) each with a separate action, or whether there is a single material that has effects on many areas of host functioning, or whether there is a combination of both.

Several investigators have obtained evidence suggesting that cancers secrete a chemical that induces extensive formation of new blood vessels by the host (Chapter 19). Furthermore, in addition to the evidence that cancers produce a material that increases the permeability of the host's tissues through effects on the ground substance (*see* Chapter 21), there is also evidence of the existence either of other cancer secretions or of other effects of a multifunctional secretion.

Probably the most extensive studies have been done on "toxo-hormone," a substance produced by cancers that interferes with the enzyme catalase in the host's liver (1-47). Some criticism of the earlier work on toxohormone has been expressed by Kampschmidt and Schultz (48) and Kampschmidt and Upchurch (49) who pointed out that the transplanted cancers used for most studies on toxo-hormone were grossly contaminated with bacteria that were carried along in successive transplantations. Indeed, one transplanted carcinoma contained 10^9 bacteria per gram. These scientists suggested that the toxohormone effects could have come from the contaminating bacteria. This was a sound criticism, which points, again, to a general disadvantage in the use of transplanted cancers. Subsequent studies, however, have shown toxohormone in extracts of non-contaminated cancers (24), and Nakahara, Hozumi and Pollard (36) have isolated toxohormone from cancers growing in germ-free mice. Furthermore, Nakahara, Tanaka, Tokuzen and Fukuoka (37) have demonstrated toxohormone in spontaneous carcinomas and chemically induced sarcomas that were never exposed to contamination. It seems clear that toxohormone is, in fact, produced by cancers, although a similar substance can be produced by some of the bacteria contaminating transplanted cancers.

Other scientists have reported that cancer extracts can hemolyse host red blood cells (50), cause death and malformations in chick embryos (51-55), damage cells in tissue culture (56), induce tolerance (57), depress DPN synthesis (58), and stimulate growth of some normal tissues (59-64). In addition, there is evidence that extracts of cancer contain a substance that stimulates the growth of other cancer cells (65-70).

There is, then, overwhelming evidence that cancers produce substances that affect host functioning, but there has never been a coordinated program designed to identify and isolate these substances.

If there proves to be one material with a wide spectrum of actions on host functions, it is probable that at least one of these actions will be to help the cancer cells invade host tissues or neutralize some of the host's defenses; if there are many materials secreted by cancer cells, it is probable that at least one will have these effects on the host.

If the chemical structure of the cancer's secretion(s) is fairly simple, pharmaceutical chemists might be able to design and synthesize a pharmacologic antidote; they have done so for other harmful or deleterious chemicals and have produced such antidotes as dimercaprol (BAL), the antihistaminic drugs and pralidoxime (Protopam), and even an antihormone, spironolactone (Aldactone), which is now in clinical use. The development of an antidote to the cancer secretion(s) could result in long-term control of cancer.

Of course it is possible that the important cancer secretion may be a toxin of such highly complex chemical nature that a specific antidote cannot be readily developed. In that case, it might be possible to develop a *toxoid* that could stimulate host resistance to the toxin. This has been done with some bacterial diseases, notably diphtheria and tetanus. The toxins produced by these bacteria are extracted, purified, modified chemically into a toxoid, and then injected into the patient who, as a result, will develop resistance not only to the toxoid but also to the original toxin. A patient who has been given an adequate series of tetanus toxoid injections usually does not develop resistance to the tetanus bacillus, but only to the *toxin* produced by that bacillus. The situation in diphtheria is parallel. It might be possible, therefore, to use the toxoid approach to circumvent the difficulties involved in trying to improve host defenses against cancer (Chapter 23). Instead of trying to induce immunity to the cancer cell itself, it may prove fruitful to try to induce immunity to the secretion(s) of the cancer cell.

It might be argued that attempts to immunize a cancer patient with toxoid would be fruitless, since the patient presumably already has substantial amounts of the cancer toxin in his body and his immune mechanisms should have been maximally stimulated by the cancer toxin, so that added toxoid could do little if any good. In terms of pure theory, this might be a valid argument. There is, however, clear evidence that the immunologic system may not function according to this theory. In the case of tetanus, two excellent examples suggest that injected toxoid may stimulate the immune system far more than circulating toxin. The horse has large numbers of tetanus bacilli in its gastrointestinal tract—more than most other animals. One might theorize then that the horse should have a high level of immunity to tetanus, but this is not the case. Horses, more so than most animals, are quite susceptible to clinical tetanus when they sustain a wound. On the other hand, appropriate injections of tetanus toxoid into horses can produce extremely high levels of immunity to the original toxin. These levels not only give the horse complete protection against tetanus, but are so high that a few cubic centimeters of the horse's serum—less than 1 per cent of the total—are enough to abort attacks of clinical tetanus in injured people who were not previously protected. Slightly larger amounts of the horse antitetanus serum have been used to cure patients who would otherwise have died of tetanus.

A second example involves patients who develop clinical tetanus. People who have not been protected and who develop clinical tetanus are sometimes saved by strenuous and prolonged medical and nursing efforts. Such patients have had nearly lethal amounts of tetanus toxin in their bodies for several days. This exposure, however, does not provide any significant protection against a subsequent attack of tetanus if another wound is incurred. By contrast, the injection of relatively small amounts of tetanus toxoid provides most persons with almost complete protection against tetanus for periods of the order of five years.

Perhaps a similiar situation would follow the injection of a cancer toxoid, if one can be developed. We cannot even estimate the likelihood of this occurrence, but in view of the tremendous value of other toxoids, this approach seems deserving of considerable effort. We will need, of course, precautions to be sure that injection of a cancer toxoid, if one is developed, will not result in enhancement of the cancer (*see* Chapter 23).

The initial research approach to identifying the cancer secretion(s) should be in two directions. Since we already have a substantial amount of information about toxohormone, intensive studies of this material may reveal what actions toxohormone exerts on the host (in addition to the effects it has on the liver enzyme). Does toxohormone influence blood vessel proliferation? Does it help change the permeability of tissue barriers? Does it cause anemia? Does it promote the establishment of metastases? Does it interfere with metabolic processes other than those involving liver catalase? Also, we ought to find out whether toxohormone exerts effects on the cancer cells. Does it increase their ameboid motility? Does it make them multiply faster? If the answer to any of these, or similar, questions is "yes," a promising avenue to the effective control of cancer may be opened. Since the existence of toxohormone has been known for over a quarter of a century (12, 13, 15-19), it is disappointing that the answers to the foregoing questions about it are not already available.

A properly coordinated national program has many advantages over our current efforts to find out more about the actions of toxohormone. Under the existing system, if several scientists at different institutions wished to study toxohormone effects, each would first produce and purify his own toxohormone. They would probably use different sources, in terms of animal species and strains and in terms of kinds of cancer from which to obtain the toxohormone. Their purification methods might also differ. As a result, there would be no valid basis on which to compare their data. Furthermore, the time, effort, and funds spent in a series of separate small-batch extractions and purifications would be enormous, and could easily prevent some scientists who are not biochemically oriented from participating in such studies.

On the other hand, in a properly coordinated national program, a team of first-rate biochemists would prepare, purify and standardize the toxohormone, using a predetermined type of cancer as the source. Then, samples of the toxohormone would be sent to the other investigators for their studies. To avoid the problems caused by contamination, the initial source of the toxohormone might be spontaneous cancers in large animals, or chemically induced cancers in laboratory animals, perhaps germ-free. Subsequently, toxohormone made from surgically removed human cancers might be used in confirmatory studies. The exact choice of the source of toxohormone should be decided by the group engaged in the study, on the basis of all the factors, including availability, existing at the time the study is started.

If toxohormone is found to influence some of the host or cancer cell functions that seem relevant to the progression of the disease, the efforts to develop an antidote or toxoid, as discussed above, should be vigorous and thorough.

We should not, however, assume that toxohormone is the most important secretion of cancer cells just because it has been the most studied. It is quite possible that another material secreted by cancers may prove to be of greater significance. Therefore, a parallel series of studies ought to be done on other possible secretions of cancer cells. The scientists engaged in these studies should, as a working hypothesis, assume the existence of a series of cancer cell secretions, each with a different action. The research teams tackling this problem ought to include biochemists who would be responsible for extracting, purifying and identifying the active agent, and other scientists, who would test the effects of extracts. These other scientists might be physiologists, pharmacologists, pathologists, microbiologists, immunologists, or general biologists, depending on the type of action being tested. If and when an active cancer secretion is isolated and identified, an antidote or toxoid should be sought as described above.

References

1. Adams, D. H. The mechanism of the liver catalase depressing action of tumors in mice. *Brit. J. Cancer 4:*183, 1950.
2. Adams, D. H. Further observations on the liver catalase depressing action of tumours. *Brit. J. Cancer 5:*115, 1951.
3. Adams, D. H. Hormonal factors influencing liver catalase activity in mice. *Biochem. J. 50:*486, 1952.
4. Appleman, D., Skavinski, E. R. and Stein, A. M. Catalase studies on normal and cancerous rats. *Cancer Res. 10:*498, 1950.
5. Endo, H., Sugimura, T., Ono, T. and Konno, K. Catalase depressing tissue factors: toxohormone and kochsaft factor. *Gann 46:*51, 1955.
6. Euler, H. V. and Heller, L. Catalase activity in liver fractions of normal and sarcomatous rats. *Ztschr. F. Krebsforsch. 56:*393, 1949.

PART IV

7. Fukunda, M., Okada, K., Akikawa, K., Matsuda, M. and Urushizaki, I. Comparative studies on the biological effect of toxohormone and bacterial lipopolysaccharide. *Gann 57:*27, 1966.
8. Fukuoka, F. and Nakahara, W. Mode of action of toxohormone. A third study on toxohormone. *Gann 42:*55, 1951.
9. Fukuoka, F. and Nakahara, W. Toxohormone and thymus involution in tumor bearing animals. A fourth study on toxohormone, a characteristic toxic substance produced by cancer tissue. *Gann 43:*55, 1952.
10. Greenfield, R. E. and Meister, A. Studies on the inhibition of liver catalase in tumor-bearing animals. *Cancer Res. 10:*222, 1950.
11. Greenfield, R. and Meister, A. The effect of injections of tumor fractions on liver catalase activity of mice. *J. Nat. Cancer Inst. 5:*997, 1951.
12. Greenstein, J. P. Titration of the liver catalase activity of normal and tumor-bearing rats and mice. *J. Nat. Cancer Inst. 2:*525, 1942.
13. Greenstein, J. P. Further studies of liver catalase activity of tumor-bearing animals. *J. Nat. Cancer Inst. 3:*397, 1943.
14. Greenstein, J. P. The *in vivo* effect on liver catalase by a tumor. *J. Nat. Cancer Inst. 15:*1603, 1955.
15. Greenstein, J. P. and Andervont, H. B. The liver catalase activity of tumor-bearing mice and the effect of spontaneous regression and removal of certain tumors. *J. Nat. Cancer Inst. 2:*345, 1942.
16. Greenstein, J. P. and Andervont, H. B. Liver catalase activity of pregnant mice and of mice bearing growing embryonic implants. *J. Nat. Cancer Inst. 4:*283, 1943.
17. Greenstein, J. P., Andervont, H. B. and Thompson, J. W. Kidney and blood catalase activity of tumor-bearing animals. *J. Nat. Cancer Inst. 2:*589, 1942.
18. Greenstein, J. P., Jenrette, W. V. and White, J. The liver catalase activity of tumor-bearing rats and the effect of extirpation of the tumors. *J. Biol. Chem. 14:*327, 1941.
19. Greenstein, J. P., Jenrette, W. V. and White, J. The liver catalase activity of tumor-bearing rats and the effect of extirpation of the tumors. *J. Nat. Cancer Inst. 2:*283, 1941.
20. Hargreaves, A. B. and Deutsch, H. F. The *in vitro* inhibition of catalase by a tumor factor. *Cancer Res. 12:*720, 1952.
21. Hozumi, M. and Ohashi, M. Effect of toxohormone on iron-protoporphyrin-chelating enzyme of liver. *Gann 52:*327, 1961.
22. Kampschmidt, R. F., Mayne, M. A., Goodwin, W. L. and Clabaugh, W. A. Duplication of some of the systemic effects of four different tumors by extracts from those tumors. *Cancer Res. 20:*368, 1960.
23. Kampschmidt, R. F. and Upchurch, H. F. Some effects of tumor implantation site on tumor-host relations. *Cancer Res. 26:*990, 1966.
24. Matsuoka, K., Hozumi, M., Koyama, K., Kawachi, T., Nagao, M. and Sugimura, T. Tumor toxohormone unrelated to bacterial contamination. *Gann 55:*411, 1964.
25. Miyajima, T. Significance of depression of activity of liver catalase in animals with cancer, in particular the influence of the ascitic fluid of patients with cancer on the activity of liver catalase. *Showa Med. J. 19:*986, 1959.
26. Miyajima, S. Studies on toxohormone prepared from human cancer ascites. *Gann 46:*111, 1955.
27. Nakagawa, S. Liver catalase reducing substance in the urine of cancer patients. *Proc. Japan Acad. 28:*305, 1952.
28. Nakagawa, S. and Nakagawa, S. Intracellular distribution of liver catalase reducing substance in malignant tumor tissues. *Proc. Japan Acad. 32:*398, 1956.

29. Nakagawa, S., Kosuge, T. and Tokunaka, H. Purification of the liver catalase-reducing substance occurring in cancer tissues, with special reference to its activity. *Gann 46:*585, 1955.

30. Nakahara, W. and Fukuoka, F. A toxic cancer tissue constituent as evidenced by its effect on liver catalase activity. *Japan Med. J. 1:*271, 1948.

31. Nakahara, W. and Fukuoka, F. Toxohormone: a characteristic toxic substance produced by cancer tissue. *Gann 40:*45, 1949.

32. Nakahara, W. and Fukuoka, F. Purification of toxic hormone. A second study on toxohormone, a characteristic toxic substance produced by cancer tissues. *Gann 41:*47, 1950.

33. Nakahara, W. and Fukuoka, F. Dialyzable form of toxohormone. A sixth study of toxohormone. *Gann 45:*67, 1954.

34. Nakahara, W. and Fukuoka, F. The newer concept of cancer toxin. *Adv. in Cancer Res. 5:*157, 1958.

35. Nakahara, W. and Fukuoka, F. *Chemistry of Cancer Toxin—Toxohormone.* Charles C Thomas, Springfield, Ill., 1961.

36. Nakahara, W., Hozumi, M. and Pollard, M. Isolation of toxohormone from tumor tissues of germfree mice. *Proc. Soc. Expt'l. Biol. and Med. 123:*124, 1966.

37. Nakahara, W., Tanaka, T., Tokuzen, R. and Fukuoka, F. Toxohormone studies in autochthonous tumor-host system. *Gann 57:*62, 1966.

38. Obara, K., Ono, S., Nishizuka, F. and Hatano, M. Study of the distribution of 1311 labeled toxohormone. *Tohoku J. Exp. Med. 89:*375, 1966.

39. Ohashi, M. Isolation of toxohormone from mouse spleen injected with Friend's virus. *Gann 52:*179, 1961.

40. Ohashi, M. and Ono, T. Purification of toxohormone by DEAE-cellulose column chromatography. *Gann 50:*347, 1959.

41. Oh-Uti, K., Maki, K., Ito, J., Aneha, Y. and Koyama, T. Liver catalase activity of patients with gastric cancer. *Tohoku J. Exp. Med. 67:*159, 1958.

42. Ono, T., Umeda, M. and Sugimura, T. Purification of toxohormone. *Gann 48:* 91, 1957.

43. Ono, T., Sugimura, T. and Umeda, M. Preparation of potent concentrates of toxohormone free from nucleic acid. *Gann 46:*617, 1955.

44. Ono, T., Sugimura, T. and Umeda, M. The purification of toxohormone. *Gann 48:*91, 1956.

45. Ralph, F. K., Mabelle, E. A. and Thomas, A. M. Some systemic effects of toxohormone. *Cancer Res. 19:*236, 1959.

46. Weil-Malherbe, W. and Schade, R. Studies on the liver catalase of normal and cancerous rats. *Biochem. J. 43:*118, 1948.

47. Yamamura, Y. Studies on the toxic substance in the cancer tissue. *Japanese J. of Cancer Clinics. 7:*85, 1961.

48. Kampschmidt, R. F. and Schultz, G. A. Absence of toxohormone in rat tumors free of bacterial contamination. *Cancer Res. 23:*751, 1963.

49. Kampschmidt, R. E. and Upchurch, H. F. Effect of bacterial contamination of the tumor-host relationships. *Cancer Res. 23:*756, 1963.

50. Reynolds, M. D. and Friedell, G. H. Further observations on tumor extracts causing hemolysis *in vitro. Proc. Soc. Expt'l. Biol. and Med. 114:*798, 1963.

51. Fiszer-Szafarz, B. Effect of human cancerous serum on the chick embryo. *Cancer Res. 27:*191, 1967.

52. Handler, A. H., Geiser, C. F. and Farber, S. Studies on mortality in chick embryos resulting from implantation of whole blood and blood fractions from patients and animals with neoplastic disease. *Proc. Nat. Acad. Sci. 48:*1549, 1962.

195

53. Handler, A. H. and Magalini, S. I. Studies on a factor(s) toxic to chick embryos in the blood of human malignancy. I. Bioassay of malignant, non-malignant, and "normal" blood in the chick embryo system. *J. Lab. Clin. Med. 68:*588, 1966.

54. Handler, A. H., Magalini, S. I. and Snegireff, S. L. Mortality in chick embryos following implantation of cells and cell fraction of heterologous leukemias. *Transplant. Bull. 28:*485, 1961.

55. Lacon, C. R. and Karnofsky, D. A. Effects of blood taken from patients with enoplastic disease on the chick embryo. *Proc. Soc. Expt'l. Biol. and Med. 115:*477, 1964.

56. Watts, J. A factor in the serum of tumour-bearing rats which is deleterious to cells in tissue culture. *Nature 197:*196, 1963.

57. Graham, J. B. and Graham, R. M. Tolerance agent in human cancer. *Surg. Gyn. Ob. 118:*1217, 1964.

58. Ono, T. and Tomaru, T. The toxic factor depressing DPN synthesis in tumor-bearing animals. *Gann 50:*37, 1959.

59. Browning, H. The action of tumors on normal tissues synchronously transplanted into the anterior chamber of the mouse eye. *Cancer Res. 12:*13, 1952.

60. Chambers, H. and Scott, G. M. A growth-promoting factor in tumour tissue. *Brit. J. Exp. Path. 7:*33, 1926.

61. Cohen, S. and Levi-Montalcini, R. Purification and properties of a nerve growth-promoting factor isolated from mouse Sarcoma 180. *Cancer Res. 17:*15, 1957.

62. Doljanski, L., Hoffman, R. S. and Tenebaum, E. The effect of tumor extracts on the growth of cells in vitro. *Growth 8:*13, 1944.

63. Ludford, R. J. and Barlow, H. The influence of malignant cells upon the growth of fibroblasts in vitro. *Cancer Res. 4:*694, 1944.

64. McLaughlin, E. D. Mitotic-stimulating effect of serum from patients with pelvic cancer. *Cancer 15:*396, 1962.

65. Flexner, S. and Jobling, J. W. On the promoting influence of heated tumor emulsions on tumor growth. *Proc. Soc. Expt'l. Biol. and Med. 4:*156, 1907.

66. Casey, A. F. The experimental alteration of malignancy with a homologous mammalian tumor material. II. Intra-cutaneous inoculation of preserved material. *Am. J. Cancer 21:*776, 1934.

67. Casey, A. F. Comparison of effect of homologous tumor material and Duran-Reynals factor on tumor growth. *Am. J. Cancer 35:*354, 1939.

68. Kaliss, N., Jonas, G. and Avnet, N. L. Growth enhancement of tumor homoio-transplants in mice following injections of homogenates and ultrafiltration sediments of mouse tumors. *Cancer Res. 10:*228, 1950.

69. Martin, J. F. and Barral, P. Reprise de la croissance du sarcome du rat a la suite d' injections d'extraits de ce même sarcome. *Bull. Assoc. Franc. l'etude Cancer 20:*370, 1931.

70. Shear, H. H., Imagawa, D. T., Syverton, J. T. and Bittner, J. J. Presence in tumor tissue of a mouse mammary cancer accelerant. *Proc. Soc. Expt'l. Biol. and Med. 78:*281, 1951.

Cancer Immunology and Host Defenses

Clinical observations on patients with cancer have convinced many doctors that the host has defenses against cancer, and that, at times, these defenses can check or even reverse the progress of the malignancy. It has seemed to many that, if there were some way to improve host defenses, cure or control of a large proportion of cancers would become practical. Host defenses may involve more than one mechanism; since the one best known is the immunologic mechanism, the hope of developing an immunologic treatment for cancer has encouraged scientists for more than half a century. Several decades ago opitmism prevailed; studies on transplantable cancers seemed to show a clear-cut way to protect an animal against cancer. Then, further experiments showed that the defenses elicited were not defenses against the cancer per se, but defenses against a foreign tissue. The techniques that could protect a mouse against a cancer transplanted from another mouse were completely useless against spontaneous cancers—the kind seen in man. For years afterwards, pessimism about immunologic approaches prevailed. Now, after many more studies have been done on cancer immunology, it appears that this field is much more complex than investigators had originally thought, but there is a guarded optimism about the possibility of unravelling these complexities and developing a useful immunologic treatment for cancer. Several excellent reviews of cancer immunology and host defenses are available (1-26).

The fundamental question to be solved is whether cancer cells possess distinctive antigens that are not found in normal cells. If the answer is negative, we cannot expect any of the regular immunologic techniques or procedures to improve host defenses. On the other hand, if cancer cells do possess distinctive antigens, the possibility of using those antigens to improve host defenses would warrant rather extensive studies.

Many scientists, using a variety of research methods, have studied cancers of different kinds in animals and man. Some of their results point to the existence of specific antigens in transplanted animal can-

cer (27-70). Two criticisms have been raised against such immunologic studies on transplantable cancers. First, there is good evidence
that most of the transplantable cancers are contaminated by saprophytic bacteria and viruses, so that the antigens in question may come
from the microorganisms, not the cancer cells. Second, even though
the mice used are inbred, they are not always perfectly syngeneic; there
may be small differences in genetic constitution, resulting perhaps
from mutations, which could confuse the interpretation of the experiments. Such criticisms have validity. However, there have been many
studies done on other types of cancer, and these, too, have pointed to
the existence of specific cancer antigens. For example, studies on
chemically induced cancers (71-86) have shown that the antigens
elaborated in these cases are specific for a particular animal. If 20
inbred mice are given a specific carcinogenic chemical, and if all of
them develop cancer, they will each have a cancer antigen, or group
of antigens, distinct from any known normal mouse antigen, and also
distinct from the cancer antigens of the other 19 mice.

There is now a large number of studies that have helped expand
our knowledge of the phenomenon of cancer immunology in animals
(103-160). A number of investigators have described different techniques and methods for isolating and identifying cancer antigens and
antibodies (161-176). It is significant that several studies have
demonstrated cancer antigens in *spontaneous* animal cancers (79,
87-102), including those of dogs (96).

Many reports on the immunology of cancer in man have also
pointed to the existence of cancer antigens (177-218). Thus, the
evidence for the existence of specific cancer antigens is impressive.
It is possible to argue that the antigens may not be qualitatively different from some normal antigens; that in cancer some normal antigens
that usually are present in amounts too small to be detected, are increased enough to be detected. This argument is, and always will be,
unanswerable. (Tiny amounts of a material will be missed by any test
whose threshold is higher than the concentration.) In our search for
practical ways of helping cancer patients, we must, however, be
guided by probabilities—and the probabilities that there are distinctive cancer antigens now seem quite high.

Although the evidence for the existence of antigens is impressive,
these antigens, compared to other antigens, are not easy to demonstrate, nor is the existence of host resistance and host antibody responses. Whereas virtually every patient who has typhoid, typhus, or
other infectious disease, after a few weeks, demonstrates high antibody titers in the serum when tested by relatively simple and direct

immunologic techniques, special, rather complex and sensitive techniques are usually needed to demonstrate cancer antigens and host antibodies to them. Some workers have interpreted this to mean that cancer antigens are "weak." Another interpretation is possible, however. It has been suggested (90) that the difficulty in demonstrating cancer antigens stems from the presence of both antigens and host antibodies in the same system before the test is run; they form complexes, so that neither is free to react with antigens or antibodies added by the researcher. In other disease conditions in which immunologic diagnosis is practical, the volume of host antibody is far greater than the volume of foreign antigen. Let us consider typhoid fever as an example. The Widal test for typhoid is positive after a few weeks in almost every patient with the disease because the volume of circulating host antibody is large, compared to the amount of typhoid antigen in the patient. Thus, most of the antibody is free to combine with any fresh typhoid antigen. Also, in the Widal test, new typhoid antigen is used, not typhoid antigen taken directly from the patient. The new typhoid antigen is free to combine with added antibody. On the other hand, typhoid antigen in the form of bacteria taken from the patient and not cultured would probably be already largely complexed with host antibody, would be unable to react with any added antibody in the test tube and, if used, would give a spurious negative response.

Unfortunately, in dealing with cancer, it is difficult to get relatively pure cancer antigen or relatively pure host antibody. A recent study by Pilch and Riggins (79) produced evidence that tends to support this finding. They worked with both spontaneous and chemically induced cancers in mice. They were unable to demonstrate any antibodies to these cancers as long as the primary growths remained. After surgical removal of the tumors, however, they were able to detect (with fluorescent antibody techniques) measurable amounts of anti-cancer antibody in the host serum for as long as three and one-half months. This study may prove to have great significance since it suggests that immunotherapy, to be optimally effective, may have to be combined with surgical removal of most of the cancer.

Attempts have also been made to treat cancer immunologically, both in animals (219-225) and man (226-232). In general, the results have been unsatisfactory, although a few reports have been optimistic.

Unfortunately, cancer immunology is complicated by a phenomenon that is not usually encountered in other immunologic relationships—the phenomenon of enhancement. Ordinarily, if an antiserum is administered to an animal or patient having a toxic or infectious material in his body, the antibodies in the antiserum neutralize the toxin or help fight the invading microorganism and thus aid the patients's recovery. For example, antiserum against snake venom will neutralize the poison of the snake against which it is directed, and antiserum against *Hemophilus influenzae* will help kill that bacterium and protect the patient. Antibodies made by the host himself (active immunity) tend to be more effective than introduced antibodies (passive immunity) in neutralizing toxins and curing infection. This, of course, is the basis of our general immunization programs against such diseases as diphtheria, tetanus, whooping cough, and so forth; the introduction of small amounts of the antigen stimulates the host to produce antibodies, and these antibodies offer protection against these infections for many years.

In cancer, however, immunologic treatment, involving either active or passive immunity, is more likely to *stimulate* than to inhibit growth and spread of the cancer. This reaction has been observed in relation to several aspects of cancer immunology. It has been found that when normal mice from a high-strain cancer are treated with cancer extract, the treatment does not retard the development of the spontaneous cancers; it usually accelerates it (233-235). If mice that are to receive transplantable cancers are pretreated with cancer antigen, the result is an increase in the incidence and spread of tumor "takes" (236-239). If one treats with cancer antigen mice that already have growing cancers, the treatment *increases* the growth rate of the cancer and shortens the life expectancy of the animal (240-244). It is of interest that this phenomenon was reported 60 years ago by Flexner and Jobling (241). Immunologic enhancement also applies to chemically induced cancers (245, 246), and to cancers of one species transplanted into another species (247).

Some investigators report that enhancement is dosage-related. One group found that small doses of antigen induced resistance to cancers, while larger ones caused enhancement (248). Another group, however, found that large amounts of antibody caused resistance to cancer and small doses caused enhancement (249). Though several studies have been done in attempts to clarify the nature of enhancement (250-277), it remains unclear. Möller (268) has stated:

It appears, therefore, that immunological enhancement is not restricted to certain tumor types or to certain antigenic systems, but is of a more general nature.

The main barrier today to effective, practical immunotherapy of cancer appears, therefore, to be the enhancement phenomenon. The National Advisory Cancer Council has stated (278):

> However, in the present state of knowledge, an important hazard is posed by the possibility that immunization of a patient with his own tumor might induce circulating antibodies of the enhancing type, causing progressive rather than regressive tumor growth.

Accordingly, if we are to develop an adequate program in cancer immunology, it seems that special attention will have to be paid to the enhancement phenomenon, and special efforts be made to solve it. One step in this direction would be a careful comparison with other immunologic phenomena, for a clue. Years ago, experienced clinicians dealing with patients having active tuberculosis warned against doing a tuberculin test on these patients. Apparently, even the minute amount of tuberculin antigen involved in the diagnostic test would be enough to make some patients worse. This situation appears to have the features of an enhancement phenomenon, and perhaps it can be investigated in animals that are susceptible to tuberculosis. Another possibility deserving exploration is that *any* antigen-antibody reaction might cause cancer growth enhancement, through the liberation of histamine and similar materials in the neighborhood of the cancer. Many antigen-antibody reactions *in vivo* cause dilation of host blood vessels, and sometimes even kill normal cells (Arthus phenomenon). It may be that the materials usually liberated following an antigen-antibody reaction make the normal cells near the cancer more vulnerable, or the cancer cells more aggressive.

An additional possibility is that the enhancement phenomenon is related in some way to the Sulzberger-Chase phenomenon in which the injection of an antigen by a "wrong" route not only fails to provoke an antibody response, but also prevents the customary antibody response to a subsequent injection of the same antigen by the "right" or usual route (279-281). For example, if a chemical antigen is given orally to a guinea pig, and if the animal receives an injection of the same antigen a few days later, antibody titers do not rise. At first, it was believed that the Sulzberger-Chase phenomenon applies only to situations in which the particular antigen is given for the first time by the "wrong" route. Frey, Geleick and deWeck, however, were able to produce a similar effect in animals that had already been sensitized to the antigen (282). They report:

201

In conclusion, the induction of the tolerance of the "Sulzberger-Chase" type is possible in previously sensitized animals.

If we assume that the host ordinarily has some immunologic defenses against cancer, then a Sulzberger-Chase type of response, by eliminating those defenses, could cause enhancement. Taliaferro and Humphrey (283) have also linked the two phenomena, stating:

The alternative must be considered that the Sulzberger-Chase phenomenon is akin to enhancement.

Each of these, and perhaps other, possible causes of enhancement deserve prompt and vigorous study.

Some other facets of the cancer immunology problem also ought to be considered. Once the enhancement problem is solved, it will be necessary to decide on the best type of immunotherapy. In general, immunotherapy may be divided into three types—heterologous, homologous and autologous.

Heterologous immunotherapy involves the injection of an antigen into a different species of animal, harvesting the antiserum, and then injecting it into the patient. There are several such antisera available in medicine, including horse antiserum for botulism, tetanus, black-widow spider bite and snake bite; and rabbit antiserum for treatment of *Hemophilus influenzae* meningitis. The heterologous antisera can be produced in reasonable quantities and potencies, but they have two major drawbacks. They are excreted by the patient at a rapid rate, so that their effect is limited to a few days. Furthermore, since they come from a foreign species, they are themselves antigenic to man. Therefore, a patient receiving an antiserum derived from horses will, in a matter of a few weeks, develop an intense allergic response to any subsequent injections. If such injections are continued, the host's allergic response to them will usually increase and lead to the host's death. Consequently, heterologous antisera can only be used effectively in acute situations, in which a cure or neutralization of toxin takes place in hours or a few days. Unfortunately, the anatomy of cancer and the dynamics of the circulation to cancer are such that any medication to have meaningful effects must be present for a long time. It is possible that a potent heterologous antiserum to cancer could prolong the lives of patients by three to four weeks, but this is too small a gain to warrant an extensive effort in this area.

Homologous immunotherapy involves the injection of an antigen into a member of the same species, harvesting the antiserum, and then injecting it into the patient. There are now available several antisera of human origin, including special gamma globulin concentrates for such conditions as cowpox (vaccinia), pertussis, and tetanus. The major advantages of homologous antiserum are that it is excreted much more slowly than heterologous antisera and it does not usually sensitize the host. Therefore, *in theory,* if a human-origin antiserum to cancer were available, it could be given to cancer patients for long periods, and could control cancer for years. There are, however, some practical drawbacks to this approach as a method of therapy. To obtain sufficient antiserum for one patient, it would be necessary to immunize and draw serum from several healthy donors. This is a procedure involving some discomfort and high cost. If the 300,000 persons who die of cancer each year in this country were to receive enough of a potent human-origin antiserum to control their cancers, a million or more healthy volunteer donors would be needed, and the cost of obtaining and processing the antiserum would be enormous. Accordingly, although homologous immunotherapy of cancer might be possible on a small-scale experimental basis, it hardly seems practical to carry it out for large numbers of cancer patients.

Autologous immunotherapy involves the injection of an antigen into a patient or potential patient who then produces his own antibodies. Autologous antisera are the most efficient of all, and appear to have none of the disadvantages of heterologous and homologous antisera. Up to now, however, our medical experience with autologous antibodies has been almost entirely in relation to prevention of disease. Antigens used in this situation, called vaccines, include those for cholera, diphtheria, virus influenza, measles, mumps, plague and poliomyelitis. Rabies vaccine is given after exposure but before development of symptoms.

In the case of patients with cancer, autologous immunotherapy would involve a novel approach—an attempt to improve host resistance to a disease that is already present by adding an antigen that presumably is also already present. Is it reasonable to expect a useful therapeutic response from such a procedure? This question cannot yet be answered but, because of its crucial importance, deserves a vigorous effort to find an answer. It would be helpful to know whether vaccination will help to combat any existing infection. One maneuver that might lead to an affirmative answer would be the use of modified antigens or modified methods of administration. It has already been demonstrated in several areas of immunology that slightly modified antigens sometimes provoke a much greater host response than the original unaltered antigen. Furthermore, the host antibodies that are produced in response to the modified antigen frequently are capable of combining with the original unaltered antigen. This may be the basis of some of the auto-immune diseases (296). There is reason to hope that a modified cancer antigen, injected into a host with cancer, could provoke a greater and more effective host response than the unmodified cancer antigens already present in the host. Several investigators have demonstrated that modified cancer antigens can improve host defenses (284-288) against transplanted cancers. Of even greater significance is the report of Czajkowski, Rosenblatt, Cushing, Vazquez and Wolf (289). They worked with both spontaneous and chemically induced cancers. Cancer cells from a mouse with cancer were modified by coupling them to an antigenic protein carrier; they were then reinjected with an adjuvant into the original animal. The growth rates of the cancers still in the animal were substantially slowed, and the investigators were able to demonstrate circulating antibodies to cancer in these animals. In control animals that were immunized with their own unmodified cancer cells, no such antibodies could be detected.

The use of adjuvants may also help improve host defenses against cancer (290, 291) since they can increase the host's responsiveness even to its own tissues (292, 293). Yet the effect of available adjuvants on host response to cancer is rather unpredictable: they may cause improvement (290, 291) or they may not (289, 294, 295). Perhaps a combination of altered antigen and adjuvant, as used by Czajkowski et al. (289), will prove more effective. The effects of adjuvants on the host's immune system may be of interest from another viewpoint. A major component of adjuvants is oil. Nakahara showed many years ago (297-300) that an injection of oil sometimes stimulates host resistance. Recently, there has been considerable public discussion of the merits of a certain unproven cancer treatment. Government authorities claimed that the only active material in the drug was creatine, a common chemical which could not influence cancer, while several patients and some public figures claimed occasional good results from the mixture. In the public discussion, little if any attention was paid to the fact that mineral oil was used as a carrier for the creatine. It is possible that the occasional good results reported were authentic, but that they came from the oil, not the alleged medication.

The recent work of Nadler and Moore (301) on transfer of sensitized lymphocytes may open another approach to the control of cancer, but as yet there is inadequate information on which to base any judgment as to the eventual value of this technique.

A substantial number of other studies have been done in the field of cancer immunology (302-338) and provide a good foundation for a major research effort in this area.

The steps that seem most likely to lead to a useful, practical control or cure for cancer are the following. First, a vigorous, intensive study of the enhancement phenomenon seems necessary. Preliminary studies can be done on mice, but confirmatory studies should also be done on dogs and larger animals, before any large-scale attempts are made to transfer the results to humans.

The kinds of experiments to be done to solve the enhancement problem will have to be worked out as the program progresses. (Some areas in which to begin have been suggested earlier in this chapter.)

A second area that ought to be developed at once is that of autologous immunotherapy, in particular of ways in which the resistance of the host to *an already existing disease* can be increased. Bacterial disease models might be used, and special attention ought to be given to the use of modified antigens, together with adjuvants of different kinds. It seems much less practical to devote any substantial amount of energy or funds to studies on heterologous immunotherapy.

References

1. Begg, R. W. Tumor-host Relations in *Adv. Cancer Res.*, 5, Academic Press, N. Y. 1958.
2. Black, M. M. and Speer, F. D. Immunology of cancer. *Surg., Gynecol., & Obstet. —Internat. Abstr. Surg. 109:*105, 1959.
3. Clerici, E. Some aspects of immunity in tumors. *Tumori 51:*369, 1965 (in Italian).
4. Elias, K. Progress in the study of host reaction to cancer. *Bull., N. Y. Acad. Med. 42:*896, 1966.
5. Furth, J. A meeting of ways in cancer research: Thoughts on the evolution and nature of neoplasms. *Cancer Res. 19:*241, 1959.
6. Furth, J. Influence of host factors on the growth of neoplastic cells. *Cancer Res. 23:*21, 1963.
7. Gorer, P. A. Some recent work on tumor immunity. *Adv. Cancer Res.* 4, Academic Press, N. Y., 1956.
8. Green, H. N. The immunologic theory of cancer. *Acta. Unio Internat. Contra Cancrum 17:*215, 1961.
9. Hauschka, T. S. Immunologic aspects of cancer: A review. *Cancer Res. 12:*615, 1952.
10. Hirsch, H. M. Some aspects of the problem of immunity against transplanted and spontaneous tumors. *Bac. Rev. 26:*336, 1962.
11. Hirsch, H. M. The antigenicity of tumor cells. *Folia Biologica* (Prague) *9:*161, 1963.
12. Klein, G. Some features of tumor-specific antigens: A general discussion. *Ann. N. Y. Acad. Sci. 101:*170, 1962.

PART IV

13. Klein, G. Tumor antigens. *Ann. Rev. Microbiol. 20:*223, 1966.
14. Koelsche, G. A. Immunologic factors in cancer: A review. *Proced. Staff Meet. Mayo Clin. 37:*219, 1962.
15. Mider, G. B. Some tumor-host relationships. In: R. W. Begg (ed.), *Proc. 1st Canad. Cancer Conf.,* p. 120, New York: Academic Press, 1955.
16. Milder, J. W. (ed.) Conference on the possible role of immunology in cancer. *Cancer Res. 21:*1165, 1961.
17. Milgrom, F. A short review of immunological investigations on cancer. *Cancer Res. 21:*862, 1961.
18. More, R. H. The relation of immunology and neoplasia. *Proc. 1st Canad. Cancer Conf. 1:*267, 1955.
19. Old, L. J., and Boyse, E. A. Immunology of experimental tumors. *Ann. Rev. Med. 15:*167, 1964.
20. Radzikhovskaia, R. M. The role of antibodies in the immunity against tumours. *Vopr. Onkol.* (Moscow) *4:*234, 1958.
21. Sinkovics, J. G., Shullenberger, C. C. and Howe, C. D. The complex pathogenic effect of tumors. *Exper. Med. and Surg. 20:*277, 1962.
22. Southam, C. M. Applications of immunology to clinical cancer: Past attempts and future possibilities. *Cancer Res. 21:*1302, 1961.
23. Witebsky, E. An immunologist's Vade Mecum. *N. Y. State J. of Med. 57:*3615, 1957.
24. Woodruff, M. F. A. Immunological aspects of cancer. *Lancet 2:*265, 1964.
25. Zilber, L. A. Specific tumor antigens. *Adv. Cancer Res.* 5, Academic Press, N. Y. 1958, p. 291.
26. Zilber, L. A. An immunological approach to tumor growth control: In: *Biological Approaches to Cancer Chemotherapy.* London and New York: Academic Press 1961, p. 231.
27. Abramoff, P., Chichinian, H., and Saunders, J. W., Jr. Detection of antigenically distinctive components of mouse melanoma S91. *J. Nat. Cancer Inst. 22:*919, 1959.
28. Andervont, H. B. Studies on immunity induced by mouse sarcoma 180. *Pub. Health Rep. 47:*1859, 1932.
29. Black, P. H., Rowe, W. P., Turner, H. C. and Huebner, R. J. A specific complement-fixing antigen present in SV40 tumor and transformed cells. *Proc. N. A. S. 50:* 1148, 1963.
30. Chambers, H. and Scott, G. M. Immunity to Jensen's rat sarcoma produced by tumour extracts. *J. Path. and Bact. 35:*284, 1932.
31. Chouroulinkov, I., Boyse, E. A., and Old, L. J. Cytotoxic activity of isoantibody on sarcoma 1. *Proc. Soc. Expt'l. Biol. and Med. 111:*263, 1962.
32. Day, E. D., Planinsek, J. A., Korngold, L. and Pressman, D. Tumor-localizing antibodies purified from antisera against Murphy rat lymphosarcoma. *J. Nat. Cancer Inst. 17:*517, 1956.
33. Adams, R. A. Specificity of the Syrian hamster's heightened susceptibility or immunity to a heterotransplanted murine leukemia. *Proc. Am. Assoc. Cancer Res. 4:* 1, 1963.
34. Dufour, D. Réaction anaphylactique locale expérimentalement produite chez le rat porteur, de la tumeur de Walker et permettant la détection de l'antigène tumorale. *Bull. Assoc. Franc. Cancer 48:*122, 1961.
35. Dufour, D. et Bao Linh, D. Etude immunologique de la tumeur de Walker. *Revue D'Immunologie 25:*64, 1961.

36. Dufour, D., Berlinguet, L. and Loiselle, J. M. Antigenic property and electrophoretic behavior of the serum albumin of rats bearing the Walker tumor. *Canadian J. of Biochem. and Physiol. 37:*1401, 1959.
37. Fink, M. A. Use of hypersensitivity techniques in the demonstration of antibody to an isologous, transplantable tumor in BALB/C mice. *Ann. N. Y. Acad. Sci. 101:* 160, 1962.
38. Flax, M. H. The action of anti-Ehrlich ascites tumor antibody. *Cancer Res. 16:* 774, 1956.
39. Foley, E. J. Immunity of C3H mice to lymphosarcoma 6-C3H-Ed following regression of the implanted tumor. *Proc. Soc. Expt'l. Biol. and Med. 80:*675, 1952.
40. Goldin, A. and Humphreys, S. R. Studies of immunity in mice surviving systemic leukemia L1210. *J. Nat. Cancer Inst., 24:*283, 1960.
41. Gorer, P. A. The role of antibodies in immunity to transplanted leukemia in mice. *J. Path. Bact. 54:*51, 1942.
42. Gorer, P. A. Antibody response to tumor inoculation in mice with special reference to partial antibodies. *Cancer Res. 7:*634, 1947.
43. Gorer, P. A. Studies in antibody response of mice to tumor inoculation. *Brit. J. Cancer 4:*372, 1948.
44. Gorer, P. A. The significance of studies with transplanted tumors. *Brit. J. Cancer 2:*103, 1948.
45. Gorer, P. A. and Mikulska, Z. B. The antibody response to tumor inoculation. *Cancer Res. 14:*651, 1954.
46. Gorer, P. A. and Kaliss, N. The effect of isoantibodies in vivo on three different neoplasms in mice. *Cancer Res. 19:*824, 1959.
47. Graff, R. J. and Kandutsch, A. A. Immunogenic properties of purified antigen preparations from a mouse sarcoma. *Transplantation 4:*465, 1966.
48. Haughton, G. Some cell-bound species specific antigens of mouse ascites tumor cells. *Ann. N. Y. Acad. Sci. 101:*131, 1962.
49. Horn, E. C. Ascites tumor development. 11. Cytotoxicity of various antisera prepared against Ehrlich ascites tumor cell components. *Cancer Res. 16:*595, 1956.
50. Kalfayan, B. and Kidd, J. G. Structural changes produced in Brown-Pearce carcinoma cells by means of a specific antibody and complement. *J. Expt'l. Med. 97:* 145, 1953.
51. Kaliss, N. The transplanted tumor as a research tool in cancer immunology. *Cancer Res. 21:*1203, 1961.
52. Kidd, J. G. A complement-binding antigen in extracts of the Brown-Pearce carcinoma of rabbits. *Proc. Soc. Expt'l. Biol. and Med. 38:*292, 1938.
53. Klein, E., and Sjögren, H. O. Humoral and cellular factors in homograft and isograft immunity against sarcoma cells. *Cancer Res. 20:*452, 1960.
54. Lewis, M. R. and Aptekman, P. M. Atrophy of tumors caused by strangulation and accompanied by development of tumor immunity in rats. *Cancer 5:*411, 1952.
55. Makari, J. G. Activity of a tumour polysaccharide substance on mice transplanted with sarcoma 180. *Nature 205:*1178, 1965.
56. Matsumoto, T. Immunological studies of tumors, 1. Differential reactions of homologous antiserum to tumor cells of different rat ascites tumors. *J. Fac. Sci. Hokkaido Univ.* Ser. VI *14:*31, 1958.
57. Matsumoto, T. Immunological studies of tumors, V. Further studies of antigenic differences between two sublines of the Yoshida sarcoma. *Gann 52:*57, 1961.
58. Mottram, J. C. and Russ, S. Observations and experiments on the susceptibility and immunity of rats toward Jensen's rat sarcoma. *Proc. Roy. Soc. London,* Series B. *90:*1, 1917-1918.

59. Nungester, W. J. and Fisher, H. The inactivation *in vivo* of mouse lymphosarcoma 6C3HED by antibodies produced in a foreign host species. *Cancer Res. 14:*284, 1954.

60. Pikovski, M. A., and Schlesinger, M. The effect of prior injections of lyophilized mouse tumor on the growth and transplantation of mouse tumor in rats. *Cancer Res. 15:*285, 1955.

61. Pressman, D., and Korngold, L. The *in vivo* localization of anti-Wagner-osteogenic sarcoma antibodies. *Cancer 6:*619, 1953.

62. Pressman, D. and Kyogoku, M. The localization in vivo of rabbit antibodies in the N-2-FAA hepatic tumors of rats. *Ann. N. Y. Acad. Sci. 101:*167, 1962.

63. Snell, G. D. The demonstration of "weak" isoantigens of transplantable tumors of mice. *Acta. Unio. Internat. Contra Cancrum 15:*924, 1959.

64. Stoerk, H. S., Budzilpvich, T. and Bielinski, T. C. Resistance to grafting with lymphosarcoma cells in rats injected with homologous lymphoid cells. *J. Mt. Sinai Hosp. 29:*169, 1952.

65. Stone, M. J., Dzoga, K. and Wissler, R. W. Combined inhibitory effect of antitumor antibody and an oncolytic virus on the solid Ehrlich tumor. *Lab. Invest. 11:* 306, 1962.

66. Trench, C. A. H., Gardner, P. S., and Green, C. A. Antibody production in tolerant rabbits to mouse lymphoma L-5178. *Brit. J. Cancer 17:*287, 1963.

67. Wallach, D. F. H. and Hager, E. B. Association of cell surface antigens with microsomal membrane fractions derived from Ehrlich ascites carcinoma cells. *Nature 196:*1004, 1962.

68. Wodinsky, I. and Kensler, C. J. Growth of L1210 leukaemia cells. *Nature 210:* 962, 1966.

69. Woodruff, M. F. A. and Symes, M. O. The use of immunologically competent cells in the treatment of cancer: Experiments with a transplantable mouse tumour. *Brit. J. Cancer 16:*707, 1962.

70. Yagi, Y., and Pressman, D. Immunologic differences between Murphy-Sturm lymphosarcoma and normal rat lymph nodes. *Proc. Soc. Expt'l. Biol. and Med. 106:*164, 1961.

71. Baldwin, R. W. Immunity to methylcholanthrene-induced tumors in inbred rats following atrophy and regression of the implanted tumors. *Brit. J. Cancer 9:*652, 1955.

72. Bubeník, J., Ivanyi, J. and Koldovsky, P. Participation of 7S and 19S antibodies in enhancement and resistance to methylcholantrene-induced tumors. *Folia Biol.* (Prague) *11:*426, 1965.

73. Foley, E. J. Antigenic properties of methylcholanthrene-induced tumors in mice of the strain of origin. *Cancer Res. 13:*835, 1953.

74. Klein, G., Sjögren, H. O., Klein, E., and Hellstrom, K. E. Demonstration of resistance against methylcholanthrene-induced sarcomas in the primary autochthonous host. *Cancer Res. 20:*1561, 1960.

75. Koldovsky, P. Isoimmunity against an induced primary tumour. *Folia Biol.* (Prague) *7:*170, 1961.

76. Matsumoto, T. Antigenicity of a crude lipopolysaccharide fraction of the methylcholanthrene-induced tumor, with special reference to isologous immunity in inbred rats. *Gann 56:*1, 1965.

77. Matsuyama, M., Maekawa, A., Horikawa, H., Suzumori, K., Soga, K., and Iwai, K. Ineffectiveness of autotransplantation on growth of the methylcholanthrene sarcoma in rats and mice. *Nature 197:*805, 1963.

78. Old, L. J., Boyse, E. A., Clarke, D. A. and Carswell, E. Antigenic properties of chemically induced tumors. *Ann. N. Y. Acad. Sci. 101:*80, 1962.

79. Pilch, Y. H. and Riggins, R. S. Antibodies to spontaneous and methylcholanthrene-induced tumors in inbred mice. *Cancer Res. 26:*871, 1966.
80. Prehn, R. T. Tumor-specific immunity to transplanted dibenz(a,h)-anthracene-induced sarcomas. *Cancer Res. 20:*1614, 1960.
81. Prehn, R. T. Specific isoantigenicities among chemically induced tumors. *Ann. N. Y. Acad. Sci. 101:*107, 1962.
82. Prehn, R. T. Cancer antigens in tumors induced by chemicals. *Fed. Proc. 24:* 1018, 1965.
83. Prehn, R. T., and Main, J. M. Immunity to methylcholanthrene-induced sarcomas. *J. Nat. Cancer Inst. 18:*769, 1957.
84. Riggins, R. S., and Pilch, Y. H. Immunity to spontaneous and methylcholanthrene-induced tumors in inbred mice. *Cancer Res. 24:*1994, 1964.
85. Weiler, E. Antigenic differences between normal hamster kidney and stilboestrol induced kidney carcinoma: Complement fixation reactions with cytoplasmic particles. *Brit. J. Cancer 10:*553, 1956.
86. Yoshida, T. O. Further evidence of immunologic reaction against methylcholanthrene-induced autochthonous tumors. *Japan. J. Exper. Med. 35:*115, 1965.
87. Attia, M. A., DeOme, K. B., and Weiss, D. W. Immunology of spontaneous mammary carcinomas in mice. 11. resistance to a rapidly and a slowly developing tumor. *Cancer Res. 25:*451, 1965.
88. Baldwin, R. W. Tumour-specific immunity against spontaneous rat tumours. *Internat. J. Cancer 1:*257, 1966.
89. Bubenik, J., Adamcova, B., and Koldovsky, P. A contribution to the question of the antigenicity of spontaneous lymphoid AKR leukaemia. *Folia Biol.* (Prague) *10:*293, 1964.
90. Cryan, W. S., Hyde, R. M. and Garb, S. Demonstration by gel diffusion of antigen in spontaneous mouse tumors. *Cancer Res. 26:*1458, 1966.
91. Gross, L. Immunological relationship of mammary carcinomas developing spontaneously in female mice of a high-tumor line. *J. Immunol. 55:*297, 1947.
92. Lavrin, D. H., Blair, P. B., and Weiss, D. W. Immunology of spontaneous mammary carcinomas in mice 111. Immunogenicity of C3H preneoplastic hyperplastic alveolar nodules in C3Hf hosts. *Cancer Res. 26:*293, 1966.
93. Lavrin, D. H., Dezfulian, M., and Weiss, D. W. The antigen responsible for acquired resistance to spontaneous mammary carcinomas in mice. *Proc. Am. Assoc. Cancer Res. 6:*38, 1965.
94. Lumsden, T. Tumour immunity 11. Antiserum treatment of spontaneous mouse carcinoma. *J. Path. and Bact. 35:*441, 1932.
95. Levi, E. Preparation of an antiserum specific to a spontaneous mouse leukaemia after the induction of artificial immunological tolerance to normal mouse tissue. *Nature 199:*501, 1963.
96. McKenna, J. M. and Prier, J. E. Some immunologic aspects of canine neoplasms. *Cancer Res. 26:*137, 1966.
97. Morton, D. L. Successful isoimmunization against a spontaneous mammary tumor in C3H/HEN mice. *Proc. Am. Assoc. Cancer Res. 3:*346, 1962.
98. Nutini, L. G., Fardon, J. C., Prince, J. E. and Duarte, A. G. Induced resistance to isologous and spontaneous tumors in inbred strains of mice. *Acta Unio. Internat. Contra Cancrum 16:*110, 1960.
99. Old, L. J., Boyse, E. A. and Stockert, E. Antigenic properties of experimental leukemias. 1. Serological studies *in vitro* with spontaneous and radiation-induced leukemias. *J. Nat. Cancer Inst. 31:*977, 1963.

PART IV

100. Podilchak, M. A. The effect of aseptic proliferative inflammation on the localization and growth of spontaneous tumors of the mammary glands in mice of the high-cancer C3HA strain. *Bull. Expt'l. Biol. Med.* (Russ.) (Eng. transl.) *46:*1389, 1958.

101. Wahren, B. Demonstration of a tumor-specific antigen in spontaneously developing AKR lymphomas. *Internat. J. Cancer 1:*41, 1966.

102. Weiss, D. W., Faulkin, L. J., Jr. and DeOme, K. B. Acquisition of heightened resistance and susceptibility to spontaneous mouse mammary carcinomas in the original host. *Cancer Res. 24:*732, 1964.

103. Abramoff, P., Saunders, J. W., Jr. and Gasseling, M. T. Cytotoxicity of heterologous immune chicken serum to normal and neoplastic mouse tissues in culture. *J. Nat. Cancer Inst. 26:*585, 1961.

104. Bashford, E., Murray, J. A. and Cramer, W. The natural and induced resistance of mice to the growth of cancer. *Proc. Roy. Soc., London,* S. B. *79:*164, 1907.

105. Bishop, D. W. Discussion on experimental tumors; the immune state involved in subcutaneous implants of prostatic tissue. *National Cancer Inst. Monograph No. 12, Biology of Prostate and Related Tissues,* 409.

106. Boyse, E. A. Immune responses to experimental tumours. *Guy's Hosp. Rep. 112:* 433, 1963.

107. Boyse, E. A., Old, L. J. and Stockert, E. Some further data on cytotoxic isoantibodies in the mouse. *Ann. N. Y. Acad. Sci. 99:*574, 1962.

108. Bubenik, J. and Koldovsky, P. Mechanism of antitumor immunity studied by means of transfers of immunity. *Folia Biol.* (Prague) *10:*427, 1964.

109. Burmester, R. B. The cytotoxic effect of avian lymphoid tumor antiserum. *Cancer Res. 7:*459, 1947.

110. Dulaney, A. D. and Arnesen, K. Cytotoxic action of antisera to cell components of normal and leukemic mouse spleens. *Proc. Soc. Expt'l. Biol. and Med. 72:*665, 1949.

111. Finney, J. W., Byers, E. H. and Wilson, R. H. Studies in tumor autoimmunity. *Cancer Res. 20:*351, 1960.

112. Fogel, M. and Sachs, L. Studies on the antigenic composition of hamster tumors induced by polyoma virus, and of normal hamster tissues *in vivo* and *in vitro. J. Nat. Cancer Inst. 29:*239, 1962.

113. Foley, E. J. Attempts to induce immunity against mammary adenocarcinoma in inbred mice. *Cancer Res. 13:*578, 1953.

114. Garvie, W. H. H. Studies on induced tumour resistance. *Brit. J. Surg. 53:*69, 1966.

115. Goldfeder, A. Studies on radiosensitivity and "immunizing" ability of mammary tumours of mice. *Brit. J. Cancer 13:*320, 1954.

116. Gorer, P. A. The antigenic structure of tumors: In *Advances in Immunology,* Vol. 1 (Taliaferro, W. H. and Humphrey, J. H. eds.). New York, Academic Press, Inc. 1961, p. 345.

117. Hirsch, H. M. Tumor isoimmunity. *Experientia 14:*269, 1958.

118. Hirsch, H. M. Tumor immunity and tissue transplantation. *Journal-Lancet 79:* 340, 1959.

119. Hirsch, H. M., Bittner, J. J., Cole, H. and Iversen, I. Can the inbred mouse be immunized against it's own tumor? *Cancer Res. 18:*344, 1958.

120. Imagawa, D. T., Syverton, J. T. and Bittner, J. J. The cytotoxicity of serum for mouse mammary cancer cells. 11. The effects upon cells in culture. *Cancer Res. 14:*8, 1954.

121. Kidd, J. G. Distinctive constituents of tumor cells and their possible relations to the phenomena of autonomy, anaplasia, and cancer causation. *Cold Spring Harbor Symposia Quant. Biol.* 11:94, 1946.

122. Klein, G., Antigenicity of tumors in genetically compatible animal hosts: In Emmelot, P. and Muhlbock, O., (ed.), *Cellular Control Mechanisms and Cancer.* Elsevier, Amsterdam, 1964, p. 236.

123. Klein, G., Sjogren, H. O. and Klein, E. Demonstration of host resistance against isotransplantation of lymphomas induced by the Gross agent. *Cancer Res.* 22:955, 1962.

124. Klein, G., Sjogren, H. O. and Klein, E. Demonstration of host resistance against sarcomas induced by implantation of cellophane films in isologous (syngeneic) recipients. *Cancer Res.* 23:84, 1963.

125. Koldovsky, P. The question of the universality of tumour antigen in isologous and homologous relationships. *Folia Biol.* (Prague) 7:162, 1961.

126. Koldovsky, P. Passive transfer of anti-tumour isoimmunity. *Folia Biol.* (Prague) 7:157, 1961.

127. Koldovsky, P. The question of the choice of method to induce antitumour isoimmunity within a group of mice with controlled antigenic homogeneity. *Folia Biol.* (Prague) 7:115, 1961.

128. Koldovsky, P. Specific tumour immunity and its use in the immunotherapy of experimental tumours. *Acta: Unio Internat. contra Cancrum* 18:187, 1962.

129. Koldovsky, P., Bubenik, J. Occurrence of tumours in mice after inoculation of Rous sarcoma and antigenic changes in these tumours. *Folia Biol.* (Prague) 10:81, 1964.

130. Koldovsky, P. and Svoboda, J. On the question of the mechanism of growth of a tumour against isoimmunity. *Folia Biol.* (Prague) 8:95, 1962.

131. Koldovsky, P., Svoboda, J. Induction of tolerance to tumour antigen. In: *Mechanisms of Immunological Tolerance.* Prague. 1962, p. 215.

132. Koldovsky, P. and Svoboda, J. Sensitivity of a tumour to immunity in relation to its antigenicity. *Folia Biol.* (Prague) 8:144, 1962.

133. Levi, E., Schechtman, A. M., Sherins, R. S. and Tobias, S. Tumor specificity and immunologic suppression. *Nature* 184:563, 1959.

134. Lumsden, T. Further observations on immunity in relation to transplantable malignant tumors. *Lancet* 2:112, 1926.

135. Lumsden, T. On the nature of immunity to implanted malignant tumors. *Lancet.* 1:116, 1927.

136. Lumsden, T. Immunity to implanted tumors. *Lancet* 1:366, 1927.

137. Lumsden, T. Tumor immunity. *Amer. J. Cancer* 15:563, 1931.

138. Lumsden, T., Macrae, T. and Skipper, E. The mechanism of homologous tumor immunity. *Lancet* 2:731, 1934.

139. Malmgren, R. A. Influence of antigenic factors in the production of antitumor cytotoxic sera. *J. Nat. Cancer Inst.* 20:417, 1958.

140. Matsuoka, Y., Nakayama, M., Hamaoka, T., Okada, Y. and Yamaumra, Y. Antibody response of the tumor-bearing animals. *Gann* 56:503, 1965.

141. Miroff, G. Localization of an inhibitor preventing mammary tumour development in mice. *Nature* 212:1259, 1966.

142. Moller, E., and Moller, G. Quantitative studies of the sensitivity of normal and neoplastic mouse cells to the cytotoxic action of isoantibodies. *J. Expt'l. Med.* 115:527, 1962.

143. Old, L. J. and Boyse, E. A. Specific antigens of tumors and leukemias of experimental animals. *Med. Clin. N. Amer.* 50:901, 1966.

PART IV

144. Old, L. J., Boyse, E. A. and Stockert, E. The G (Gross) leukemia antigen. *Cancer Res. 25:*813, 1965.
145. Pikovski, M. A. and Witz, I. P. Antigenic composition of normal tissues and tumours in an inbred strain of mice. Changes in certain globulins associated with tumour growth. *Brit. J. Cancer, 15:*584, 1961.
146. Osler, A. B. Immunologic studies of autochthonous cancer—An evaluation of several procedures. *Cancer Res. 21:*1187, 1961.
147. Russell, B. R. G. The manifestation of active resistance to the growth of implanted cancer. *Fifth Scientific Report, Imperial Cancer Research Fund,* London, 1912. (p. 1).
148. Schrek, R. and Preston, F. W. An anti-tumor factor in the blood of tumor immune rats. *Surg. Forum 5:*631, 1954.
149. Schrek, R. and Preston, F. W. Cytotoxicity of a homologous immune serum to a transplantable rat tumor by the method of unstrained cell counts. *Cancer Res. 17:*102, 1957.
150. Sekla, B. and Holeckova, E. Production of antitumour factors in homologous and heterologous immune systems. *Acta Unio Internat. Contra Cancer 18:*76, 1962.
151. Spar, I. L., Bale, W. F., Goodland, R. L., Caserett, G. W. and Michaelson, S. W. Distribution of injected 1131-labeled antibody to dog fibrin in tumor-bearing dogs. *Cancer Res. 20:*1501, 1960.
152. Stuck, B., Boyse, E. A., Old, L. J., and Carswell, E. A. ML: A new antigen found in leukaemias and mammary tumours of the mouse. *Nature 203:*1033, 1964.
153. Stuck, B., Old, L. J. and Boyse, E. A. Occurrence of soluble antigen in the plasma of mice with virus-induced leukemia. *Proc. N. A. S. 52:*950, 1964.
154. Takeda, K., Tsuji, Y. Maruyama, K. and Maki, T. Immunological correlation between DAB hepatoma and MC sarcoma induced in an identical rat. *Gann 51: (suppl.)* 273, 1960.
155. Wigzell, H. Immunological depression of tumor growth in F_1 hybrid/parental strain systems. *Cancer Res. 21:*365, 1961.
156. Wissler, R. W. and Flax, M. H. Cytotoxic effects of antitumor serum. *Ann. N. Y. Acad. Sci. 69:*773, 1957-1958.
157. Witz, I., Hermann, G., Pikovski, M. and Gross, J. The antigenic composition of tumours, sera and urines of tumour-bearing mice and the partial purification of two antigens present in increased amounts. *Brit. J. Cancer 18:*397, 1964.
158. Woglom, W. H. Immunity to transplantable tumours. *Cancer Rev. 4:*129, 1929.
159. Yoshida, T. O. and Southam, C. M. Attempts to find cell associated immune reaction against autochthonous tumors. *Japan J. Exp. Med. 33:*369, 1963.
160. Martin, D. S., Fugmann, R. A. and Hayworth, P. Surgery, cancer chemotherapy, host defenses, and tumor size. *J. Nat. Cancer Inst. 29:*817, 1962.
161. Abelev, G. I. and Zvetkov, V. S. The method of isolation of specific antigens of tumour and normal tissue. *Acta Unio Internat. Contra Cancer 18:*91, 1962.
162. Afonso, E. Electrophoretic patterns of tumour tissue proteins. *J. Clin. Path. 16:*375, 1963.
163. Day, E. D. and Pressman, D. Purification of tumor-localizing antibodies. *Ann. N. Y. Acad. Sci. 69:*651, 1957.
164. Engelhardt, N. V. Study of monospecific antitumour sera by the method of fluorescent antibodies. *Acta Unio Internat. Contra Cancer 18:*94, 1962.
165. Gardashyan, A. M., Avenirova, Z. A. and Brondz, B. D. Analysis of the anaphylaxis-desensitization reaction for the study of tumor antigens. *Acta Unio Internat. Contra Cancer 18:*83, 1962.
166. Gluck, E. Fluorescent antibodies in cancer research: A review. *Cancer Res. 22:*895, 1962.

CHAPTER 23

167. Goster, B. S. The immunochemistry of malignant change in tissues. *Herald of the Academy of Med. Sci.* (Moscow) *15:*41, 1960.
168. Makari, J. G. The polysaccharide behaviour of cancer antigens. *Brit. M. J. 1:* 355, 1958.
169. McKenna, J. M., Sanderson, R. P., and Blakemore, W. S. Extraction of distinctive antigens from neoplastic tissues. *Science,* 135, 1962.
170. McKhann, C. F. Methods of detecting cancer antigens and anti-tumor antibody. *Fed. Proc. 24:*1033, 1965.
171. Perez-Cuadrado, S., Haberman, S. and Race, G. J. Cancerous and normal tissue antigens studies by immunohistochemical and ultrastructural methods. *Cancer 18:* 73, 1965.
172. Phelan, J. T. Some aspects of localizing antitumor antibodies as applied to regional perfusion. *Can. Chem. Rep.* Dec. 1960, p. 131.
173. Rapport, M. M. and Graf, L. Immunochemical studies of organ and tumor lipids I. The production of antibodies against a lipid haptene by injection of the mitochondrial fraction of rat lymphosarcoma. *Cancer 8:*538, 1955.
174. Rapport, M. M., Graf, L. and Alonzo, N. Immunochemical studies of organ and tumor lipids. II. Organ and species specificity of the lipid antigens of the lymphosarcoma. *Cancer 8:*546, 1955.
175. Sjoegren, H. O. Transplantation methods as a tool for detection of tumor-specific antigens. *Prog. Exper. Tumor Res. 6:*289, 1965.
176. Wissler, R. W., Barker, P. A., Flax, M. H., LaVia, M. F. and Talmage, D. W. A study of the preparation, localization and effects of antitumor antibodies labeled with 1131. *Cancer Res. 16:*761, 1956.
177. Adelsberger, L. and Zimmerman, H. M. Skin sensitizing properties of antihuman tumor sera. *Internat. Arch. Allergy 21:*249, 1962.
178. Aizawa, M. and Southam, C. M. Serum antibodies following homotransplantation of human cancer cells. *Ann. N. Y. Acad. Sci. 87:*293, 1960.
179. Bergol'ts, V. M. and Shersul'skaia, L. V. The antigenetic properties of "human leukemic factor" cultivated on the choriollantoic membrane of the chick embryo. *Biull. Eksptl. Biol.* 1 Med. (Moscow) *45:*84, 1958.
180. Björklund, B. and Björklund, V. Antigenicity of pooled human malignant and normal tissues by cyto-immunological technique: presence of an insoluble, heat-labile tumor antigen. *Internat. Arch. Allergy and Appl. Immunol. 10:*153, 1957.
181. Blakemore, W. S. and McKenna, J. M. Presence in patients with malignancies of antibodies reactive with antigens derived from HeLa and J-111. *Surgery 52:*213, 1962.
182. Björklund, B., Björklund, V. and Hedlof, I. Antigenicity of pooled human malignant and normal tissues by cytoimmunological technique. 111. Distribution of tumor antigen. *J. Nat. Cancer Inst. 26:*533, 1961.
183. Blakemore, W. S. and McKenna, J. M. Antigenic distinction of human tumors. *Acta Unio. Internat. Contra Cancer 19:*151, 1963.
184. Day, E. D., Lassiter, S., Woodhall, B., Mahaley, J. L. and Mahaley, M. S., Jr. The localization of radioantibodies in human brain tumors 1. Preliminary exploration. *Cancer Res. 25:*773, 1965.
185. DeCarvalho, S. Segration of antigens from human leukemic and tumoral cells by fluorocarbon extraction. 1. Detection by a gel diffusion method. *J. Lab. Clin. Med. 56:*333, 1960.
186. DeCarvalho, S. Preparation of antigens specific of human breast carcinoma by an immunochromatographic method. *Nature 203:*1186, 1964.

187. DeCarvalho, S. and Rand, H. J. Antigens in human tumors revealed in suppressed rabbits rendered tolerant to normal human tissues. *Exper. and Molecular Path. 2:*32, 1963.
188. Enneking, W. F. Immunological aspects of osteogenic sarcoma. *J. Bone and Joint Surg. 44(A):*1027, 1962.
189. Fujiwara, E. The relationship between the peptide structure and the immunological activity of the serum albumin of patients with carcinoma. *Gann 53:*159, 1962.
190. Gorodilova, V. V. Specific antigen of breast cancer. *Problems Oncol.* (Moscow) *5:*59, 1959.
191. Grace, J. T., Jr. and Kondo, T. Investigation of host resistance in cancer patients. *Ann. Surg. 148:*633, 1958.
192. Grace, J. T., Jr. and Lehoczky, A. Tumor-host relationship factors in man. *Surgery 46:*238, 1959.
193. Gragerova, P. E. Antigens of malignant tumors of the human stomach. *Prob. Oncol.* (Moscow) *7:*36, 1961.
194. Graham, J. B. and Graham, R. M. Antibodies elicited by cancer in patients. *Cancer 8:*409, 1955.
195. Hughes, L. E. and Lytton, B. Antigenic properties of human tumours: Delayed cutaneous hypersensitivity reactions. *Brit. Med. J. 1:*209, 1964.
196. Itakura, K. Studies on human cancer antigens by gel diffusion method. *Gann 54:* 93, 1963.
197. Kolmylova, V. N. and Yeroshkina, A. M. Similarities and differences in the antigenic composition of human sarcoma and leukaemic tissues. *Prob. Oncol.* (Moscow) *5:*1, 1959.
198. Korngold, L. The distribution and immunochemical properties of human tissue and tumor antigens. *Ann. N. Y. Acad. Sci. 69:*681, 1957.
199. Korngold, L. The distribution and immunochemical properties of human tissue and tumor antigens. *Ann. N. Y. Acad. Sci. 69:*681, 1957-1958.
200. Korngold, L. Antigenic specificity of myeloma globulins. *J. of the Nat. Cancer Inst. 30:*553, 1963.
201. Korngold, L. and VanLeeuwen, G. Immunological and electrophoretic studies of human tissue and tumor antigens. *Cancer Res. 17:*775, 1957.
202. Loisillier, F. et al. Immunologic studies on mammary epitheliomas in humans. *Ann. Inst. Pasteur 109:*1, 1965.
203. Mahaley, M. S., Jr., Mahaley, J. L. and Day, E. D. The localization of radioantibodies in human brain tumors 11. Radioautography. *Cancer Res. 25:*779, 1965.
204. Makari, J. G. Detection of antigens in sera of patients with neoplastic disease by Schultz-Dale test. *Brit. Med. J. 2:*358, 1958.
205. Marchbanks, R. M. The "full" antigen of cancerous and normal human tissues. *Internat. Abstr. Biol. Sci. Immunol. & Exper. Path. 23:*86, 1961.
206. McKenna, J. M., Sanderson, R. P. and Blakemore, W. S. Demonstration of a soluble antigen in some human tumors. *Fed. Proc. 23:*351, 1964.
207. McKenna, J. M., Sanderson, R. P. and Blakemore, W. S. Studies of the antigens of human tumors. 1. Demonstration of a soluble specific antigen in HeLa cells and some human tumors. *Cancer Res. 24:*754, 1964.
208. McKenna, J. M., Sanderson, R. P., Davis, F. E. and Blakemore, W. S. Studies on the antigens of human tumors. 11. Demonstration of a soluble specific antigen (G) in cell lines derived from malignant human tissue. *Cancer Res. 26:*984, 1966.
209. Miller, D. G. and Hsu, T. C. The action of cytotoxic antisera on the HeLa strain of human carcinoma. *Cancer Res. 16:*306, 1956.

210. Mountain, I. M. Cytopathogenic effect of antiserum to human malignant epithelial cells (strain HeLa) on HeLa cell culture. *J. Immunol. 75:*478, 1955.
211. Perez-Cuadrado, S., Haberman, S. and Race, G. J. Production of specific antisera to human cancer cell nuclear antigens. *Fed. Proc. 23:*451, 1964.
212. Perez-Cuadrado, S., Haberman, S. and Race, G. J. Production of specific antisera to human cancerous tissues. 1. Use of differential centrifugation and nucleic acid enzymes in antigen preparation. *Dallas M. J. 50:*77, 1964.
213. Takayanagi, N., Asakura, S., Kenbe, M. and Isikawa, T. Antigen analysis of body fluid in cancer patients. *Gann 50:*232, 1959.
214. Takayanagi, N. and Miyaki, Y. Immunological analysis of the paraprotein fractions in the sera from patients with malignant tumors. *Gann 51:(Suppl.)* 265, 1960.
215. Takayanagi, N. Antigen analysis of sera from patients with malignant tumors by immunodiffusion methods. *Gann 56:*317, 1965.
216. Tee, D. E. H., Wang, M. and Watkins, J. Antigenic properties of human tumours. *Nature 203:*987, 1964.
217. Wilson, R. H., Byers, E. H., Schram, A. C. and Delaney, L. R. Common immunochemical properties of tumors. *Clin. Res. 11:*62, 1963.
218. Wilson, R. H., Byers, E. H., Schram, A. C. and Shields, W. F. Host resistance to cancer. 111. Studies in human tumor autoimmunity. In: *Conceptual Advances in Immunology and Oncology.* Hoeber Medical Division, Harper and Row, N. Y., 1962, p. 521.
219. Aizawa, M., Imamura, T., Motoyama, T., Kasai, S., Tozawa, T., Abe, H., Sasage, S. and Ikeda, K. On immunological therapy of Yoshida sarcoma. *Gann 42:*138, 1952.
220. Delorme, E. J. and Alexander, P. Treatment of primary fibrosarcoma in the rat with immune lymphocytes. *Lancet 2:*117, 1964.
221. Kidd, J. G. Suppression of growth of the Brown-Pearce tumor by a specific antibody. *Science 99:*348, 1944.
222. Kidd, J. G. Suppression of growth of Brown-Pearce tumor cells by a specific antibody; with a consideration of the nature of the reacting cell constituent. *J. Expt'l. Med. 83:*227, 1946.
223. Koldovsky, P. Combined surgical removal and specific immunotherapy of experimental tumours. *Folia Biol.* (Prague) *8:*90, 1962.
224. Motoyama, T., Tozawa, T., Aizawa, M. and Imamura, T. The therapeutic effect upon Yoshida sarcoma of immune sera against Yoshida sarcoma of rabbit absorbed with several methods. *Gann 43:*248, 1952.
225. Nettleship, A. Regression produced in the Murphy lymphosarcoma by the injection of heterologous antibodies. *Am. J. Pathology 21:*527, 1945.
226. Bogomolets, A. A. Anti-reticular cytotoxic serum as a means of pathogenetic therapy. *Am. Rev. Soviet Med. 1:*101, 1943, also *Brit. M. J. 2:*203, 1943.
227. Bogomolets, A. A. New trends in therapy and prophylaxis of cancer. *Soviet Med. 9:*3, 1944.
228. DeCarvalho, S. Preliminary experimentation with specific immunotherapy of neoplastic disease in man. 1. Immediate effects of hyperimmune equine gamma globulin. *Cancer 16:*306, 1963.
229. Graham, J. B. and Graham, R. M. The effect of vaccine on cancer patients. *Surg., Gyn. and Obst. 109:*131, 1959.
230. Klein, G. Recent trends in tumor immunology. *Israel J. Med. Sci. 2:*135, 1966.
231. Sacks, J. H. and Hume, D. M. Attempts to induce immunity to cancer with autogenous tumor nucleoprotein. *Clin. Res. 11:*46, 1963.

PART IV

232. von Leyden, E. and Blumenthal, F. Attempts to immunize humans by inoculation of their own cancer. *Deutsch. Med. Wochensch. 28:*637, 1902.
233. Attia, M. Enhancement of a spontaneous tumor in the strain of origin following vaccination with a tumor membrane fraction. *Proc. Am. Assoc. Cancer Res. 4:* 3, 1963.
234. Hirsch, H. M. and Iversen, I. Accelerated development of spontaneous mammary tumors in mice pretreated with mammary tumor tissue and adjuvant. *Cancer Res. 21:*752, 1961.
235. McHugh, R. B., Faulkner, J. E. and Hirsch, H. M. A multivariate analysis of some experiments in tumor immunity. *Folia Biol. 9:*171, 1963.
236. Kaliss, N. Acceptance of tumor homografts by mice injected with antiserum. 11. Effect of time of injection. *Proc. Soc. Expt'l. Biol. and Med. 91:*432, 1956.
237. Kaliss, N. and Kandutsch, A. A. Acceptance of tumor homografts by mice injected with antiserum. 1. Activity of serum fractions. *Proc. Soc. Expt'l. and Med. 91:*118, 1956.
238. Miroff, S., Martinez, C. and Bittner, J. J. Acceleration in the transplantation and killing time of mammary tumors in mice pretreated with a heat stable tumor tissue preparation. *Cancer Res. 15:*437, 1955.
239. Snell, G. D., Cloudman, A. M., Factor, E. and Douglass, P. Inhibition and stimulation of tumor homotransplants by prior injections of lyophilized tumor tissue. *J. Nat. Cancer Inst. 6:*303, 1946.
240. Castellanos, H., Ketchel, M. M. and Sturgis, S. H. Immunologic acceleration of death in animals with transplanted tumors. *Cancer Res. 26:*1921, 1966.
241. Flexner, S. and Jobling, J. W. On the promoting influence of heated tumor emulsions on tumor growth. *Proc. Soc. Expt'l. Biol. and Med. 4:*156, 1907.
242. Gitlitz, G. F., Ship, A. G., Glick, J. L. and Glick, A. H. Local inhibition and enhancement of growth of transplanted tumor cells in mice. *J. Surg. Res. 3:*370, 1963.
243. Kaliss, N. and Bryant, B. F. Factors determining homograft destruction and immunological enhancement in mice receiving successive tumor inocula. *J. Nat. Cancer Inst. 20:*691, 1958.
244. Moller, E. Interaction between tumor and host during progressive neoplastic growth in histoincompatible recipients. *J. Nat. Cancer Inst. 35:*1053, 1965.
245. Bubeník, J., Iványi, J. and Koldovský, P. Participation of 7S and 19S antibodies in enhancement and resistance to methylcholanthrene-induced tumours. *Folia Biol.* (Prague) *6:*426, 1965.
246. Wodinsky, I., Helinski, A. and Kensler, C. J. Enhancement of transplantability of 3, 4, 9, 10-Dibenzpyrene-induced fibrosarcoma in random-bred mice. *Nature 209:*414, 1966.
247. Adams, R. A. Enhancing agent in the plasma of Syrian hamsters bearing a heterotransplantable murine leukemia. *Fed. Proc. 22:*514, 1963.
248. Bubenik, J. and Koldovsky, P. The mechanism of antitumour immunity studied by means of transfers of immunity. *Folia Biol.* (Prague) *10:*427, 1964.
249. Phillips, M. E. and Stetson, C. A. Passive transfer of immunity to Sarcoma 1 with serum. *Proc. Soc. Expt'l. Biol. and Med. 111:*265, 1962.
250. Batchelor, J. R. The mechanisms and significance of immunological enhancement. *Guy's Hosp. Rep. 112:*345, 1963.
251. Berne, B. H. Immunological homograft enhancement. Interactions of antiserum and skin and tumor homografts. *Proc. Soc. Expt'l. Biol. Med. 118:*228, 1965.
252. Billingham, R. E., Brent, L., and Medawar, P. B. "Enhancement" in normal homografts, with a note on its possible mechanism. *Transplantation Bull. 3:*84, 1956.

CHAPTER 23

253. Boyse, E. A., Old, L. J. and Stockert, E. Immunological enhancement of a leukemia. *Nature 194:*1142, 1962.
254. Bubenik, J., Ivanyi, J. and Koldovsky, P. Heterogeneity of antitumour antibodies. *Folia Biol.* (Prague) *11:*240, 1965.
255. Green, H. N. and Wilson, R. Further observations on tumor-enhancing factors: their bearing on the immunological theory of cancer. *Nature 182:*1054, 1958.
256. Green, H. N. and Wilson, R. Nature of the tumor-enhancing factor. *Nature 178:* 851, 1956.
257. Halasz, N. A. and Orloff, M. J. The passive transfer of enhancement as applied to skin homografts. *J. Immunol. 94:*253, 1965.
258. Haskova, V. and Svoboda, J. Relationship between transplantation immunity and immunological enhancement. In: *Mechanisms of Immunological Tolerance.* Hasek, M., Lengerova, A. and Vojtiskova, M., Eds. *Czech. Acad. Sci.* Praha, 1962, p. 431.
259. Haskova, V., Svoboda, J. and Matousek, V. Relationships between transplantation immunity and immunological enhancement. *Folia Biol.* (Prague) *8:*16, 1962.
260. Ichihashi, H. Influence of immune responses on tumor growth. *Gann 56:*223, 1965.
261. Kaliss, N. Immunological enhancement of tumor homografts in mice: A review. *Cancer Res. 18:*992, 1958.
262. Kaliss, N. The elements of immunologic enhancement: A consideration of mechanisms. *Ann. N. Y. Acad. Sci. 101:*64, 1962.
263. Kaliss, N. The induction of the homograft reaction in the presence of immunological enhancement of tumor homografts. In: *Mechanisms of Immunological Tolerance.* Hasek, M., Lengerova, A. and Vojtiskova, M., Eds. *Czech. Acad. Sci.* Praha, 1962, p. 413.
264. Kaliss, N. Immunological enhancement the immunologically induced prolongation of tumor homograft survival. In: *Proc. 10th Congr. Intern. Soc. Blood Transf.:* Karger. Basel, 1964, p. 91.
265. Kaliss, N. Immunological enhancement and inhibition of tumor growth: relationship to various immunological mechanisms. *Fed. Proc. 24:*1024, 1965.
266. Kaliss, N. Immunological enhancement: Conditions for its expression and its relevance for grafts of normal tissues. *Ann. N. Y. Acad. of Sci. 129:*155, 1966.
267. Möller, G. Studies on the mechanism of immunological enhancement of tumor homografts. 1. Specificity of immunological enhancement. *J. Nat. Cancer Inst. 30:*1153, 1963.
268. Möller, G. Studies on the mechanism of immunological enhancement of tumor homografts. 11. Effect of isoantibodies on various tumor cells. *J. Nat. Cancer Inst. 30:*1177, 1963.
269. Möller, G. Studies on the mechanism of immunological enhancement of tumor homografts. 111. Interaction between humoral isoantibodies and immune lymphoid cells. *J. Nat. Cancer Inst. 30:*1205, 1963.
270. Movitz, D., Saphir, O. and Strauss, A. A. Effects of an antireticular cytotoxic serum on the Brown-Pearce carcinoma of the rabbit. *Cancer Res. 9:*17, 1949.
271. Ruszkiewicz, M. Relationship between enhancing and sensitizing properties of transplantation antigens in the mouse. *Conf. on Tumor Antigens,* Sukhumi, 1965.
272. Snell, G. D. The suppression of the enhancing effect in mice by the addition of donor lymph nodes to the tumor inoculum. *Transplantation Bull. 3:*83, 1956.
273. Snell, G. D., Winn, H. J., Stimpfling, J. H. and Parker, S. J. Depression by antibody of the immune response to homografts and its role in immunological enhancement. *J. Exp. Med. 112:*293, 1960.

217

PART IV

274. Voisin, G. A. Greffes tumorales et facilitation immunologique ("immunological enhancement"). *Rev. Franc. Etudes Clin. et Biol. 8:*927, 1963.
275. Wheatley, D. N. and Easty, G. C. The growth and infiltration of Ehrlich's ascites tumour in mice with reduced immunological responses. *Brit. J. Cancer 18:*743, 1966.
276. Southam, C. M. Relationship of immunology to cancer: A review. *Cancer Res. 20:*271, 1960.
277. Feldman, M. and Globerson, A. Studies on the mechanism of immunological enhancement of tumor grafts. *J. Nat. Cancer Inst. 25:*631, 1960.
278. National Advisory Cancer Council—*Progress Against Cancer, 1966.* U. S. Dept. of H. E. W., Washington, p. 63.
279. Sulzberger, M. B. Arsphenamine hypersensitiveness in guinea pigs. I. Experiments in prevention and in desensitization. *Arch. Dermat. and Syph. 20:*669, 1929.
280. Sulzberger, M. B. Arsphenamine hypersensitiveness in guinea pigs. II. Experiment demonstrating the role of the skin, both as originator and as site of the hypersensitiveness. *Arch. Derm. and Syph. 22:*839, 1930.
281. Chase, M. W. Inhibition of experimental drug allergy by prior feeding of the sensitizing agent. *Proc. Soc. Expt'l. Biol. and Med. 61:*257, 1956.
282. Frey, J. R., Geleick, H. and deWeck, A. Immunologic tolerance induced in animals previously sensitized to simple chemical compounds. *Science 144:*853, 1964.
283. Taliaferro, W. H. and Humphrey, J. H. *Advances in Immunology,* Vol. 1, Academic Press, N. Y., 1961, p. 49.
284. Apffel, C. A., Arnason, B. G. and Peters, J. H. Induction of tumour immunity with cells treated with iodoacetate. *Nature 209:*694, 1966.
285. Jutila, J. W., Weiser, R. S. & Evans, C. A. Immunization of the A/Jax mouse with irradiated cells of its indigenous tumour, Sarcoma 1. *Nature 195:*301, 1962.
286. Molomut, N., Gross, L. and Padnos, M. Immunological properties of tumours. *Nature 198:*38, 1963.
287. Polglase, W. J. Immunization against Ehrlich's ascites carcinoma with streptomycin complexes from tumour cells. *Nature 197:*301, 1963.
288. Revesz, L. Detection of antigenic differences in isologous host-tumor systems by pretreatment with heavily irradiated tumor cells. *Cancer Res. 20:*443, 1960.
289. Czajkowski, N. P., Rosenblatt, M., Cushing, F. R., Vasquez, J. and Wolf, P. L. Production of active immunity to malignant neoplastic tissue. Chemical coupling to an antigenic protein carrier. *Cancer 19:*739, 1966.
290. Fink, A. M., Smith, P. and Rothlauf, M. V. Antibody production in BALB/c mice following injection of lyophilized tumor S621 in Freund's adjuvant. *Proc. Soc. Expt'l. Biol. and Med. 90:*590, 1955.
291. Freund, J. The mode of action of immunologic adjuvants. *Advances in Tuberc. Res. 7:*130, Karger. Basel, Switzerland and New York, N. Y., 1956.
292. Kabat, E. A., Wolf, A. and Bezer, A. E. The rapid production of acute disseminated encephalomyelitis in rhesus monkeys by injection of heterologous and homologous brain tissue with adjuvants. *J. Expt'l. Med. 85:*117, 1947.
293. Waksman, B. H. and Adams, R. D. Allergic neuritis: An experimental disease of rabbits induced by the injection of peripheral nervous tissue and adjuvants. *J. Expt'l. Med. 102:*213, 1955.
294. Rhodes, E. L. An attempt to obtain auto-immunity to tumours with Freund's adjuvant and tetanus toxoid. *Nature 193:*1091, 1962.
295. Schoenberg, M. D. and Moore, R. D. The failure of Freund's adjuvant to affect the survival of mice with transplanted sarcoma 180. *Cancer Res. 20:*1505, 1960.
296. Harwin, S. M., Paterson, P. Y. and Didakow, N. C. Antibodies against autologous brain in rats with allergic encephalomyelitis. *Nature 189:*322, 1961.

297. Nakahara, W. Studies on lymphoid activity. VI. Immunity to transplanted cancer induced by injection of olive oil. *J. Expt'l. Med. 35:*493, 1922.
298. Nakahara, W. Studies on lymphoid activity. VII. Suppression of induced immunity to transplanted cancer by large doses of olive oil. *J. Expt'l. Med. 38:*315, 1923.
299. Nakahara, W. Effect of fatty acids on the resistance of mice to transplanted cancer. *J. Expt'l. Med. 40:*363, 1924.
300. Nakahara, W. Resistance to spontaneous mouse cancer induced by injections of oleic acid. *J. Expt'l. Med. 41:*347, 1925.
301. Nadler, S. H., and Moore, E. G. Clinical immunologic study of malignant disease: Response to tumor transplants and transfer of leukocytes. *Ann. Surg. 164:*482, 1966.
302. Brondz, B. D., Antibodies to the specific antigen of tumor cell membrane. *Prob. Oncol.* (Moscow) *10:*81, 1964.
303. Bullock, F. D. and Rohdenburg, G. L. Fluctuations in concomitant immunity. *J. Cancer Res. 5:*129, 1920.
304. Caspari, W. *Tumor and Immunitat.* Strahlentherap. *15:*831, 1923.
305. Chambers, H. and Russ, S. Immunity to tumor growth and other experimental investigations—a reply to recent criticism. *J. Cancer Res. 10:*109, 1926.
306. Chambers, H. and Scott, G. M. Experiments upon immunity to tumour growth. *Lancet 1:*212, 1922.
307. Chambers, H. and Scott, G. M. Experiments on immunity to tumor growth. *Brit. J. Expt'l. Path. 5:*1, 1924.
308. Cinader, B. Perspectives and prospects of immunotherapy autoantibodies and acquired immunological tolerance. *Canad. Cancer Conf. 5:*279, 1963.
309. Goldstein, M. N. and Hiramoto, R. Cytotoxicity of a horse antihuman cancer serum for normal and malignant cells *in vitro. J. Nat. Cancer Inst. 27:*487, 1961.
310. Greenspan, I., Brown, E. R. and Schwartz, S. O. Immunologically specific antigens in leukemic tissues. *Blood 21:*717, 1963.
311. Haddow, A. Immunology of the cancer cell: Tumour-specific antigens. *Brit. Med. Bull. 21:*133, 1965.
312. Kampschmidt, R. F. and Upchurch, H. F. Effect of bacterial contamination of the tumor on tumor-host relationships. *Cancer Res. 23:*756, 1963.
313. Kellock, T. H., Chambers, H. and Russ, S. An attempt to procure immunity to malignant disease in man. *Lancet 1:*217, 1922.
314. Kidd, J. G. Does the host react against his own cancer cells? *Cancer Res. 21:* 1170, 1961.
315. Martin, D. S. Evidence for a host defense adjuvant to chemotherapy against spontaneous cancer. *Proc. Amer. Assoc. Cancer Res. 3:*341, 1962.
316. McKenna, J. M., Sanderson, R. P. and Blakemore, W. S. Specificity of antigens in extracts from HeLa and J-111 cells. *Fed. Proc. 20:*150, 1961.
317. Mikulska, Z. B., Smith, C. and Alexander, P. Evidence for an immunological reaction of the host directed against its own actively growing primary tumor. *J. Nat. Canc. Inst. 36:*29, 1966.
318. Molomut, N. A hypothesis of progression of malignancy based on immune responses. *Neoplasma 10:*155, 1963.
319. Murray, G. Experiments in immunity in cancer. *Canad. Med. Assn. J. 79:*249, 1958.
320. Nairn, R. C., Philips, J., Ghose, T., Porteous, I. B. and Fothergill, J. E. Production of a precipitin against renal cancer. *Brit. Med. J. 1:*1702, 1963.
321. Nairn, R. C., Richmond, H. G. and McEntegard, M. G. Immunological differences between normal and malignant cells. *Brit. Med. J. 2:*1335, 1960.

PART IV

322. Old, L. J., Benacerraf, B., Clarke, D. A., Carswell, E. A. and Stockert, E. The role of the reticuloendothelial system in the host reaction to neoplasia. *Cancer Res. 21:*1281, 1961.
323. Prehn, R. T. Failure of immunizations against tumorigenesis. *J. Nat. Cancer Inst. 26:*223, 1961.
324. Rapport, M. M. and Graf, L. Cancer antigens: How specific should they be? *Cancer Res. 21:*1225, 1961.
325. Sachs, L. Immunogenetic properties of tumour cells. *Abstracts of Papers, 7th Internat. Cancer Congress, 1958,* London, p. 11.
326. Russ, S. New attempts to procure immunity to malignant disease in man. *Canad. Med. Assn. J. 12:*841, 1922.
327. Southam, C. M. Immunopathology of cancer. *Fed. Proc. 24:*1007, 1965.
328. Spencer, R. R. Tumor immunity. *J. Nat. Cancer Inst. 2:*317, 1942.
329. Stern, K. Immunological approaches to the cancer problem. *Chicago Med. School Quart. 14:*68, 1953.
330. Stern, K. A new approach to tumor immunity. *Nature 185:*787, 1960.
331. Stern, K. Host factors in neoplastic disease: A review of current concepts and trends in cancer research. *Hebrew Med. J. 1 & 2:*1, 1962.
332. Takeda, K., Kikuchi, K., Itakura, K. and Tanigaki, N. Studies on the localization of the specific antigen in tumor cells. *Gann 51:(Supp.)*272, 1960.
333. Tyler, A. An immunological analysis of cancer. *J. Nat. Cancer Inst. 25:*1197, 1960.
334. Tyzzer, E. E. Tumor immunity. *J. Cancer Res. 1:*125, 1916.
335. Vaughan, J. W. and Eppler, H. H. The immune mechanism in cancer. *Trans. Amer. Surg. Assn. 41:*421, 1923.
336. Witebsky, E., Rose, N. R. and Shulman, S. Studies of normal and malignant tissue antigens. *Cancer Res. 16:*831, 1956.
337. Zil'ber, L. A. Specific component of malignant tumors. *Uspekhi Sovremennoi Biologii 30:*188, 1950. Translated at N. I. H., Bethesda, Md.
338. Zilber, L. A. Studies on tumor antigens. *J. Nat. Cancer Inst. 18:*341, 1957.

Factors Affecting Metastases

One of the most important characteristics of cancer cells is their ability to migrate to distant sites in the body and there to continue multiplying and invading. This is referred to as "metastasis"; a secondary growth that is the result is also called metastasis (plural: metastases). The metastases cause most of the deaths from cancer. Our surgeons are capable of removing almost all primary cancers. However, after the primary cancer has been removed, metastases grow in distant organs, including lungs, liver and brain. Usually, metastases are multiple, and there is little chance of removing them surgically.

At times, migrating cancer cells lodge in a distant organ and remain dormant; for years, they neither multiply nor invade. Then, they may suddenly begin to grow and invade. Dormancy is an important feature of some metastases, but we do not know which factors promote dormancy and which tend to oppose it.

If metastasis could be controlled, it would be possible to save over 90 per cent of cancer patients; accordingly, this phenomenon deserves intensive study.

(Metastasis occurs not only in cancer but also in several bacterial diseases. The bacteria migrate from the original site to other, distant sites, and set up new foci of infection.)

More than 50 years ago, Weil (1) and Takahashi (2) demonstrated that only a small proportion of wandering cancer cells actually become metastases. More recently, Engell (3), and Cole and his associates (4) have demonstrated the same thing.

Some general studies have examined several of the factors that may promote or hinder the establishment and growth of metastases, and have tentatively evaluated them (5-39). The work of several investigators suggests that the nature and behavior of the host tissue in which the cancer cells lodge is of considerable importance (40-42). In contrast, at least one group of scientists (43) considered the role played by the host tissue to be minor.

There is one aspect of the relationship of host tissue to metastasis that seems of great practical importance. It has been proven beyond

221

doubt that trauma greatly increases the likelihood that a particular area may become the site of a metastasis. The nature of the trauma may vary. Metastasis formation is promoted by surgical trauma (44, 45), even by manipulation of internal organs (14), by inflammation (46), by local trauma and ischemia (47), by injection of irritant or toxic chemicals (48, 49), and by disease in an organ or tissue (50). It seems that anything that disrupts the normal functioning of a tissue or organ may increase the likelihood of metastases forming there.

It has also been observed (52-55) that there is a relationship between the clotting tendency of the blood and the incidence of metastasis. If the blood is more coagulable than normal, small clots may form in peripheral vessels; when a wandering cancer cell becomes attached to a clot, it is much more likely to produce a metastasis than if there is no clot to which it can be become attached. The effects of our current drugs on metastasis are unclear. Deductively, we might conclude that the anti-cancer agents that are used in the treatment of some primary cancers ought to be helpful in preventing or retarding the growth of metastases. The study of Cruz and his associates in 1956 (57) suggested that this might occur. However, subsequent studies by four different teams of investigators (58-61) seem to show that the presently available anti-cancer drugs increase the production of metastases. Clearly, our understanding of the mechanisms that influence the development and growth of metastases is woefully deficient, even though the experimental techniques and equipment needed to clarify these points have been available to us for almost half a century.

The questions about metastasis that ought to be answered without any further delay may be divided into two main groups: those that are directly related to our present clinical management of cancer patients, and those that may lead to new therapeutic approaches.

1. Let us first consider the aspects of metastasis that are directly related to the primary current treatment of cancer—surgery. The main question to be answered is whether a better understanding of the factors influencing metastasis could significantly improve the survival rate after surgery.

Some patients are fortunate enough not to have any circulating cancer cells before or during surgery. These patients will probably be completely cured by the operation, and we need not consider them further.

It seem clear, however, that most cancer patients have circulating cancer cells even before their disease is diagnosed. There is evidence that, during and immediately after the operation on the primary cancer, the stresses on the patient may induce some of the wandering cancer cells to become metastases. How can we reduce the chances of this happening?

Surgeons are well aware of the need for careful, gentle handling during surgery, but, realistically, no surgical operation could possibly avoid trauma and stress completely. The question then is whether different kinds of trauma might involve significantly different risks of metastasis. There might be a difference in the incidence of metastasis if the operative trauma were produced by heat from a cautery, rather than by scalpel, scissors and hemostat.

The type of anesthesia used could also be an important factor in two respects. It has been shown that the presence of chemicals may increase the likelihood of metastases in a particular area (48, 49). Fisher and Fisher (68) have reported that, when chloroform in mineral oil is injected subcutaneously into experimental animals, the incidence of metastases in the liver increases. Presumably, the chloroform is absorbed from the injection site and carried to the liver by the circulation. Inhaled chloroform would probably have a similar effect. Chloroform is rarely used as an anesthetic today, but the fact that one anesthetic agent has been shown to increase metastases should be enough to make us suspect others of also having this action and to warrant further studies in this area. In most operations for cancer, inhalation anesthesia is used, and the gases involved might act as foreign chemicals. Is it possible that the incidence of lung metastases after cancer surgery is high because some of the inhaled gases produce a type of chemical trauma, and cause the wandering or dormant cancer cell to become a metastasis? If this were the case, a change to other types of anesthetics might reduce the high incidence of lung metastasis.

Many of the anesthetic agents in general use tend to lower the blood pressure. Shivas and Finlayson (51) have suggested that a fall of blood pressure (hypotension) may induce metastasis formation. They say:

Turning to the practical management of malignant disease it seems immediately necessary to question the use of hypotensive anesthesia in the patient suffering from a malignant neoplasm.

Thus, we ought to know whether any particular anesthetic agent increases or decreases the likelihood of metastasis, either by acting as a foreign chemical, or by changing the blood pressure, or through any other mechanism.

It is common during and after cancer surgery to give the patient various fluids intravenously. Might they have an effect on metastasis? Garvie and Matheson (56) have presented evidence that suggests that solution of dextrans—both high and low molecular weight—promote the development of metastases from circulating cancer cells. On the other hand, Wood, Baker and Johnson (67) report that the low molecular weight dextrans do not increase lung metastasis in animals. Which report is applicable to metastasis in man? Apparently, metastases are not increased by solutions of dilute glucose or physiologic saline. What effect on metastasis do other intravenous medications have, particularly blood and its derivatives? We do not know.

2. Another group of studies is needed to clarify the mechanisms involved in metastasis. Hopefully, such studies could lead to ways of preventing, controlling or slowing metastatic growth. Some of the questions that need to be answered are:

a. What is the relationship between the growth of the primary cancer and the growth of metastases? Will surgical removal of a primary cancer slow the growth of existing metastases, speed it, or have no significant effect? This question should be answered for all the different kinds of cancers (62-64). How might a combination of surgery and radiation therapy of the primary cancer affect the growth of existing metastases?

b. What effects do our currently available anti-cancer drugs have on the growth rate of existing metastases? Some studies (58-61) suggest that at least some of these drugs have an undesirable effect on metastasis. What about the possible effects of other drugs on metastasis?

c. Which factors increase and which decrease the hospitality of various organs to metastases?

d. Why do some metastases remain dormant for years? Can we make them revert to dormancy? (65, 66)

Most of the studies on metastasis thus far have been done on transplantable cancers, which, as pointed out in Chapter 14, may not furnish answers applicable to metastasis of spontaneous cancers in man. Accordingly, studies on metastasis of spontaneous animal cancers ought to be expanded. Technical problems may make it excessively difficult to do some of these studies. For example, some studies require prolonged intravenous infusion into animals as small as a mouse, and this procedure is technically difficult to carry out.

Unfortunately, spontaneous cancers in rats and rabbits are exceedingly rare. Probably the most suitable animals for such studies would be dogs or pigs with spontaneous cancers. Their availability and advantages are discussed in Chapter 29.

In summary, many facets of the metastasis problem deserve prompt and intensive study. All of the proposed studies can be performed properly with our existing techniques and personnel. Indeed, most of these questions could, and should, have been answered years ago.

References

1. Weil, R. Intravascular implantation of rat tumors. *J. Med. Res. 28:*497, 1913.
2. Takahashi, M. An experimental study of metastasis. *J. Path. Bact. 20:*1, 1915.
3. Engell, H. C. Cancer cells in the circulating blood. *Acta Chir. Scand. (Suppl.) 20:*1, 1955.
4. Cole, W. H., Roberts, S., Watne, A., McDonald, G., and McGrew, E. The dissemination of cancer cells. *N. Y. Acad. Med. Bull. 34:*163, 1958.
5. Levin, I. The mechanism of metastasis formation in experimental cancer. *J. Exp. Med. 18:*397, 1913.
6. Tyzzer, E. E. Factors in the production and growth of tumor metastases. *J. Med. Res. 23:*309, 1913.
7. Cliffton, E. E., and Agostino, D. Factors affecting the development of metastatic cancer. *Cancer 15:*276, 1962.
8. Coman, D. R. Mechanisms responsible for the origins and distribution of bloodborne tumor metastases: A review. *Cancer Res. 13:*397, 1953.
9. Fisher, E. R. and Fisher, B. Experimental studies of factors influencing hepatic metastases. I. Effect of number of tumor cells injected and time of growth. *Cancer 12:*926, 1959.
10. Fisher, B., and Fisher, E. R. Experimental studies of factors influencing hepatic metastases. II. Effect of partial hepatectomy. *Cancer 12:*929, 1959.
11. Fisher, E. R., and Fisher, B. Effect of reticuloendothelial interference on experimental metastases. *Surg. Forum 11:*55, 1960.
12. Fisher, E. R. and Fisher, B. Experimental studies of factors influencing hepatic metastases. V. Effect of cortisone and adrenalectomy. *Cancer Res. 20:*492, 1960.
13. Fisher, E. R., and Fisher, B. Experimental studies of factors influencing hepatic metastases. VII. Effect of reticuloendothelial interference. *Cancer Res. 21:*275, 1961.
14. Fisher, E. R. and Fisher, B. Experimental studies of factors influencing development of hepatic metastases from circulating tumor cells. *Acta Cytol. 9:*146, 1965.
15. Fisher, B. and Fisher, E. R. Experimental studies of factors influencing hepatic metastases. XVI. Rheologic alterations. *Cancer Res. 26:*183, 1966.
16. Fisher, E. R. and Fisher, B. Experimental studies of factors influencing development of hepatic metastases. XVII. Role of thyroid. *Cancer Res. 26:*2248, 1966.
17. Fisher, B., Fisher, E. R., and Lee, S. H. The effect of alteration of liver blood flow upon experimental hepatic metastases. *Surg. Gyn. & Obst. 112:*11, 1961.

18. Fisher, E. R. and Turnbull, R. B., Jr. The cytologic demonstration and significance of tumor cells in the mesenteric venous blood in patients with colorectal carcinoma. *Surg. Gyn. & Obst. 100:*102, 1955.
19. Folkman, J., Long, D. M. and Becker, F. F. Growth and metastasis of tumor in organ culture. *Cancer 16:*453, 1963.
20. Greene, H. S. N. and Harvey, E. K. Metastasis of heterologously transplanted tumors. *Cancer Res. 24:*1678, 1964.
21. Griffin, C. H. Metabolism of cancer cell *in Fundamental Aspects of Normal and Malignant Growth* (Nowinski, ed.). Elsevier Publ. Co., New York, 1960.
22. Karrer, K., Humphreys, S. R. and Golden, A. An experimental model for studying factors which influence metastasis of malignant tumors. *Internat. J. Cancer 2:*213, 1967.
23. Madden, R. E. and Karpas, C. M. Arrest of circulating tumor cells versus metastases formation. *Arch. Surg. 94:*307, 1967.
24. Martinez, C. and Bittner, J. J. Effect of cortisone on lung metastasis production of a transplanted mammary adenocarcinoma. *Proc. Soc. Exptl. Biol. and Med. 89:* 569, 1955.
25. Molomut, N., Spain, D. M., Gault, S. D. and Kreisler, L. Preliminary report on the experimental induction of metastases from a heterologous cancer graft in mice. *Proc. Nat. Acad. Sci. 38:*991, 1952.
26. Selecki, E. E. A study of the metastatic distribution of Ehrlich ascites tumour cells in mice. *Australian J. Exp. Biol. Med. Sci. 37:*489, 1959.
27. Vinogradova, V. D., Podzei, L. K., Mandrik, E. V. and Saraeva, Z. M. Body resistance and some peculiarities of the metastatic process. *Acta Unio. Internat. Contra Cancr. 18:*6, 1962.
28. von Essen, C. F. and Kaplan, H. S. Further studies on metastasis of a transplantable mouse mammary carcinoma after roentgen irradiation. *J. Nat. Cancer Inst. 12:*883, 1952.
29. Watanabe, S. The metastasizability of tumour cells. *Cancer 7:*215, 1954.
30. Willis, R. A. *The Spread of Tumours in the Human Body.* London, J. and A. Churchill, 1934 (p. 162).
31. Willis, R. A. *The Spread of Tumours in the Human Body.* London, Butterworth and Co. 1952 (p. 447).
32. Wissler, R. W. Effects of cytotoxic antibodies on tumour cells and their possible role in controlling metastases. *Bull. of Swiss Acad. Med. Sci. 20:*122, 1964.
33. Wood, J. S., Holyoke, E. D., Clason, W. P. C., Sommers, S. C. and Warren, S. An experimental study of the relationship between tumor size and number of lung metastases. *Cancer 7:*437, 1954.
34. Wood, J. S., Holyoke, E. D., Sommers, S. C. and Warren, S. Influence of pituitary growth hormone on growth and metastasis formation of a transplantable mouse sarcoma. *Bull. Johns Hopkins Hosp. 96:*93, 1955.
35. Wood, J. S., Holyoke, E. D., and Yardley, J. H. An experimental study of the influence of adrenal steroids, growth hormone and anticoagulants on pulmonary metastasis formation in mice. *Proc. Amer. Assoc. Cancer Res. 2:*149, 1956.
36. Young, J. S. and Griffith, H. D. The dynamics of parenchymatous embolism in relation to the dissemination of malignant tumours. *J. Path. and Bact. 62:*293, 1950.
37. Zeidman, I. Metastasis: A review of recent advances. *Cancer Res. 17:*157, 1957.
38. Krain, L. S. The alteration of blood-borne metastases by oriented electric fields. *J. Surg. Res. 7:*115, 1967.
39. Fisher, E. R., and Fisher, B. Recent observations on concepts of metastasis. *Arch. Path. 83:*321, 1967.

40. Boyd, W. Tissue resistance in malignant disease. *Surg. Gyn. & Obst. 32:*306, 1921.
41. Fisher, B. and Fisher, E. R. Experimental studies of factors influencing hepatic metastases. XVIII. Significance of trapped tumor cells. *Proc. Soc. Exptl. Biol. and Med. 124:*881, 1967.
42. Southam, C. M., Babcock, V. I. and Bailey, R. B. Selective tissue localization of human cancer transplants in newborn rats. *Transplantation. 5:*1, 1967.
43. Coman, D. R., deLong, R. P. and McCutcheon, M. Studies on the mechanisms of metastasis. The distribution of tumors in various organs in relation to the distribution of arterial emboli. *Cancer Res. 11:*648, 1951.
44. Fisher, B. and Fisher, E. R. Experimental studies of factors influencing hepatic metastases. III. Effect of surgical trauma—with special reference to liver injury. *Ann. Surg. 150:*731, 1959.
45. Fisher, E. R., and Fisher, B. Experimental studies of factors influencing the development of hepatic metastases. XIII. Effect of hepatic trauma in parabiotic pairs. *Cancer Res. 23:*896, 1963.
46. Podilchak, M. D. The influence of an inflammatory process on the growth and metastasizing behaviour of the Brown-Pearce tumour (in Russian). *Vopr. Onkol. 4:*734, 1958.
47. Robinson, K. P. and Hoppe, E. The development of blood-borne metastases—effect of local trauma and ischemia. *Arch. Surg. 85:*720, 1962.
48. Crowley, J. D. and Still, W. J. S. Metastatic carcinoma at the site of injection of iron-dextran complex. *Brit. Med. J. 1:*1411, 1960.
49. Black, J. W. The localization of metastatic Brown-Pearce carcinoma in granulation tissue. *Brit. J. Cancer 18:*143, 1964.
50. Fisher, E. R. and Fisher, B. Experimental studies of factors influencing hepatic metastases. IV. Effect of cirrhosis. *Cancer 13:*860, 1960.
51. Shivas, A. A. and Finlayson, N. D. C. The resistance of arteries to tumor invasion. *Brit. J. Cancer 19:*486, 1965.
52. Agostino, D. and Cliffton, E. E. Anticoagulants and the development of pulmonary metastases. Anticoagulant effect on the Walker 256 carcinosarcoma in rats. *Arch. Surg. 84:*449, 1962.
53. Agostino, D. and Cliffton, E. E. Decrease in pulmonary metastases: potentiation of nitrogen mustard effect by heparin and fibrinolysin. *Ann. Surg. 157:*400, 1963.
54. Waterbury, L. S. and Hampton, J. W. Hypercoagulability with malignancy. *Angiology 18:*197, 1967.
55. Yamada, T. Mutual adhesiveness of tumor cells in "hepatoma islands" of the rat ascites hepatoma. Studies on the mechanism of tumor metastasis. *Z. Krebsforsch. 65:*75, 1962.
56. Garvie, W. H. H., and Matheson, A. B. The effect of intravenous fluids on the development of experimental tumour metastases: Their effect on tumour cell aggregation. *Brit. J. Cancer 20:*838, 1966.
57. Cruz, E. P., McDonald, G. O. and Cole, W. H. Prophylactic treatments of cancer and use of chemotherapeutic agents to prevent tumor metastases. *Surgery 40:* 291, 1956.
58. Kondo, T. and Moore, G. E. Production of metastases by treatment with carcinostatic agents. I. Effects of carcinostatic agents on the host. *Cancer Res. 21:*1396, 1961.
59. Hitchings, G. H., and Elion, G. B. Chemical suppression of the immune response. *Pharmacol. Rev. 15:*365, 1963.
60. Humphreys, S. R., Glynn, J. P. and Goldin, A. Suppression of the homograft response by pretreatment with antitumor agents. *Transplantation 1:*65, 1963.

PART IV

61. Fisher, B. and Fisher, E. R. Effect of experimental perfusion upon the biologic and pathologic behavior of tumors. *Surgery 56:*651, 1964.
62. Mann, L. T. Spontaneous disappearance of pulmonary metastases after nephrectomy for hypernephroma: Four year followup. *J. Urol. 59:*564, 1948.
63. Jenkins, G. Regression of pulmonary metastasis following nephrectomy for hypernephroma: Eight year followup. *J. Urol. 82:*37, 1959.
64. Schatten, W. E. An experimental study of postoperative tumor metastases. I. Growth of pulmonary metastases following total removal of primary leg tumor. *Cancer 11:*455, 1958.
65 Hadfield, G. The dormant cancer cell. *Brit. Med. J. 2:*607, 1954.
66. Fisher, B. and Fisher, E. R. Experimental evidence in support of the dormant tumour cell. *Science 130:*918, 1959.
67. Wood, S. Jr., Baker, R. R. and Johnson, J. H. Failure of low molecular weight dextrans to alter the frequency of lung metastasis. *Cancer 20:*281, 1967.
68. Fisher, B. and Fisher, E. R. Metastases of Cancer Cells in *Methods in Cancer Research* edited by Busch, H. Academic Press, N. Y., 1967, p. 272.

Treatment of Cancer with Bacteria and Bacterial Products

The author's interest in the possible effects of bacteria and bacterial products on cancer began in 1959 while carrying out a project that involved testing the effects of some plant extracts on mice with spontaneous cancers. A number of soluble extracts had been tested with no apparent benefit, and there were seven materials left that were rather insoluble in saline. These materials were either suspended or dissolved in highly alkaline solution for injection at a site distant from the cancer. The mice receiving these plant materials showed a significant increase in sloughing out of the cancers. Ordinarily, the incidence of sloughing, or so-called spontaneous cure, of the cancers in our mice had been about the figure reported by Haddow, 8 per 1,000. In the mice treated with injections of the relatively insoluble materials, however, the incidence of complete sloughing out of the cancers ranged from 70 to 200 per 1,000. Many of the animals appeared to be cured. The chances that these diverse chemicals had had a direct, anti-cancer effect were so small that we looked for other explanations. It was noted that many of the mice had developed local infections at the injection sites, and all the available evidence suggested that the sloughing of the cancers resulted from the bacterial infections. Unfortunately, we were unable to follow this up, for various reasons, but informal inquiries disclosed that other investigators had observed regressions and cures in animals following infections.

DeWerdt (1), who worked in the laboratories of the New York State Health Department, observed that after an infection by a strain of *Salmonella,* a substantial number of mice were cured of their cancers. He was able to make extracts of the bacterial cultures, and these, too, affected mouse cancers. However, his findings aroused little if any interest.

The literature on cancer research contains a substantial number of reports of anti-cancer effects of several microorganisms on animal

229

cancers of various types (2-31, 202-204). The species involved include: *Bacillus prodigiosus,* now known as *Serratia marcescens* (2) (see also, mixed toxins); *Streptococcus pyogenes* (3, 5, 6, 7, 15, 19, 20, 23, 24); *Escherichia coli* (8, 17); *Proteus* (12); *Corynebacterium parvum* (13, 31); *Bordetella pertussis* (21); *Mycobacterium tuberculosis* (25, 28); *B. enteritidis,* now *Salmonella enteritidis* (27, 28); and mixed bacterial toxins (11, 14, 16, 58-139, 171, 172).

Some of the comments of the scientists who have studied these bacterial products are striking. Duran-Reynals (8) observed that fast-growing malignant tumors were more susceptible to the bacterial toxin than slow-growing ones, and he suggested (9)

... that the newly formed vessels of malignant growth, either as a consequence of an excessive permeability or through some other cause, are extremely sensitive to injections of blood-carried bacterial toxins, and it is this fact which creates a very special state, the tumor vulnerability which is responsible for the regression of malignant growths.

Shwartzman (27, 28) reported that:

... both spontaneous infection with *B. enteritidis* and deliberately induced infection with a strain of this species exerted a "striking" inhibitory influence on mouse sarcoma 180.

Weiss *et al.* (30) studied several kinds of mouse cancers and found that various fractions of tubercle bacilli had anti-cancer effects, *depending on the type of tumor studied.*

There have also been negative reports (33-40), but they do not contradict the basic premise that bacteria and bacterial products have anti-cancer activity. Instead, they delineate some of the boundaries of the effects, both in terms of the bacterial strain used and the type of cancer tested. For example, Christensen (35) states that his streptococci preparations, which were effective against rabbit cancers, were not effective against mouse cancers. Also, he reported (36) that one preparation (phage lysates of hemolytic streptococci) inhibited the growth of a particular cancer (Brown-Pearce) while another preparation (mixed bacterial toxins) had no effect on its growth. These reports alone are enough to warrant a major effort to seek a useful cancer treatment from bacteria and bacterial extracts. But more information is available to us. There are many excellent clinical reports on the effects of bacteria and bacterial products on cancers in man. These reports have not received adequate attention, for reasons that we will consider later.

Beginning in the late 19th century, many reports have been made of apparently incurable cancers that regressed after the patient had an attack of erysipelas (41-52, 179-195), a serious streptococcal infection of the skin—one of the most active organs in maintaining body defenses. In the early 1880's Fehleisen was the first physician to report the artificial induction of erysipelas in an attempt to help incurable cancer patients (45, 46). Today, the availability of sulfonamides and antibiotics has made erysipelas a rarity.

Among the physicians who observed the regression of cancer after erysipelas was William B. Coley (1862-1936), whose work appears to be unfamiliar to many people. Born in Westport, Connecticut, he graduated from Harvard Medical School and became a surgeon, specializing in cancer. He was on the staff and chief of the bone cancer section of Memorial Hospital in New York. From 1909 to 1930 he was clinical professor of surgery and cancer research at Cornell University Medical College (32). All of Dr. Coley's discoveries, claims, formulae and procedures were announced to the medical profession through publication in leading medical journals. He always encouraged critical trial and evaluation of his procedures. He never had any financial interest in his discoveries; they were made freely available. His life was devoted to attempts to save the lives of patients with cancer.

In 1891, having lost his first cancer patient despite early and radical surgery, Dr. Coley sought to learn more about the disease and to discover, if possible, better means of controlling it. He searched the New York Hospital records for all cases of the type he had failed to cure and found the history of a man with incurable recurrent sarcoma of the neck whose disease had progressed despite repeated and radical surgery; the patient had then developed erysipelas, and the sarcoma had disappeared. This had occurred in 1884. Dr. Coley succeeded in tracing this man in 1891, and found him in good health and free from any further evidence of sarcoma, seven years after the disappearance of his sarcoma (54). Dr. Coley then decided to try to imitate nature, i.e., to induce erysipelas in such cases. His first patient had an inoperable (three times recurrent) myxosarcoma of the tonsil and neck. After several unsuccessful attempts, because the cultures had been attenuated, erysipelas developed, and the extensive growth disappeared (55, 56). Other attempts to induce erysipelas in cancer patients were largely unsuccessful, and Dr. Coley then tried injecting filtered or heat-killed cultures of streptococci isolated from erysipelas. When these also proved ineffective, he began to use a mixture of *Streptococcus pyogenes* and *Bacillus prodigiosus* (now known as

231

Serratia marcescens), and thereafter continued to experiment with variations of this mixture.

Dr. Coley, using his mixed toxins, achieved a substantial number of cures of advanced inoperable cancers (57-95, 198, 199). Other physicians here and abroad also were able to cure patients with these mixtures (96-129). Coley's mixed toxins were produced by a major drug manufacturer from 1900 to 1950, and were prescribed rather widely, mostly in the United States and England. Nevertheless, this method of therapy has fallen into disuse. Why? Let us consider carefully all the relevant information.

One possible reason is that Coley's toxins may have given a temporary, illusory benefit only. This has been true of several proposed cancer treatments that were widely heralded when first used but that proved to have little long-term effect. Could this have been the case with Coley's toxins? Apparently not. Follow-up studies on cases treated by Coley and his colleagues (130-137, 200, 201), and a few other examples may serve to show the duration of anti-cancer effect of the mixed toxins.

The first of Coley's patients to receive the mixed toxins was a 16-year-old boy with inoperable spindle cell sarcoma of the abdominal wall and pelvis, involving the bladder. After treatment with Coley's toxins, the sarcoma regressed and the patient remained in good health for 26 years when he died of a heart attack.

The outcomes in nine other patients treated by Coley were reported on in one publication (135). All had inoperable, far-advanced cancers. Their histories after treatment were as follows: 25-year survival with death from heart attack; alive and well 10 years later; alive and well 46 years later; 38-year survival with death from a second cancer; alive and well 44 years later; 31-year survival with death from stroke; 1-year survival with death from original disease; alive and well 37 years later; and alive and well 35 years later. Furthermore, follow-up of patients of other doctors using Coley's toxins revealed similarly long survivals (135).

These are admittedly selected cases. The earlier studies gave much less information about the patients who were not helped by Coley's toxins. However, there have been subsequent studies that included the failures as well as successes of this method (130, 137). For example, since 1953, workers at the New York Cancer Research Institute have abstracted and analyzed over 1,000 cases of microscopically proven, usually inoperable, cases of cancers treated by bacterial toxin therapy. More than half (540) of these patients were traced from 5 to 66 years after onset of their cancers. Seventy-seven of these five-year survivals died of their original cancers more than five years after onset; 63 developed an entirely different kind of neoplasm from 6 to 59 years after recovery from the first. Most of the rest of these 540 patients died of some type of cardiovascular disease.

There is, of course, the possibility that some of Coley's patients simply had spontaneous regressions, unrelated to his treatment with toxins. This seems most unlikely, however. Spontaneous long-term regressions of advanced cancers are rare in man—much rarer than in mice. Exact figures are not available, but we may estimate that there have been only 100 to 300 reported authentic cases of spontaneous long-term regressions of advanced cancers in all the medical literature (167). There is less than one chance in 1,000 that any single physician will encounter in his lifetime one true case of spontaneous cure or long-term regression of advanced cancer. The chances against his encountering two would be less than one in a million. The chances against encountering three would be less than one in a billion. The chances of a physician encountering 10 such cases are much too small to have any meaning. Thus, we must assume that Dr. Coley's patients did not have spontaneous regressions. There is a corollary possibility: so-called spontaneous remissions reported by other doctors may not have been spontaneous at all. Some may have been caused by bacterial infections (154).

Furthermore, it must be pointed out that Coley and the other physicians using his method probably cured more patients than those reported in the literature. The cases reported in the article referred to earlier (135) were patients who could be traced and examined after many years. In all likelihood, many who could not be traced a quarter to half a century after treatment had also been cured; they could have moved, or died of causes unconnected with cancer.

Another possibility to be considered is that Coley and others using his method may have diagnosed some of the cases incorrectly. Their patients may have had some benign disease that simulated cancer. But in every case that was used for end-result studies the diagnosis was confirmed by microscopic study by a highly qualified pathologist. Indeed, the pathologists who did the microscopic diagnoses on Coley's patients were among the most distinguished in the nation, including W. F. Whitney of Massachusetts General Hospital, H. T. Brooks of Post-Graduate Hospital in New York, William H. Welch of Johns Hopkins Hospital, John Funke of Jefferson Medical College in Philadelphia, James Ewing of Memorial Hospital in New York, and A. C. Broders of the Mayo Clinic. In many cases, sections of a

tumor were sent to several pathologists for their opinions, and all
agreed on the cancerous nature of the growth (135).

Another question that may arise is whether the favorable response
of the patients came from some other therapeutic agent, such as
surgery or radiation. A reading of the histories eliminates this possibility. The majority of the patients treated by Coley's method were
either inoperable or had had major recurrences of their cancers when
the toxin treatments were begun.

Accordingly, after a careful scrutiny of the work done on the
effects of bacteria and bacterial products in patients with advanced
cancer, the conclusion seems inescapable that these agents have, in
fact, cured or controlled a significant number of patients who would
otherwise have died of their disease in a short time. Indeed, the results reported for these bacterial products appear to be more encouraging than those being reported for the highly toxic anti-cancer
drugs developed in our screening program and used in patients today
(164).

In considering why Coley's method of treating cancer with toxins
fell into disuse, it should be noted that before the advent of antibiotics, the concept of a "spectrum of activity" was not widely understood. Today, we are well aware that an antibiotic can affect some
kinds of bacteria but not others. Similarly, the concept that an anti-
cancer drug may have a selective action is now generally accepted;
vinblastine, for instance, can cure some human cancers without having any useful effects on others. When Coley developed his treatment,
these concepts were less widely comprehended. Accordingly, Coley's
toxins were, for a time, used in most kinds of human cancer. But a
careful scrutiny of the cases that were reported to benefit from this
treatment (54-138) indicates that sarcomas and lymphomas, including reticulum-cell sarcoma of bone, appeared to respond more dramatically than others. Complete and permanent regression also
occurred in some malignant melanomas, neuroblastomas, testicular
cancers, and carcinoma of the rectum and colon. Coley's toxins
appeared to have less effect on most carcinomas, although a few
dramatic and long-lasting results did occur even in such cases. Sarcomas are much less common than carcinomas, and the larger percentage of negative results in the carcinomas treated may have
obscured the good results obtained in the sarcomas.

Furthermore, in the majority of patients receiving toxin therapy,
the cancers were far advanced and inoperable, often with obvious
multiple metastases, when the toxin treatments were begun. Such
cases could hardly be expected to respond to any type of therapy, and

the favorable response of even a small percentage of such patients can be considered a major therapeutic achievement. The results might have been much better in all types of neoplasms if toxin therapy had been started earlier in the course of the disease. Another point is that few physicians, including Coley himself at first, realized the importance of continued treatment for long periods (135).

Finally, the preparations of Coley's toxins were crude and variable. Many different preparations were made available over a period of years; unfortunately, many were apparently ineffective. The science of bacteriology was still young in those days, and the techniques were not adequately developed. Some of the bacterial strains used were probably of low effectiveness.

It appears likely that a combination of these factors, and perhaps others, accounts for the loss of interest in Coley's toxins. Nevertheless, the studies and reports on it, though old, still have validity. If various types of cancer, incurable by surgery or radiation, were permanently benefited by bacterial toxins in the past, it is difficult to see why they could not be cured by the same, or more effective, bacterial toxins today.

The evidence available suggests that the bacterial toxins that Coley used were effective only in certain kinds of cancer. This does not mean that bacterial therapy must always be limited to those kinds of cancer. From the animal studies cited earlier, there is evidence that other species of bacteria might produce substances capable of controlling or curing other kinds of cancer.

Some additional evidence to help support the concept that bacteria can produce substances antagonistic to cancer has come from an unexpected quarter. In recent years, surgeons have at times utilized antibiotics or mechanical flushing when operating on patients with cancer of the gastrointestinal tract. Their purpose was to reduce markedly the bacterial flora of the intestines and thus reduce the chances of postoperative infection. An unexpected result, however, has been reported—the reduction of the bacterial flora increases the incidence of local recurrence of the cancer (140-143). Apparently, the bacteria normally present in the intestinal tract have some inhibiting effect on the growth of cancer; when that inhibition is removed, even for a short time, local recurrence of cancer becomes more common.

The ways in which bacteria and their products exert an effect on cancer are not clear. There is no reason to believe that the same mechanism operates in all bacteria. Several mechanisms have been suggested (144-153). Corollary evidence from other fields points to an immunologic adjuvant action of some bacterial toxins (156, 163).

235

There is also good evidence that certain bacteria and their toxins, notably streptococci and staphylococci, are able to confer strong antigenicity on substances that normally are not antigenic to a particular host, or only weakly so (196, 197).

Accordingly, it seems clear that the search for bacterial agents to help cure or control cancer warrants a major effort. Several approaches should be followed more or less simultaneously. Basic research on the mechanisms whereby various bacterial toxins exert their effects may lead to useful therapeutic developments. For example, there is excellent evidence that a major action of the extract of *Bacillus prodigiosus* (*Serratia marcescens*) is its toxicity to the walls of the blood vessels supplying the cancer (144). On the other hand, Hirsch (162) has emphasized the possibility of stimulation of host defenses by bacterial endotoxins, and considers further studies in this area to be promising. Perhaps Coley's toxins, consisting of extracts of two separate bacteria, involve two entirely different mechanisms of action, which give additive, or potentiation, effects. With a better understanding of the mechanisms, it may be possible to choose more effective combinations of bacteria.

More animal studies are needed, testing the effects of different bacteria and their products on a variety of cancers. Wherever possible, these studies should be performed on spontaneous cancers, including those in larger animals. Some studies should be done on mice bearing transplantable cancers, but negative results in such studies should not be given too much weight. Over the course of multiple transplantations—sometimes as frequent as one every 10 days—all transplantable cancers have been exposed to bacteria, and most of them carry contaminating bacteria along to succeeding mice. Through the many generations of cancer cells, evolutionary changes have occurred in the transplantable cancers, adapting them to these bacteria. This process is analogous to the development of antibiotic resistance by bacteria after exposure to antibiotics. Accordingly, we may expect transplantable cancers to be more resistant to most bacteria than would be the case with spontaneous or induced cancers.

It would also be worthwhile to test various bacterial extracts against a wide variety of human cancers growing in the hamster cheek pouch.

Some trials in patients with apparently hopeless cancers seem appropriate, even before completion of the animal studies. Preparations similar to Coley's toxins should be made available for clinical testing. With the advances in bacteriology, it should be possible to develop and standardize preparations at least as effective as the best ones available to Coley. As the testing proceeds, even more effective preparations could be developed. In planning such clinical trials, two points should be emphasized. First, careful selection of patients and analysis of results by type of cancer are essential if poor results in one type of common cancer are not to obscure the cure or excellent control in other types. Second, the treatment should be continued for long periods, even if no beneficial results are seen at first.

If bacterial preparations can be obtained that will give results in patients with advanced incurable cancer, equivalent to the results reported by Coley and the other doctors of his era, serious consideration should be given to employing these preparations in patients having the disease in an earlier stage. The evidence suggests that perhaps bacterial preparations should be given to some patients before and after surgery. If so, a controlled experiment could be developed in which one group of patients with the specified cancers is treated by standard operative and adjuvant measures, while a matched group receives, in addition, a full course of bacterial toxins, before and after surgery. The differences in survival between the two groups should give a clearer picture of the value of the bacterial toxins as adjuvants in the surgical treatment of specified cancers.

The use of bacterial products to try to cure or control cancer is a promising approach, supported by scores of scientific and medical reports on animals and patients and deserves much greater support than it has been receiving recently. Cameron (178) has expressed a similar idea. He states:

> It is high time the whole question of Coley's fluid was reexamined. The disillusionment and condemnation appear to have arisen from the impression current at the time that here at last had been discovered the cure-all for cancer. Coley made no such claims. He merely reported that a proportion of patients treated by this method obtained striking regression of their tumours and that the treatment appeared to have some palliative influence on the remainder. In a retrospective survey of Coley's work, it has been shown that out of 312 patients with various inoperable tumours of histologically-proven malignancy, no fewer than 134 were alive and well five years after the commencement of their treatment.

Evidence from many sources points to this research area as one with considerable chance for success in a reasonable period of time.

PART IV

References

1. DeWerdt, J. Personal communication.
2. Beebe, S. P. and Tracy, M. The treatment of experimental tumors with bacterial toxins. *J.A.M.A. 49:*1493, 1907.
3. Christensen, E. A. Infection and malignant tumours: Inhibition of Brown-Pearce carcinoma by cell-free extract of haemolytic streptococci prepared by grinding the bacteria with alumina. *Acta Path. et Microbiol. Scand. 59:*1, 1963.
4. Christensen, E. A. and Kjems, E. Infection and malignant tumours. 2. *Acta Path. Et. Microbiol. Scand. 46:*296, 1959.
5. Christensen, E. A. Infection and malignant tumours. 5. Inhibition of Brown-Pearce carcinoma by cell-free extract of haemolytic streptococci prepared by grinding the bacteria with alumina. *Acta. Path. et. Microbiol. Scand. 59:*1, 1963.
6. Christensen, E. A. Infection and malignant tumours. 6. The heat stability of the tumour-inhibiting factor in extract from haemolytic streptococci, and a comparison of extracts from a streptococcal, a staphylococcal and a coli strain in their effect on Brown-Pearce carcinoma. *Acta. Path. et Microbiol. Scand. 59:*465, 1963.
7. Minami, M. Experimental anticancer studies. Part 29. Relation between anticancer activity of hemolytic streptococci and the type of suspending medium. *Ann. Rep. Inst. TB Kanazawa Univ. 23:*15 and 163, 1966. (Abstr. No. 66-1561 in *Cancer Abstr.)*
8. Duran Reynals, F. Reaction of transplantable and spontaneous tumors to blood-carried bacterial toxins in animals unsusceptible to the Shwartzman phenomenon. *Proc. Soc. Exptl. Biol. and Med. 31:*341, 1933.
9. Duran Reynals, F. Reaction of spontaneous mouse carcinomas to blood carried bacterial toxins. *Proc. Soc. Exptl. Biol. and Med. 32:*1517, 1935.
10. Duran Reynals, F. Reactions of spontaneous mouse carcinomas to blood carried bacterial toxins. *Proc. Soc. Exptl. Biol. and Med. 32:*1517, 1935.
11. Donnelly, A. J., Havas, H. F. and Groesbeck, M. E. Mixed bacterial toxins in the treatment of tumors. II. Gross and microscopic changes produced in sarcoma 37 and in mouse tissues. *Cancer Res. 18:*149, 1958.
12. Fogg, L. C. Effect of certain bacterial products upon the growth of mouse tumor. *Pub. Health Rep. 51:*56, 1936.
13. Halpern, B. N., Biozzi, G., Stiffel, C. and Mouton, D. Inhibition of tumour growth by administration of killed Corynebacterium parvum. *Nature 212:*853, 1966.
14. Havas, H. F. and Donnelly, A. J. Mixed bacterial toxins in the treatment of tumors. IV. Response of methylcholanthrene-induced, spontaneous, and transplanted tumors in mice. *Cancer Res. 21:*17, 1961.
15. Havas, H. F., Donnelly, A. J. and Porreca, A. V. The cytotoxic effects of hemolytic streptococci on ascites tumor cells. *Cancer Res. 23:*700, 1963.
16. Havas, H. F., Groesbeck, M. E. and Donnelly, A. J. Mixed bacterial toxins in the treatment of tumors. I. Methods of preparation and effects on normal and sarcoma 37-bearing mice. *Cancer Res. 18:*141, 1958.
17. Ikawa, M., Koepfli, J. B., Mudd, S. G. and Niemann, C. An agent from E. coli causing hemorrhage and regression of an experimental mouse tumor. III. The component fatty acids of the phospholipide moiety. *J. Am. Chem. Soc. 75:*1035, 1953.
18. Jordan, R. T., Rasmussen, A. F. and Bierman, H. R. Effect of group A streptococci on transplantable leukemia of mice. *Cancer Res. 18:*943, 1958.
19. Koshimura, S. and Shoin, S. Experimental anticancer studies. Part 13. On the streptolysin-S-synthetixing and anticancer activities of cell-free extract from living haemolytic streptococci. *Gann 51:*309, 1960.

238

20. Koshimura, S., Shimiza, R., Fujimura, A. and Okamoto, H. Experimental anti-cancer studies XXI. Effect of penicillin treatment of hemolytic streptococcus on its anticancer activity. *Gann 55:*233, 1964.
21. Malkiel, S. and Hargis, B. J. Influence of B. pertussis on host survival following S-180 implantation. *Cancer Res. 21:*1461, 1961.
22. Marsh, H. C. The synergic activity of staphylococcus toxin. *Yale J. Biol. and Med. 17:*359, 1944.
23. Okamoto, H., Shoin, S., Koshimura, S., and Shimizu, R. Experimental anticancer studies Part XXVII. Effect of penicillin treatment of hemolytic streptococci, grown in RNase-Core broth, on their anticancer activity. *Japan J. Exp. Med. 35:* 249, 1965.
24. Okamoto, H., Minami, M., Shoin, S., Koshimura, S. and Shimizu, R. Experimental cancer studies. Part XXXI. On the streptococcal preparation having potent anti-cancer activity. *Japan J. Exp. Med. 36:*175, 1966.
25. Old, L. J., Clarke, D. A. and Benacerraf, B. Effect of bacillus Calmette-Guerin infection on transplanted tumors in the mouse. *Nature 184:*291, 1959.
26. Pannett, C. A. Inhibition of the growth of implanted mouse carcinoma by an irradiated bacterial culture. *Nature 201:*404, 1964.
27. Shwartzman, G. Effect of spontaneous and induced infections upon the development of mouse sarcoma 180. (Preliminary report) *Proc. Soc. Expt'l. Biol. and Med. 32:*1603, 1935.
28. Shwartzman, G. Reactivity of malignant neoplasms to bacterial filtrates. I. The effect of spontaneous or induced infections on the growth of mouse sarcoma 180. *Arch. Path. 21:*284, 1936.
29. Watanabe, T. Regression of mouse ascites tumors by the treatment with bacterial extracts. *Japan J. Exp. Med. 36:*453, 1966.
30. Weiss, D. W., Bonhag, R. S. and DeOme, K. B. Protective activity of fractions of tubercle bacilli against isologous tumours in mice. *Nature 190:*889, 1961.
31. Woodruff, M. F. A. and Boak, J. L. Inhibitory effect of injection of Corynebac-terium parvum on the growth of tumour transplants in isogenic hosts. *Brit. J. Cancer 20:*345, 1966.
32. *American Men of Science.* Science Press, New York, 1927, p. 194.
33. Zahl, P. A. Action of bacterial toxins on tumors. VIII. *J. Nat. Cancer Inst. 11:* 279, 1950.
34. Shear, J. J. Effect of a concentrate from Bacillus prodigiosus filtrate on sub-cutaneous primary induced mouse tumors. *Cancer Res. 1:*731, 1941.
35. Christensen, E. A. Infection and malignant tumours. 8. Studies on the effect of preparations of streptococci on mouse tumours. *Acta. Path. et Microbiol. Scand. 60:*343, 1964.
36. Christensen, E. A. Infection and malignant tumours. 4. Comparison between the effect of phage lysates of haemolytic streptococci and "Coley Mixed Toxins" on Brown-Pearce carcinoma. *Acta. Path. et Microbiol. Scand. 58:*43, 1963.
37. Christensen, E. A. Infection and malignant tumours. 3. Further studies on the effect on tumours of phage lysates of haemolytic streptococci. *Acta. Path. et Microbiol. Scand. 57:*175, 1963.
38. Christensen, E. A. and Kjems, E. Infection and malignant tumours. Comparison between extract (intracellular products) and culture-filtrate (extracellular products) of haemolytic streptococci, in their effect on Brown-Pearce carcinoma in young rabbits. *Acta. Path. et Microbiol. Scand. 60:*182, 1964.
39. Christensen, E. A. Infection and malignant tumours; growth of Brown-Pearce carcinoma in rabbits treated with living or killed haemolytic streptococci. *Acta. Path. et Microbiol. Scand. 46:*285, 1959.

PART IV

40. Weilbaecher, D. A., Bornside, G. H. and Cohn, I., Jr. Growth of Brown-Pearce carcinoma in the presence of intestinal bacteria. *Arch. Surg. 94:*8, 1967.
41. Bruns, P. Die Heilwirkung des Erysipels auf Geschwülste. *Beiträge f. Klin. Chir. 3:*443, 1887-1888.
42. Bolognino, G. Maligne Geschwülste und erysipelatöse Infection. *Ztschr. f. Krebsf. 6:*261, 1907-1908.
43. Czerny, V. Über Heilversuche bei malignen Geschwülsten mit Erysipeltoxinen. *Münch. Med. Woch. 36:*833, 1895.
44. De Gaetano, L. Un caso di epithelioma della bozza frontale sinistra, dapprima guarito per attacco di erysipela—riproduzione resistente ad ulteriori attachi di erysipela, asportazione e plastica col metodo Italiano a lembo autoplastico dal braccio destro; guarigigione. *Gior. Internat. D. Sci. Med. Napoli 25:*117, 1903.
45. Fehleisen, F. Über Erysipel. *Deutsch. Ztschr. f. Chir.* (Leipzig) *16:*391, 1881-1882.
46. Fehleisen, F. Über die Züchtung der Erysipel-kokken auf künstlichem Nährboden und ihre Übertragbavkeit auf den Menschen. *Deutsch. Med. Woch. 8:*553, 1882.
47. Kleeblatt, D. Ein Beitrag zur Heilwirkung des Erysipels bei malignen Tumoren. *Münch. Med. Woch. 37:*107, 1890.
48. Koch, R. and Petruschky, J. Beobachtungen über Erysipel—Impfungen am Menschen. *Zeitsch. f. Hyg. u. Inf. Kr. 23:*477, 1896.
49. Roger, H. Contribution a l'étude expérimentale du streptocoque de l'érysipèle. *Rev. de Med. 12:*929, 1892.
50. Watson, A. L. A case of recurrent sarcoma with apparent spontaneous cure and gradual shrinking of the tumors. Lancet *1:*300, 1902.
51. Wyeth, J. A. Sarcoma cured by acute inflammation. *Med. Rec. 57:*125, 1900.
52. Nadeau, O. E. Case of carcinoma of the bladder apparently cured by erysipelas. *Surg. Clin. North Amer. 11:*57, 1931.
53. Personal communication from New York Cancer Research Institute, 1225 Park Ave., New York 10028.
54. Coley, W. B. Contribution to the knowledge of sarcoma. *Ann. Surg. 14:*119, 1891.
55. Coley, W. B. The treatment of malignant tumors by repeated inoculations of erysipelas, with a report of original cases. *Am. J. Med. Sc. 105:*487, 1893.
56. Coley, W. B. Treatment of malignant tumors by repeated inoculations of erysipelas, with a report of 10 cases. *Med. Rec. 43:*60, 1893.
57. Coley, W. B. A preliminary note on the treatment of inoperable sarcoma by the toxic products of erysipelas. *Post-graduate 8:*278, 1893.
58. Coley, W. B. Treatment of inoperable malignant tumors with toxins of erysipelas and the Bacillus prodigiosus. *Trans. Amer. Surg. Assn. 12:*183, 1894.
59. Coley, W. B. The treatment of inoperable malignant tumors with the toxins of erysipelas and Bacillus prodigiosus. *Med. Rec. 47:*65, 1895.
60. Coley, W. B. The therapeutic value of the mixed toxins of erysipelas and Bacillus prodigiosus in the treatment of inoperable malignant tumors. *Am. J. M. Sc. 112:* 251, 1896.
61. Coley, W. B. Further observations upon the treatment of malignant tumors with the mixed toxins of erysipelas and Bacillus prodigiosus, with a report of 160 cases. *Bull. Johns Hopkins Hosp. 65:*157, 1896.
62. Coley, W. B. Recurrent round celled sarcoma of the lip treated with the mixed toxins. *Post-graduate 12:*346, 1897.
63. Coley, W. B. Inoperable sarcoma cured by mixed toxins of erysipelas. *Ann. Surg. 25:*174, 1897.
64. Coley, W. B. Spindle-celled sarcoma of the abdominal wall successfully treated by the mixed toxins of erysipelas and Bacillus prodigiosus. *Ann. Surg. 26:*232, 1897.

65. Coley, W. B. A case of recurrent inoperable spindle-celled sarcoma of the parotid successfully treated with the mixed toxins of erysipelas and Bacillus prodigiosus. *Ann. Surg. 28:*244, 1898.

66. Coley, W. B. The treatment of inoperable sarcoma with the mixed toxins of erysipelas and Bacillus prodigiosus: immediate and final results in one hundred and forty cases. *J.A.M.A. 31:*389-395, 456-465, 1898. (see also Med. Rec. *54:*294, 1898)

67. Coley, W. B. The treatment of inoperable cancer. *St. Paul Med. J. 2:*365, 1900.

68. Coley, W. B. Mixed toxins of erysipelas and Bacillus prodigiosus in treatment of sarcoma. *J.A.M.A. 34:*906, 1900.

69. Coley, W. B. Late results of the treatment of inoperable sarcoma with the mixed toxins of erysipelas and Bacillus prodigiosus. *Phila. Med. Journ. 7:*1013, 1901.

70. Coley, W. B. Late results of the treatment of inoperable sarcoma with the mixed toxins of erysipelas and Bacillus prodigiosus. *Trans. Amer. Surg. Assn. 19:*27, 1901.

71. Coley, W. B. Small round cell sarcoma of the parotid successfully treated by the mixed toxins of erysipelas and Bacillus prodigiosus. *Ann. Surg. 35:*421, 1902.

72. Coley, W. B. Observations upon the symptomatology and treatment of sarcoma. *Trans. Lehigh Valey Med. Assn. 1:*55, 1903.

73. Coley, W. B. Treatment operative and by the mixed toxins. *Brooklyn M. J. 20:* 313, 1906.

74. Coley, W. B. Late results of the treatment of inoperable sarcoma by the mixed toxins of erysipelas and Bacillus prodigiosus. *Am. J. Med. Sc. 131:*375, 1906.

75. Coley, W. B. Inoperable sarcoma. A further report of cases successfully treated with the mixed toxins of erysipelas and Bacillus prodigiosus. *Med. Rec. 72:*129, 1907.

76. Coley, W. B. Sarcoma of the long bones: the diagnosis, treatment and prognosis with a report of sixty-nine cases. *Ann. Surg. 45:*321, 1907.

77. Coley, W. B. Inoperable round cell sarcoma of the back; with metastatic tumor involving a large portion of the lower jaw; entire disappearance under 2½ months' treatment with the mixed toxins. *Ann. Surg. 48:*465, 1908.

78. Coley, W. B. The treatment of sarcoma with mixed toxins of erysipelas and Bacillus prodigiosus. *Boston M. and S. J. 158:*175, 1908.

79. Coley, W. B. The treatment of inoperable sarcoma by bacterial toxins. *Proc. Royal Soc. Med., Surg. Sect. 3:*1, 1909-1910.

80. Coley, W. B. The treatment of inoperable sarcoma with the mixed toxins of erysipelas and Bacillus prodigiosus. *Trans. New Hampshire M. Soc.* 225, 1910.

81. Coley, W. B. A report of recent cases of inoperable sarcoma successfully treated with mixed toxins of erysipelas and Bacillus prodigiosus. *Surg. Gyn. and Obst. 13:* 174, 1911.

82. Coley, W. B. Disappearance of a recurrent carcinoma after injections of mixed toxins. *Ann. Surg. 55:*897, 1912.

83. Coley, W. B. Inoperable adenocarcinoma of the soft palate, rendered operable by the use of the mixed toxins. *Ann. Surg. 58:*559, 1913.

84. Coley, W. B. *The Treatment of Malignant Inoperable Tumors with the Mixed Toxins of Erysipelas and Bacillus Prodigiosus with a Brief Report of 80 Cases Successfully Treated with the Toxins from 1893-1914.* Brussels: M. Weissenbruch. 1914.

85. Coley, W. B. Inoperable recurrent tumor of nasopharynx, involving ethmoid, sphenoid, frontal and superiod maxillae bones (carcinoma); disappearance under six weeks' treatment with the mixed toxins. *Ann. Surg. 62:*353, 1915.

86. Coley, W. B. Inoperable spindle-celled sarcoma of the superior maxilla; disappearance under 2½ months' treatment with the mixed toxins of erysipelas and Bacillus prodigiosus. *Ann. Surg. 62:*504, 1915.
87. Coley, W. B. Primary neoplasms of the lymphatic glands, including Hodgkin's disease. *Trans. Amer. Surg. Assn. 33:*499, 1915. (See also *Ann. Surg. 63:*34, 1916.)
88. Coley, W. B. and Hoguet, J. P. Melanotic Cancer; with a report of 90 cases. *Trans. Amer. Surg. Assn. 34:*319, 1916.
89. Coley, W. B. and Coley, B. L. End results in 169 operable cases of periosteal ostenogenic sarcoma and endothelioma, including a small group of malignant central sarcoma. *Trans. Amer. Surg. Assn. 43:*857, 1925.
90. Coley, W. B. Sarcoma of the long bones. Clinical lecture on end results. Exhibition of patients illustrating end results of treatment. *Surg. Clin. North Amer. 9:* 583, 1929.
91. Coley, W. B. Treatment of bone sarcoma. *Cancer Review 4:*426, 1929.
92. Coley, W. B. Endothelial myeloma of tibia; long-standing cure by toxin treatment. *Ann. Surg. 93:*447, 1931.
93. Coley, W. B. The treatment of sarcoma of the long bones. *Trans. Amer. Surg. Assn. 50:*383, 1932.
94. Coley, W. B. and Blum, D. M. Large malignant tumor (sarcoma) of the uterus with multiple bone metastases (femur, pelvic bones and skull); Case successfully treated by hysterectomy and Coley's toxins (erysipelas and Bacillus prodigiosus). *Am. J. Surg. 23:*47, 1934.
95. Coley, W. B. Diagnosis and treatment of bone sarcoma. *Glasgow, M. J. 126:* 49-86, 128-164, 1936.
96. Andrews, E. A study of a few suggestive cases. *Chicago Med. Rec. 8:*1, 1895.
97. Battie, W. H. A case illustrating the advantage of Coley's fluid in the treatment of inoperable tumours. *Trans. Med. Soc. London 21:*362, 1897-1898.
98. Christian, S. L. and Palmer, L. A. An apparent recovery from multiple sarcoma with involvement of both bone and soft parts treated by toxin of erysipelas and Bacillus prodigiosus (Coley). *Amer. J. Surg. 4:*188, 1928. (See also Apparent recovery from multiple sarcomata. *Military Surg. 61:*42, 1927.)
99. Czerny, V. Über Heilversuche bei malignen Geschwülsten mit Erysipeltoxinen. *Münch. Med. Woch. 36:*833, 1895.
100. Emerson, F. P. Sarcoma of the tonsil treated with Coley's Toxins. *Laryngoscope,* St. Louis *17:*212, 1907.
101. Green, R. M. The use of Coley toxins in the treatment of sarcoma. *Boston M. and S. J. 165:*1, 1911.
102. Greenwood, H. H. Note on a case of melanotic sarcoma treated by Coley's fluid. *Lancet 2:*881, 1912. (See also *1:*25, 1912.)
103. Harmer, T. W. A study of the efficiency of mixed toxins (Coley) in inoperable sarcoma. A critical analysis of 134 microscopically proven cases. *Boston M. and S. J. 173:*331-338, 373-377, 411-416, 440-448, 1915.
104. Harmer, T. W. Remarks upon the effects observed in the use of the mixed toxins (Coley) in certain cases of sarcoma. *Boston M. and S. J. 171:*253, 1914.
105. Johnson, W. B. A case of sarcoma of the palate successfully treated with the toxins of erysipelas. *Med. Rec. 46:*616, 1894.
106. Lagueuz, P. Le sérum de Coley dans les cas de sarcome ou carcinome ou dans les cas de récidive après operation. *Bull. Méd. de Quebec 10:*469, 1908.
107. Large, S. H. Four cases of sarcoma of the nose and throat treated with Coley's toxins. *Cleveland Med. J. 10:*318, 1911.

108. Lilienthal, H. Mediastinal sarcoma—treated with Coley's fluid. *Ann. Surg. 85:* 615, 1927.
109. Matagne, J. H. J. Premiers essais de traitement des tumeurs malignes inopérables par les toxines de Coley: Un cas de cancer guéri. *Gaz. Med. Liège 8:*401, 1896.
110. Matagne, J. H. J. Traitement des tumeurs malignes inopérables par l'érysipèle et les toxines de Coley. *Gaz. Méd. Belge. 12:*375, 1899-1900.
111. Matagne, J. H. J. Les toxines de Coley employées dans le but de prévenir la récidive du cancer. *Presse Med. Belge. 53:*1, 1902.
112. Matagne, J. H. J. Presentation de cancereux guéris par les toxines de Coley, employées conjointement avec intervention chirurgicale. *Presse Méd. Belge. 57:*173, 1905.
113. Meriweather, F. T. Some remarks upon Coley's treatment of malignant growths. *Louisville Monthly J. M. and S. 6:*173, 1900.
114. Moullin, H. M. *The Treatment of Sarcoma and Carcinoma by Injections of Mixed Toxins.* London: John Bale Sons and Danielsson, 1898.
115. Mynter, H. Sarcoma of the abdominal cavity cured by the toxins of erysipelas. *Med. Rec. 47:*167, 1895.
116. Nicholson, C. M. Report of four cases of sarcoma treated by injection of erysipelas and prodigiosus toxins. *Amer. J. Surg. and Gyn.* (St. Louis) *13:*10, 1899.
117. Odier, R. Traitement des affections sarcomateuses par les toxins de M. Coley. *Rev. Med. de la Suisse Rom.* (Geneva) *28:*649, 1908.
118. Oliver, J. C. Results obtained from the use of Coley's toxins in the treatment of sarcoma. *Ohio M. J. 7:*483, 1911.
119. Palmer, C. W. Treatment of sarcoma with the mixed toxins of erysipelas and Bacillus prodigiosus. *J. Ophthal. Otol. and Laryng. 12:*214, 1900.
120. Repin, C. La toxithérapie des tumeurs malignes. *Rev. de Chir. 15:*465, 1895.
121. Shields, E. H. Coley's toxins in sarcoma. *Lancet-Clinic,* Cincinnati, *111:*701, 1914.
122. Spencer, C. G. A case of sarcoma treated with Coley's fluid. *J. Royal Army M. Corps. 12:*449, 1909. (See also Lancet *2:*1127, 1912.)
123. Spencer, C. G. A case of sarcoma treated by Coley's fluid. *Proc. Royal Med. Clin. Sect. 2:*152, 1908-1909.
124. Stewart, F. T. Sarcoma of psoas muscle treated by Coley's fluid. *Ann. Surg. 51:* 285, 1910.
125. Tosier, F. L. Non-operative sarcoma; a treatment. *Vermont M. Monthly 15:*217, 1909.
126. Tupper, P. V. The treatment of inoperable sarcoma with Coley's mixed toxins: report of cases. *Med. Rev. 39:*425, 1899.
127. Ward, G. S. Mixed cell sarcoma treated by local excision and Coley's fluid. No recurrence after three years. *Brit. M. J. 2:*1484, 1913.
128. Warthin, A. S. Multiple primary neoplasms in one individual (spindle cell sarcoma of forearm, adenocarcinoma of pylorus, myomata of stomach wall); treatment with Coley's mixture. *Phila. M. J. 8:*701, 1901.
129. Winberg, O. K. Inoperable round celled sarcoma of the upper jaw with metastases. Successfully treated with the mixed toxins of erysipelas and Bacillus prodigiosus. *Med. Rec. 41:*681, 1902.
130. Fowler, G. A. *Beneficial Effects of Acute Bacterial Infections or Bacterial Toxin Therapy on Cancer of the Colon or Rectum.* N. Y. Cancer Res. Inst., N. Y., 1966.
131. Fowler, G. A. and Nauts, H. C. *Effects of Acute Concurrent Infection on Cancer in Man.* Series A. Pyogenic infection—152 cases. N. Y. Cancer Res. Inst., N. Y., 1964.

PART IV

132. Fowler, G. A. and Nauts, H. C. *Effects of Acute Concurrent Infections on Cancer in Man.* Series B. Non-pyogenic infections. N. Y. Cancer Res. Inst., N. Y., 1966.
133. Nauts, H. C. and Coley, B. L. A review of the treatment of malignant tumors by Coley bacterial toxins. In: *Approaches to Tumor Chemotherapy,* A.A.A.S., Lancaster, Pa., The Science Press Printing Co., 1947 (pp. 217-335).
134. Nauts, H. C. and Fowler, G. A. *Host Resistance Mechanisms Against Cancer.* Vol. 1. Monograph No. 5. N. Y. Cancer Research Inst., N. Y., 1958.
135. Nauts, H. C., Fowler, G. A. and Bogatko, F. H. A review of the influence of bacterial infection and of bacterial products (Coley's toxins) on malignant tumors in man. *Acta Medica Scand. 145 (Suppl. 276):*5, 1953.
136. Nauts, H. C., Swift, W. E. and Coley, B. L. Treatment of malignant tumors by bacterial toxins as developed by the late William B. Coley, M.D., reviewed in the light of modern research. *Cancer Res. 6:*205, 1946.
137. Micholson, J. T. and Fowler, G. A. *End Results in Reticulum Cell Sarcoma of Bone Treated by Toxin Therapy Alone or Combined with Surgery and/or Radiation* (46 cases) or with concurrent infection (5 cases). N. Y. Cancer Res. Inst., N. Y., 1966.
138. Richardson, M. H. A case of apparently hopeless infiltration of left axilla and scapula by round cell sarcoma; extirpation attempted and abandoned; extensive and severe wound infection, followed by disappearance of the tumor. *Trans. Amer. Surg. Assn. 16:*309, 1898. (See also Ann. Surg. *28:*741, 1898.)
139. Spronck, C. H. H. Tumeurs malignes et maladies infectieuses. *Ann. Inst. Pasteur. 6:*683, 1892.
140. Beal, J. M. and G. N. Cornell. A study of the problem of recurrence of carcinoma and the anastomotic site following resection of the colon for carcinoma. *Ann. Surg. 143:*1, 1956.
141. Cohn, I., Jr. and Atik, M. The influence of antibiotics on the spread of tumors of the colon: An experimental study. *Ann. Surg. 151:*917, 1960.
142. Cole, W. H. and Webb, R. S., Jr. Factors in the dissemination of cancer. *J. Am. Geriatrics Soc. 11:*35, 1963.
143. Vink, M. Local recurrence of cancer in the large bowel: The role of implantation metastases and bowel disinfection. *Brit. J. Surg. 41:*431, 1954.
144. Algire, G. H., Legallais, F. Y. and Park, H. D. Vascular reactions of normal and malignant tissues in vivo. II. The vascular reaction of normal and neoplastic tissues of mice to a bacterial polysaccharide from Serratia marescens (Bacillus prodigiosus) culture filtrates. *J. Nat. Cancer Inst. 8:*53, 1947.
145. Campbell, D. H., Farr, R. S. and Rinderknecht, H. The production of hemorrhage in sarcoma 180 in mice by anaphylaxis and the inhibitory effect of cortisone on the hemorrhage-producing factor from E. Coli. *J. Nat. Cancer Inst. 15:* 1651, 1953.
146. Creech, H. J., Hamilton, M. A., Nishimura, E. T. and Hankwitz, R. F. The influence of antibody-containing fractions on the lethal and tumor-necrotising actions of polysaccharides from Serratia marcescens (Bacillus prodigiosus). *Cancer Res. 8:*330, 1948.
147. Duran Reynals, F. Reaction of transplantable and spontaneous tumors to blood-carried bacterial toxins in animals unsusceptible to the Shwartzman phenomenon. *Proc. Soc. Exptl. Biol. and Med. 31:*341, 1933.
148. Duran Reynals, F. Reaction of spontaneous mouse carcinomas to blood carried bacterial toxins. *Proc. Soc. Exptl. Biol. and Med. 32:*1517, 1935.
149. Landy, M. and Shear, M. J. Host responses elicited by polysaccharides of bacterial and mammalian derivation. *Fed. Proc. 16:*857, 1958.

150. Shear, M. J. and Andervont, H. B. Chemical treatment of tumors. III. Separation of hemorrhage-producing fraction of B. coli filtrate. *Proc. Soc. Exptl. Biol. and Med. 34:*323, 1936.

151. Shear, M. J. Chemical treatment of tumors. IV. Properties of hemorrhage-producing fraction of B. coli filtrate. *Proc. Soc. Exptl. Biol. and Med. 34:*325, 1936.

152. Shear, M. J. Chemical treatment of tumors; reactions of mice with primary subcutaneous tumors to injection of hemorrhage-producing bacterial polysaccharide. *J. Nat. Cancer Inst. 4:*461, 1944.

153. Zahl, P. A., Starr, M. P. and Hutner, S. H. Effect of bacterial toxins on tumors. VII. Tumor-hemorrhagic factor in bacteria. *Am. J. Hyg. 41:*41, 1945.

154. Seligman, A. M. Review of Everson, T. C. and Cole, W. H. Regression of cancer. *J.A.M.A. 198:*680, 1966.

155. Wynne, E. S. and Irvine, L. A. Bacteriological approaches to cancer research. *R. Texas Rep. Biol. and Med. 20:*532, 1962.

156. Maculla, E. S. The immunochemistry of mouse tissue components. II. The comparative antigenic composition of homologous and heterologous mouse tumor transplants. *Yale J. Biol. and Med. 20:*343, 1947.

157. Klyueva, N. G. and Roskin, G. I. *Regression of Malignant Tumours under the Influence of Products of Microbial Metabolism.* Moscow, L. A. Tarasevicha Inst., 1957.

158. Holloman, L. Reactions of patients and of tumors to injection of S. marcescens polysaccharide in eight cases of malignant disease. In: *Approaches to Tumor Chemotherapy.* 1947, p. 273. Publication of the American Association for the Advancement of Science, Pennsylvania.

159. Brues, A. M. and Shear, J. M. Chemical treatment of tumors. X. Reactions of four patients with advanced malignant tumors to injections of a polysaccharide from Serratia marcescens culture filtrate. *J. Nat. Cancer Inst. 5:*195, 1944.

160. Janes, D. W., Goldschmidt, M. E., Cash, H. P. and Williams, R. P. Production of purple pigment by a mutant of Serratia marcescens. *Texas Rep. Biol. and Med. 24:*489, 1966.

161. Gregory, P. Bacillus subtilis as an antibiotic in the treatment of cancer. *Southern M. J. 43:*397, 1950.

162. Hirsch, H. M. Some aspects of the problem of immunity against transplanted and spontaneous tumors. *Bact. Rev. 26:*336, 1962.

163. Balner, H., Old, L. J. and Clarke, D. A. Accelerated rejection of male skin isografts by female C57BL mice infected with Bacillus Calmette-Guerin (B.C.G.). *Proc. Soc. Expt'l. Biol. and Med. 109:*58, 1962.

164. Hyman, G. A. and Cassileth, P. A. Efficacy of cyclophosphamide in the management of reticulum cell sarcoma. *Cancer 19:*1386, 1966.

165. Schwartzman, G. Phenomenon of local tissue reactivity to Serratia marcescens (B. prodigiosus). Immunological relationships between Serratia mascescens culture filtrates and Shear polysaccharide. *Cancer Res. 4:*191, 1944.

166. Gellhorn, A. A critical evaluation of the current status of clinical cancer chemotherapy. *Cancer Res. 13:*205, 1953.

167. Everson, T. C. and Cole, W. H. *Spontaneous Regression of Cancer.* Saunders, Philadelphia, 1966.

168. Bunting, M. I., Robinow, C. F. and Bunting, H. Factors affecting elaboration of pigment and polysaccharides by Serratia marcescens. *J. Bact. 58:*114, 1949.

169. Podilchak, M. D. Vliyanie stafilokokkovoi infektsii na eksperimentalnyi rak. (The influence of staphylococcal infection on experimental cancers). *Med. Zhur. 21:*72, 1951.

170. Pike, R. M. The production of hyaluronic acid and hyaluronidase by some strains of group A streptococci. *Ann. N. Y. Acad. Sci. 52:*1070, 1950.

171. Pelner, L. and Fowler, G. A. Host-tumor antagonism. XIII. Sarcoma of the soft tissues treated by bacterial toxins: successful series. *J. Amer. Geriat. Soc. 7:*624, 1959.

172. Pelner, L. Host-tumor antagonism. XV. The apparently beneficial effects of acute concurrent infections or of toxin therapy on the course of malignant melanoma. *J. Amer. Geriat. Soc. 8:*378, 1960.

173. O'Malley, W. E., Achinstein, B. and Shear, M. J. Action of bacterial polysaccharide on tumors. II. Damage of Sarcoma 37 by serum of mice treated with Serratia marcescens polysaccharide, and induced tolerance. *J. Nat. Cancer Inst. 29:*1169, 1962.

174. Koshimura, S., Hirata, R. and Shoin, S. On the streptolysin S synthesising and anticancer activities of cell-free extract from living haemolytic streptococci. *Cancer Chemother. Rep. 13:*107, 1961.

175. Huth, E. F. Zum Antagonismus zwischen bakteriellen Infektionen und malignen Enkrankungen. *Med. Klin. 53:*2173, 1958.

176. Havas, H. F., Donnelly, A. J. and Levine, S. I. Mixed bacterial toxins in the treatment of tumors. III. Effect of tumor removal on the toxicity and mortality rate in mice. *Cancer Res. 20:*393, 1960.

177. Grabchenko, E. M. and Podilchak, M. D. Vliyanie stafilokokkovoi i streptokokkovoi infektsii na rakovuyu opukhol. (The effect of straphylococcal and streptococcal infections on malignant tumours.) *Vopr. Onkol. 21:*233, 1952.

178. Cameron, E. *Hyaluronidase and Cancer.* Pergamon Press, Oxford, England, 1966, p. 177.

179. Mishtolt, A. D. On the curative action of erysipelas in cases of tumors. *Lond. Med. Rec. 12:*11, 1884.

180. Selva, J. A study of erysipelas: its infectious nature; the depression upon the vital powers; septicaemia as a complication; the curative influence upon granulating surfaces and upon sarcomatous growths. *N. Y. Med. J. 60:*815, 1894.

181. Mosengeil, K. Alteration des Charakters einer Geschwulst nach Auftreten von Erysipelas. *Arch. f. klin. Chir. 12:*68, 1871.

182. Mosengeil, K. Fall von gleichzeitig über eine sehr grosse Hautpartie ausgebreitetem Erysipel. *Arch. f. klin. Chir. 12:*107, 1871.

183. O'Keef, P. A case of recurring multiple sarcoma cured by contracting erysipelas. *Trans. Med. Soc. Wisconsin 32:*102, 1898.

184. Plenio, C. J. O. Über einen Fall von Totalresorption eines grossen Melanosarkoms. *Arch. f. Klin. Chir. 34:*398, 1887.

185. Reding, R. L'équilibre acide base et l'équilibre ionique dans le cancer et le précancer. Contribution a l'étude des mechanismes biologiques régulateurs de la division cellulaire. *Cancer* (Bruxelles) *5:*97, 1928.

186. Sell, A. Maligne Nydannelsers Paavirkning af Erysipelas. (The erysipelas treatment of malignant tumors.) *Hospitalstidende,* Kopenhagen *4:*389, 1895.

187. Stein, J. Ischeznovenie opucholi nod vlijaniem rochi (erysipele salutaire). (Disappearance of a tumor under the influence of erysipelas.) *Vrach. St. Petersburg 3:*262, 1882. (Abstract in *London Med. Rec. 11:*186, 1883.)

188. Viliavine, G. D. Case of cancer cured after erysipelas (in Russian). *Vestnik khir. 14:*151, 1928.

189. Watson, A. L. A case of recurrent sarcoma with apparent spontaneous cure and gradual shrinking of the tumours. *Lancet 1:*300, 1902.

190. Bidlot, A. Un cas remarquable de guérison d'un cancer uterin à la suite de l'apparition d'un erysipèle. *Gazette médicale de Liège 5:*232, 1893.

191. Biedert, P. (Vorläufige) Heilung einer ausgebreiteten Sarkomwucherung in einem Kinderkopf durch Erysipel. *Deutsch med. Zeit. 4:*45, 1886.

192. Galloway, J. Erysipele Salutarie in Kaposi sarcoma in Mycosis Fungoides. *Practitioner 9:*601, 1899.

193. Hanszel, F. Involution eines Rhinolaryngoscleroms durch Erysipel der Gesichtshaut und eines Sarcoms des Rachens durch Streptococcen und Staphylococcen Infection. *Monatschr. f. Ohrenh.* Berlin *36:*249, 1902.

194. Marchetti, L. Sarcoma soprajoideo a rapido sviluppo, recidivato due volte e guarito in seguito ad infezione eresipelatosa. *Gazz. Med. Lomb.* (Milan) *62:*51, 1903.

195. Martin, H. A case of untreated basal cell carcinoma of the face which regressed during an attack of erysipelas. *Bull. Memorial Hospital, N. Y. 1-2:*49, 1929-30.

196. Glynn, L. E. and Holborrow, E. J. The production of complete antigens from polysaccharide haptenes by streptococci and other organisms. *J. Path. & Bact. 64:* 881, 1952.

197. Burky, E. L. The production in the rabbit of hypersensitive reactions to lens, rabbit muscle, and low ragweed extracts by the action of staphylococcus toxins. *J. Allergy 5:*466, 1933-34.

198. Coley, W. B. Malignant tumors of the testicle in an infant. *Trans. South. Surg. Assn. 30:*126, 1918.

199. Coley, W. B. End results in malignant disease of the testis. *Trans. Amer. Surg. Assn. 35:*370, 1923.

200. Fowler, G. A. *The Beneficial Effects of Concurrent Infection, Inflammation or Fever, and of Bacterial Toxin Therapy on Neuroblastoma.* New York Cancer Research Institute, N. Y., 1966.

201. Fowler, G. A. *The Beneficial Effects of Acute Concurrent Infections, Inflammation or Bacterial Toxin Therapy on Malignant Melanoma.* New York Cancer Research Institute, N. Y., 1966.

202. Heneghan, J. B. and Cohn, I., Jr. Ehrlich ascites tumor growth in gnotobiotic animals. *Proc. Am. Assn. Cancer Res. 7:*30, 1966.

203. Navashin, S. M., Fomina, I. P. and Terent'eva, T. G. Induced tolerance for antitumor action of bacterial polysaccharides. *Fed. Proc.* (Translation Supplement) *25:*T1083, 1966.

204. Okamoto, H., Minami, M., Shoin, S., Koshimura, S. and Shimizu, R. Experimental anticancer studies. XXXI. On the streptococcal preparation having potent anticancer activity. *Jap. J. Exp. Med. 36:*175, 1966.

205. Okamoto, H., Shoin, S., Minami, M., Koshimura, S. and Shimizu, R. Experimental anticancer studies. XXX. Factors influencing the streptolysin s-forming ability of streptococci having anticancer activity. *Jap. J. Exp. Med. 36:*161, 1966.

206. Chandler, J. J., Stark, D. B., Allen, C. V. and Fletcher, W. S. Observations on the treatment of cancer by bacterial toxins. *Amer. Surg. 31:*443, 1965.

207. Cole, D. R., Dreyer, B., Rousselot, L. M. and Tendler, M. D. The radioprotective and antitumor effects of mixed bacterial toxins and anthramycin. *Amer. J. Roentg. Radium. Ther. & Nuclear Med. 47:*997, 1966.

Anti-Cancer Medication from the Sea

One of the most promising leads in cancer research is being developed by Sister M. Rosarii Schmeer, O.P., Chairman of the Biology Department at the College of St. Mary of the Springs in Columbus, Ohio. Sister Rosarii has been doing her experiments during vacations and in whatever odd moments are left after her teaching and administrative duties have been performed. She became aware of the fact that, although cancers have been reported as occurring in almost all kinds of animals, there were no verified cytological reports of spontaneous cancer in animals without backbones. The few reports of "tumors" in these animals all seem to describe benign growths rather than cancer (1-6). She also had read reports (7) that extracts of certain ocean animals had anti-tumor properties, and, further, that extracts of mollusks had anti-viral actions (9). She wondered whether mollusks might contain some anti-cancer factor, and planned and performed a series of experiments to find out. Starting with some simple studies, she has developed an impressive series of results and observations.

First, she studied extracts of different kinds of mollusks, testing them against sarcoma 180 transplanted into mice. The results showed anti-cancer activity in all the species tested, but by far the greatest activity was found in extracts of the common clam, *Mercenaria mercenaria* (10, 11) (also called quahog and cherrystone). Accordingly, she concentrated her efforts on the clam. She ground up fresh clams in a Waring blendor, made extracts with sterile water, and, in a series of controlled experiments, used the extracts to treat mice with several different kinds of transplanted cancer, including sarcoma 180 and Krebs 2 ascites carcinoma (10-18, 22).

In a typical experiment, mice were given subcutaneous injections of cancer cells. After four days, all the mice were examined, and those without palpable tumors were discarded. Those with tumors were divided into "treated" and control groups. The control groups were given injections of saline, while the treated groups were given injections of clam extract. All the control mice died of their cancers within 28 days. Between 80 and 100 per cent of the treated groups in several sets of experiments lived in apparently good health for 180 days, and many of them delivered normal litters in that period. At the end of 180 days, the mice were sacrificed and the experiment was terminated. It is noteworthy that, in the doses needed to exert this effect, the clam extract was nontoxic. Sister Rosarii has named the active extract mercenene.

Sister Rosarii has also shown that mercenene is effective against human cancer cells in tissue culture, but not against noncancerous human cells (13, 16).

Of particular interest is the observation that injections of mercenene for periods of one to three weeks apparently produced complete cures in most of the animals. It was not necessary to continue treatment beyond a few weeks in order to keep the mice free of cancer for the remainder of the trial.

These basic observations on the anti-cancer effects of mercenene have now been confirmed by two independent investigators, Hegyeli (19) and Szent-Gyorgyi (20), the Nobel prize winner. In addition, Li and his colleagues (8) have reported that clam extracts inhibited the development of virus-induced cancers in hamsters.

Having established the anti-cancer effects of mercenene in mouse cancer, Sister Rosarii has done further studies on the material. She observed that high concentrations of the clam extract had some toxic effects, but that after dialysis the toxicity was gone. This has been interpreted as an indication that the toxicity was due to potassium which is removed by dialysis. Although crude mercenene is heat-labile (10), purified mercenene is quite stable at the boiling point of water and at lower temperatures, and it can be lyophilized to a powder that remains potent after storage (16).

In some recent experiments, Sister Rosarii has tested fractions of the crude clam extract and has been able to pinpoint one of the fractions which contains most of the activity. She has made a good start toward identifying the active anti-cancer material (12, 16), has been able to concentrate the active principle tenfold (16), and has worked out the approximate anti-cancer potency of clam extracts. She assigns one unit to the amount that will produce 50 per cent inhibition of cancer growth in a mouse. On this basis, a kilogram of clams (without shells) in summer months would produce about 10,000 units of mercenene (10). This is an immensely important and practical point. If we are unable to synthesize mercenene or obtain it from other sources, we now have reason to think that the amount present in clams is high enough to make it possible eventually to use that source for producing a drug with which to treat substantial numbers of human patients.

It had been noted that clams taken in the winter had much less anti-cancer activity than those taken in the summer. Hegyeli (19) has performed some studies that showed that clams taken in winter would regain the summer level of anti-cancer potency if warm sea water was circulated through their tank for several weeks. Sister Rosarii investigated a related clam, *Mercenaria campechiensis,* which inhabits more southerly waters. She found that extracts of this clam also had a high level of anti-cancer activity (14).

Let us now consider the significance of these studies, and how subsequent experiments in this area might fit into a national cancer research program. Although the studies on mercenene are encouraging, a certain degree of caution is still needed in interpreting them. Thus far, most of the work on mercenene has utilized transplanted cancers. As pointed out in Chapter 14 scores of materials have been found that cure transplanted cancers but are largely ineffective in spontaneous cancers of mice and men. To be sure, the low toxicity of mercenene and its biological origin are reasons for encouragement. Nevertheless, an important step would be the demonstration that mercenene has a significant effect on spontaneous cancers in mice, preferably random-bred mice. It would be helpful if the cooperation of veterinarians (as discussed in Chapter 29) could be secured to assist in developing evidence that mercenene can cure or control spontaneous cancers in larger animals: such studies could be designed so that, within a year, we would know the answer. Let us assume that these studies are done and do show that mercenene has a useful curative or controlling effect against the spontaneous cancers. It would then be advisable to start a whole series of simultaneous studies. This would involve a greater cost than doing the studies sequentially, but the time saved would more than compensate for the extra cost.

One series of studies should be performed, in several cooperating institutions, on the effects of mercenene on various kinds of human cancers grown in the hamster cheek pouch. This study should tell us which human cancers are likely to respond to mercenene, and which are not. Then, in the early years of mercenene production, when there may well be a shortage, the available medication could be used for those who are likely to be helped by it. Research scientists could then concentrate on finding treatments for the kinds of cancer that do not respond to mercenene.

Chemists and biochemists should, at the same time, be studying the chemical composition of mercenene. Once its composition is known, possibly it can be synthesized and made available at a reasonable cost. Furthermore, if and when its composition is known, it may be possible to design and synthesize modifications of the basic molecule, in order to improve the potency and broaden the spectrum of anti-cancer effects.

On the other hand, it may take chemists a long time to determine the chemical structure of mercenene, or it may not be possible to synthesize it. In that case, all supplies of mercenene would have to come from the sea. Accordingly, as soon as mercenene has been shown to be effective in spontaneous cancers, studies should be started on natural sources of this agent. It would be important to find out where mercenene itself originates. There seem to be two good possibilities.

First, mercenene may be synthesized by the clam, either completely or from precursors in its food. If so, we may for a long time be dependent on clams for this material. In that event, it would be most important to study other species of clams, particularly those in southern waters, to see if they contain comparable amounts of mercenene. Also, animals that prey on clams, such as the starfish, should be studied to find out if they, too, concentrate mercenene. If they do, they may be another source of the material. Studies should also be started on ways to increase the clam harvest sufficiently to provide mercenene for all patients needing it.

A second possibility is that mercenene originates in the ocean plankton and is concentrated by the clam. Sister Rosarii has pointed out that the nature of the clam makes this a reasonable possibility to consider (14). Clams are animated filters that pass large volumes of water through their mantle, straining out the microscopic plankton on which they feed. They are known to concentrate chemicals that are produced by the plankton, including some toxins. If it can be shown that mercenene comes from a planktonic organism, it may be possible to cultivate that organism in artificial media and obtain the mercenene from it directly as we now obtain antibiotics from cultures in artificial media.

The several studies proposed would require a substantial effort from teams of investigators drawn from a number of scientific disciplines. Unfortunately, there is not yet available sufficient extract for clinical testing. Some patients with cancer have, however, been placed on a supplementary whole clam diet, and have been reported to show considerable improvement (21).

Another aspect of the mercenene story is also of interest. Sister Rosarii's work was first supported by a fellowship from the National Science Foundation. Since then, the costs of her research have been borne by grants from voluntary agencies, particularly the American Cancer Society. This is an excellent demonstration of the value of the voluntary health research agencies in supporting investigators during the early stages of their work.

References

1. Ryder, J. A. On a tumor in the oyster. *Proc. Acad. Nat. Sci. of Phila.* Jan. 25, 1887, p. 25.
2. Collinge, W. E. Note on a tumour in Anodonta cygnaea, linn. *J. Anat. Physiol.* 22:154, 1890.
3. Williams, J. W. A tumour in the fresh-water mussel. *J. Anat. Physiol.* 24:307, 1890.
4. Smith, G. M. A mesenchymal tumor in an oyster (Ostrea virginica). *Am. J. Cancer* 22:838, 1934.
5. Garrison, W. Nun's battle against cancer. *Sign,* July 1965.
6. Schmeer, M. R. In: *Antibiotic News 2:*4, 1965 (Oct. 13).
7. Sullivan, T. D. and Nigrelli, R. F. Antitumorous action of biologics of marine origin. I. Survival of Swiss mice inoculated with Krebs-2 ascites tumor and treated with Holuthurin, a steroid saponin from the sea cucumber Actinopyga agassizi. *Proc. Am. Assoc. Cancer Res. 2:*151, 1956.
8. Li, C. P., Prescott, B., Eddy, B., Caldes, G., Green, W. R., Martino, E. C. and Young, A. M. Antiviral activity of paolins from clams. *Ann. N. Y. Acad. Sci. 130:* 374, 1965.
9. Signoret, P. Mise en évidence, chez certains bivalves marins, de systemes inhibiteurs agissant sur le virus de la mosaique du Tabac. *C. R. Acad. Sc. Paris 259:*3892, 1964.
10. Schmeer, M. R. Growth-inhibiting agents from mercenaria extracts: chemical and biological properties. *Science 144:*413, 1964.
11. Schmeer, M. R. and Huala, C. V. Mercenene: In vivo effects of mollusk extracts on the sarcoma 180. *Ann. N. Y. Acad. Sci. 118:*603, 1965.
12. Schmeer, M. R. Chemical and biological characteristics of growth-inhibiting agents from Mercenaria mercenaria extracts II. *Biol. Bull. 127:*388, 1964.
13. Schmeer, M. R. and Beery, G. Mercenene: A preliminary investigation of the cytological effects of this anti-tumor agent extracted from Mercenaria mercenaria on the Krebs-2 carcinoma. *Biol. Bull. 129:*420, 1965.
14. Schmeer, M. R. and Beery, G. Mercenene-growth-inhibitor extracted from the clam Mercenaria campechiensis. A preliminary investigation of *in-vivo* and *in-vitro* activity. *Life Sciences 4:*2157, 1965.
15. Schmeer, M. R. and Beery, G. Mercenene: Growth-inhibitor extracted from Mercenaria campechiensis. *In vivo* and *in vitro* activity. *Biol. Bull. 129:*420, 1965.

16. Schmeer, M. R., Horton, D. and Tanimura, A. Mercenene, a tumor inhibitor from *Mercenaria:* Purification and characterization studies. *Life Sciences 5:*1169, 1966.
17. Schmeer, M. R. and Cassidy, J. D. Mercenene: Preliminary analysis of induced focal changes in the Krebs-2 carcinoma fine structure. *Biol. Bull. 131:*405, 1966.
18. Schmeer, M. R. Mercenene: cytopathologic effects on Krebs-2 carcinoma in CF1 mice and HeLa (At1) and human amnion (FL) cell lines. *Cancer Chemotherapy Rep. 50:*655, 1966.
19. Hegyeli, A. Temperature dependence of the activity of the antitumor factor in the common clam. *Science 146:*77, 1964.
20. Szent-Gyorgyi, A. Cell division and cancer. *Science 149:*34, 1965.
21. Schmeer, M. R. Unpublished communication, 1967.
22. Schmeer, M. R. Mercenene: growth-inhibiting agent of Mercenaria extracts. Further chemical and biological characterization. *Ann. N. Y. Acad. Sci. 136:*211, 1966.

Leukemia and Ascorbic Acid

There is a possibility that some of the more distressing and dangerous symptoms of leukemia may be due to a relative deficiency of ascorbic acid (Vitamin C). Some deductions from the available information suggest that the leukemic cells may take up virtually all the available ascorbic acid, leaving such small amounts in the plasma and the tissues that the patient develops the symptoms of scurvy, a condition caused by ascorbic acid deficiency. Furthermore, it appears that administration of usual doses of ascorbic acid would have virtually no therapeutic effect because the avidity of the leukemic cells for this vitamin would keep it from the deficient tissue cells. Accordingly, experimental treatment with unusually large doses of ascorbic acid, aimed at correcting the deficiency in plasma and tissues, might have a good chance of relieving some of the most distressing symptoms of leukemia and, possibly, of prolonging the patient's life. Let us examine some of the relevant information.

In leukemia, the symptoms and signs that are reminiscent of scurvy include bleeding, especially from the gums, x-ray changes in the bones, and lowered resistance to infection. This leads us to query whether there might be some relationship between the *symptoms* of leukemia and the levels of ascorbic acid. We are not implying that ascorbic acid deficiency is related to the *cause* of leukemia, only that it may, in some fashion, be involved in certain leukemic *signs* and *symptoms*. Since some of these symptoms frequently lead to death, leukemia patients might be helped if the symptoms could be alleviated.

In searching for a possible relationship between leukemia and ascorbic acid, we find one that is readily apparent. All white blood cells (leukocytes), normal and leukemic, have a high affinity for ascorbic acid. In health, the leukocytes contain from 20 to 45 *times* the serum concentration of ascorbic acid, depending on the population sample studied and the investigator (1-4). (The platelets contain about the same levels as the leukocytes.) In ascorbic acid deficiency in otherwise normal persons, the ascorbic acid level in the leukocytes is about 100 *times* the level in the plasma. This, of course, suggests a partition effect, with the leukocytes drawing the ascorbic acid out of the serum. The significance of this observation lies in the probability that the leukocytes will, in a sense, hoard the available ascorbic acid, even when the plasma concentrations fall to scurvy levels.

The actual levels of ascorbic acid in leukemic leukocytes are roughly comparable to the levels in normal leukocytes. The potential affinity of leukemic cells for ascorbic acid, however, may be even greater than the affinity of normal leukocytes. Barkham and Howard (4) found ascorbic acid levels of over 60 mgm per 100 cc in packed leukemic cells, after giving the patients large doses of ascorbic acid. (The normal plasma concentration is 0.7 to 1.4 mgm per 100 cc.)

In patients with leukemia, the concentration of ascorbic acid ranged from 45 to over 100 *times* the concentration in the plasma, according to different observers (1, 3, 4).

Let us consider next the total number of leukocytes that may be involved. In leukemia, there are two obvious departures from normal, a marked increase in the numbers of white blood cells, and an abnormality in those cells. For many decades, it was believed that the increase in white blood cells in leukemia came about because of increased multiplication rates of the parent cells in the bone marrow. Recent studies (5-7) suggest that this is not the case, and that leukemic cells may not be produced at more rapid rates than normal leukocytes. Instead, the large numbers of leukemic cells may be explained by long survival times of the immature leukemic cells, whereas the normal, mature white blood cells have short survival times (6 to 12 hours).

The total number of white blood cells in the entire body, whether in health or in leukemia, is far greater than the number in the blood. Despite their name, only a small fraction of the white cells are actually in the blood stream at any particular time. Most are scattered throughout the body tissues. This distribution of the white blood cells exists, in general, in leukemia as well as in health, although the exact ratios may differ somewhat. One estimate is that in health there are 36 times as many lymphocytes, a type of white blood cell, outside the blood as inside (8). Similarly, a very small proportion of the granulocytes, another type, are actually in the blood stream at any one time (9, 10). Let us assume—conservatively—that the total number of white cells in the entire body is 30 times the number in the blood. In health, the leukocyte volume in the blood is approximately 1 per cent of the total blood volume, or about 50 cc of white blood cells in 5 liters of blood. Accordingly, in a condition of health, we should expect 30 times that amount, or about 1,500 cc of leukocytes, distributed throughout the body.

In leukemia, not only does the leukocyte content of the blood rise, but the number of leukocytes in the tissues also rises—perhaps even to a proportionately higher level. Thus in leukemia, with white blood cell counts of 10 times normal (a level which is not unusual), the total volume of white blood cells in the body may rise to 10 and even 15 liters.

If these white blood cells require 60 mgm of ascorbic acid per 100 cc of packed cells, as suggested by the studies of Barkham and Howard (4), then 15 liters, or 15,000 cc, of such cells could require 60 mgm × 150 or 9,000 mgm, which is 9 grams.

In the normal body, there are about 4 grams of ascorbic acid (11), and about 1 gram of this is held by the white blood cells. However, in leukemia, 4 grams of ascorbic acid are not enough to saturate the large volume of white blood cells; up to 9 grams may be needed. In other words, there is a potential deficit of about 8 grams of ascorbic acid insofar as the leukocytes are concerned; until that deficit is made up, virtually none of the ingested or administered ascorbic acid would get to the other body cells requiring it. Furthermore, it appears that much of the ascorbic acid that is taken up by the leukocytes is not released in an active form when the leukocytes are destroyed. Thus, the daily requirement of ascorbic acid in leukemia would probably be several times the normal requirement, even if the initial deficit were made up.

As an initial estimate, subject to experimental testing, it seems that in patients with leukemia, from 5 to 15 *grams* of ascorbic acid might be needed to bring the leukocytes up to a sufficient degree of saturation to allow the other cells of the body to obtain an adequate supply of ascorbic acid. (Barkham and Howard (4) found that in one of their patients, approximately 15 *grams* of ascorbic acid were needed to produce saturation.) Afterwards, from 0.5 to 1 *gram* of ascorbic acid per day would probably be needed to maintain reasonable plasma and tissue levels. However, the usual ascorbic acid intake in a good diet is only 75 *mgm* per day. When ascorbic acid is prescribed as a supplement, the dose is usually 100 to 250 *mgm* per day. With such doses, in leukemia, one would expect practically all the absorbed ascorbic acid to be sequestered by the leukocytes, leaving virtually none for the tissues. Accordingly, the subsequent development of symptoms resembling scurvy may simply represent actual scurvy in the affected tissues.

This problem seems worthy of further study. Ascorbic acid balance studies should be done in patients with leukemia. Techniques of administration will probably have to be modified, since one cannot give high concentrations of ascorbic acid without a considerable loss in the urine, even when a deficiency exists. A suggested modification would be the administration of 500 mgm every two hours for six doses per day, until saturation occurs. Then, measurements of plasma and leukocyte levels of ascorbic acid should be continued while the patient receives the usual recommended dietary amount of the vitamin, 75 mgm. The rate of fall in plasma levels may provide some indication of the rate of destruction of this vitamin in leukemias. Care must be taken that the plasma does not contain debris from broken down leukocytes or platelets.

In leukemic patients who tend to bleed and who exhibit other signs reminiscent of scurvy, a clinical trial of large doses (5 grams per day in divided doses) of ascorbic acid seems justifiable. Should it be shown that such large doses relieve the symptoms of ascorbic acid deficiency, then we suggest that the leukemia patient might receive more benefit from the chemotherapeutic agents currently available if ascorbic acid were added to the therapeutic regimen.

References

1. Butler, A. M. and Cushman, M. Distribution of ascorbic acid in the blood and its nutritional significance. *J. Clin. Invest. 19:*459, 1940.
2. Bodansky, O., Wroblewski, F. and Markardt, B. Concentrations of ascorbic acid in plasma and white blood cells of patients with cancer and noncancerous chronic disease. *Cancer 5:*678, 1952.
3. Waldo, A. L. and Zipf, R. E. Ascorbic acid level in leukemic patients. *Cancer 8:* 187, 1955.
4. Barkham, P. and Howard, A. N. Distribution of ascorbic acid in normal and leukaemic blood. *Biochem. J. 70:*163, 1958.
5. Gavosto, F., Maraini, G. and Pileri, A. Proliferative capacity of acute leukaemia cells. *Nature 187:*611, 1960.
6. Vladimirskaya, E. B., Simonov, E. E., Balakhovskii, I. S., and Ivanova, I. E. Proliferative activity of leukemic cells in acute leukemia. *Fed. Proc.* (Trans. Suppl.) *24:*633, 1966.
7. Astaldi, G. Differentiation, proliferation, and maturation of haemopoietic cells studies in tissue culture. *Ciba Foundation Symposium on Haemopoiesis.* London, 1960, p. 99.
8. Price, D. *Dynamics of Proliferating Tissues.* U. of Chicago Press, Chicago, 1958, p. 66.
9. *Ibid.,* p. 71.

PART IV

10. Osgood, E. E. Number and distribution of human hemic cells. *Blood 9:*1141, 1954.

11. Lowry, O. H., Bessey, O. A., Brock, M. J. and Lopez, J. A. The interrelationship of dietary, serum, white blood cell, and total body ascorbic acid. *J. Biol. Chem. 166:*111, 1946.

PART V

MOBILIZATION OF OUR NATIONAL RESOURCES AGAINST CANCER

A major component of our efforts to cure or control cancer must be the efficient utilization of all persons who are willing and able to contribute to the national program. We must include not only the cancer scientists who are currently engaged in research, but also many scientists who could be productive in cancer research, but are not doing such research now. Some cancer scientists of proven ability are not working on cancer because they cannot obtain the research grants they need. Then, there are scientists in such fields as immunology, pharmacology, and pathology who would be willing to work in the cancer area, but are not doing so because they happen not to have original ideas upon which to base a cancer research program. Many would be willing to join programs initiated by other scientists.

There are also several groups of scientists, who are not usually thought of when the term "cancer researcher" is used. These scientists have specialized skills, abilities and training which could be invaluable in many facets of a well-coordinated national program. A few members of such groups are doing cancer research, but most are not and, indeed, may themselves be unaware of the extent to which they could help.

In this section several groups of scientists and technicians will be considered, and examples given of the ways in which they could help reach the goal of a cure or control for cancer.

Increasing the Supply of Cancer Research Scientists and Technicians

A major expansion of our research program would, of course, require a corresponding increase in the number of scientists and technicians working on the cancer problem. These extra people can be obtained, however, within a fairly short period of time and without any serious disruption of other important programs. Let us first consider the scientists.

Cancer Research Scientists

As of November 1965, more than half the research applications to the National Cancer Institute (NCI) were being turned down, and of those that were being approved less than half were being funded. Let us consider the applications that have been approved but not funded. Each of these represents a scientist whose work and ideas have passed critical scrutiny at his own institution and in Washington. Each represents a scientist who wants to do cancer research and who is capable of doing it, but who cannot because he cannot obtain the needed funds. It seems a logical conclusion, therefore, that by furnishing these people with the needed support, we can practically double the number of cancer research scientists almost immediately. Of course, the longer we delay, the less effective will be our efforts at keeping these men in cancer research, or bringing them back into it after they have gone into other fields of endeavor.

Among the applications that have been rejected by the NCI, there have probably been a substantial number that came from competent scientists, but that had one or another flaw, in the eyes of the reviewing committees. Flaws can be corrected, however, if someone who knows what they are is willing to correct them. Perhaps some of these rejected applications were written unskillfully; others, perhaps, asked for too much money; in still others the review of the literature may not have been satisfactory. Perhaps, in some cases, the ideas and approaches just did not appeal to the review committees. Within the group of unsuccessful applicants, we should be able to find many who can do worthwhile cancer research. If we add their number to that of the scientists involved in projects that were approved but not funded, the number of immediately competent researchers may turn out to be three times the number now engaged in cancer research.

The question may be raised as to whether the cancer research scientists who were unable to obtain financial support for their own projects would be willing to work on projects suggested by some person or group in Washington. I believe most of them would be willing, and would do an excellent job, especially if they were permitted to choose from several projects. Cancer research is different from scientific research that does not involve so many human lives. There is less feeling of "ownership" of ideas and approaches when cancer is involved. The primary desire of most cancer scientists is to help save lives, and they could be expected to work on their own ideas or on a joint program as long as they would feel that the project was worthwhile.

Other Scientists

There are many scientists who do not think of themselves as cancer researchers, but who could, and would, contribute a great deal to a coordinated cancer research program if they were invited to do so. Training in the basic medical, biological and chemical sciences, at the Ph.D. level, is discipline-oriented; the student is trained to do competent work within a fairly wide area of such particular scientific disciplines as microbiology and immunology, pharmacology, and biochemistry. After receiving their degrees, these scientists think of themselves as microbiologists and immunologists, pharmacologists, biochemists and so forth. They may, and often do, have special interests within their disciplines, but they remain broadly competent within their disciplines. An immunologist or biochemist who had never worked with cancer would probably find it difficult to complete a cancer research project by himself, but if invited to work with a team and contribute his own special knowledge and skills, he could fit in quickly and do valuable work. After a few years, most of these scientists would have learned enough about cancer to carry on independent research if they wished to do so. In the past, a substantial number of cancer researchers have come from these ranks. Whether this trend will continue depends on what we do.

Although most of these scientists are working on research problems of their own, many of them would be willing to defer their own research to help find a cure or control for cancer. They are not likely to do so, however, until our cancer research program is revitalized and reorganized. Certainly, few of these scientists are likely, under the present circumstances, to try to break into cancer research by applying for research support. The prospect of spending many months preparing a research grant application that has less than 25 per cent chance of approval and funding is simply not attractive.

On the other hand, if we had a series of task forces aimed at attacking discrete parts of the cancer problem, and if the task forces would invite the scientists to join them and would assure the scientists of reasonable support for their work, a large proportion would join. This method of recruitment has been used with great success by the national space program; it could also succeed in a national cancer research program.

Scientists over 65

Qualified scientists who have been involuntarily retired after reaching an arbitrary age—sometimes 65, sometimes 68, and sometimes 70—are another source of supply. Many of these scientists want desperately to continue doing constructive work and yet are denied the opportunity to do so simply because they were born in a particular year. Most of them are still intellectually capable of doing important work if they were allowed to do so. The extent to which brains and experience are lost by forced retirements and, reciprocally, the extent to which older scientists can continue to make contributions has not been adequately studied. Some examples may be revealing, however.

In 1966, one of the two recipients of the Nobel Prize in medicine was Francis Peyton Rous, who was eighty-seven at the time, and still actively engaged in research at Rockefeller University.

Another example is Eugene Opie who, in 1942, took over the chairmanship of the pathology department at Cornell University Medical College when the man who had held that position went into military service. Although well past the retirement age, Dr. Opie remained chairman for the duration of the war. He had had a distinguished career: He had published key articles on the pathology of tuberculosis; his study of the pathology of diabetes had led to the discovery of insulin; he had been a dean of a leading medical school. The students at Cornell were pleased to have so distinguished and capable a teacher, and quickly realized that Dr. Opie had plenty of vigor and ability. At the end of the war, Dr. Opie went to Rockefeller University to undertake full-time research, which he is continuing today. Even after he had reached his 90th year, he made contributions (1-4) that any scientist half Dr. Opie's age would be happy to have to his credit.

It is no coincidence that both Dr. Rous and Dr. Opie are at Rockefeller University. That institution is one of very few that allow older scientists to keep up their research. Surely humanity has gained much from this wise policy. In planning a major cancer research program, we ought to include provisions that will permit us to utilize the services of all capable scientists, regardless of how old they are.

Objections to this proposal have often been directed at the possibility that older scientists may have had one or more "silent" strokes which would sharply reduce their capabilities. In reply to such objections, we point out that the life of one famous scientist suggests that even an overt stroke need not, by itself, disqualify a scientist from contributing to medical research. At the age of forty-four, Louis Pasteur suffered a major stroke which almost proved fatal. Although he recovered, his entire left side, arm, hand, leg and tongue, remained paralyzed for the rest of his life. Nevertheless, Pasteur kept working, and the major discoveries for which he is honored today were all made after the stroke (5). How fortunate we are that no one forced Pasteur to stop his experiments because of a stroke!

Technicians

In cancer research today, many senior investigators are doing tasks that they could readily delegate to technicians, if they had the technicians. There is a shortage of competent, college-trained cancer research technicians today, and the shortage could become more severe with an expansion of the program unless preventive steps are taken. The main problem is a financial one. The salaries of medical research technicians, in terms of the salaries offered to educated people for highly skilled work, generally are at, or close to, the bottom of the scale. In some large institutions, the beginning yearly salary for a college-trained medical technician who works a 40-hour week, 50 weeks a year, is as low as $4,000. Increases are infrequent, and the ceiling is low. How are these jobs filled today? Some cancer technicians are young men interested in the field and eager to make a contribution to humanity. It may take six months to a year to train a technician adequately. Soon afterwards, he recognizes that he cannot support himself, and even less a family, on a medical research technician's income. He then leaves—with regrets—for a field in which salaries are more reasonable.

Some cancer research technicians are young women who take the position until they marry and raise a family, or until their husbands finish school. While working, they do a fine job, but seldom consider returning to research when their children have reached school age. In part, this is so because of unwise and unfair income tax regulations.

There are very few career research technicians—people who intend to keep up their work for 20 or more years—and they are priceless. In cancer research laboratories one usually finds a succession of technicians, each staying for a rather brief period, while the scientists spend a disproportionate amount of time looking for, and training, their replacements.

Two major steps must be taken in order to correct this situation. First, cancer research technicians—and other medical technicians—ought to receive a reasonable income, commensurate with their training and with the job requirements. In negotiating research grants and contracts with universities and institutes, the Federal Government should require a salary range for technicians that is comparable to the salaries paid to technicians working for NASA and similar agencies. A reasonable salary structure should lead to the development of a corps of experienced career technicians.

A second step that needs to be taken is a revision of income tax regulations in relation to working mothers. Such a revision would not only increase the supply of cancer research technicians, but would also help relieve the shortages of nurses, teachers and other skilled people. Many women would like to return to the work for which they trained, once their children have reached school age, but find it economically impossible to do so. If they went to work, they would have to pay an income tax on their salaries, but would not be allowed to deduct the cost of a maid or housekeeper whom they would have to hire. Considering the other expenses connected with holding a job, such as carfare, lunches, and clothing, she may actually lose money by returning to work. So in many cases she does not go back to work, and valuable and scarce skills are lost to the nation.

The U.S. Treasury would not lose money by fair treatment of working mothers; it would gain, since many more would return to work and have an income on which to pay taxes. Furthermore, the maids and housekeepers would also pay income taxes on their wages. A fair policy would not deprive men of jobs, since the positions in which women are paid substantially more than the wages of a housekeeper require specialized skills and training, and are positions that often are unfilled.

References

1. Opie, E. L. On the relation of inflammation to the chemical constitution of injurious agents. On the pharmacology of inflammation. *J. Exptl. Med. 117:*425, 1963.
2. Opie, E. L. Inflammation in serous cavities. *A.M.A. Arch. Pathol. 78:*1, 1964.
3. Opie, E. L. The relation of the inflammation to the molecular structure of carbon compounds soluble in the fluids of the body. *J. Expt'l. Med. 121:*487, 1965.
4. Opie, E. L. The normal and pathological movement of water in tissues and its relation to the colligative properties of solutions and to inflammation. *Proc. N.A.S. 56:*426, 1966.
5. Dubos, R. *Pasteur and Modern Science.* Doubleday and Co., Garden City, N. Y., 1960, p. 104.

The Potential Contributions of the Veterinary Profession to Cancer Research

Since the bulk of cancer research is being, and will probably continue to be, conducted on animals, one might expect that veterinarians, who are expert in diseases of animals, would be playing a major role in the research program. But the members of the veterinary profession, thus far, have not been given the support they need to make a major contribution to the national cancer research effort. There were first-class veterinary colleges in 1966 that did not have a single grant for cancer research from the National Cancer Institute. To be sure, individual veterinarians are on the staffs of some hospitals and medical schools, in charge of the animal quarters and the general health and well-being of the animals therein. Obviously, this is only a small fraction of the contribution that veterinarians could make if an adequate program were in existence.

The potential importance of a program that includes the veterinarians is based not only on the training and experience of veterinarians in terms of animal diseases, but also on the access veterinarians have to large animals, and on the current emphasis on comparative medicine as well as on the facilities existing in the nation's 18 colleges of veterinary medicine. In several areas, the veterinary profession can perform studies that would be almost impossible for any other group to undertake.

Dr. Cotchin, of the Royal Veterinary College in London, has studied cancers in animals in great detail and has commented (17):

Further, therapeutic studies on the spontaneous tumours of animals should be extended. Such studies would exploit the property that distinguishes them from the experimental tumours of laboratory animals usually employed—that is, that these neoplasms are spontaneous. A transplanted tumour might well behave differently in such trials from a spontaneous tumour. The dosage rate, too, applicable to small laboratory animals may be such that results obtained are different from what they would be in an animal that is big enough, both absolutely and relatively to the tumour it bears, to receive a dosage rate and treatment regime that are more comparable with what can be given to humans.

Let us consider some of the areas in which the veterinary profession could contribute greatly to finding a cure or control for cancer.

All of the species of mammals known to us develop cancer. The domestic animals develop certain types of cancer that are admirably suited for some important research projects. The person who is accustomed to thinking of cancer research in terms of hundreds or thousands of mice may find it hard to accept the suggestion that a cow might be more suitable for some studies. Nevertheless, for some studies, cows would be not only more suitable but also more economical than mice—provided that the cows were handled and kept at a veterinary school, not in a hospital or medical school in a large city. For some studies, in which the experimenter intends to make and study extracts of cancers, a large mass of cancer tissue is needed. It may be easier and more economical to obtain this material from one or two cows than from a thousand mice.

A few years ago, in connection with some research the author was doing in leukemia, a substantial volume of leukemic cells was needed. For one part of the study, human leukemic cells were used; they were obtained, with permission, from patients with leukemia. We hoped to make some comparisons with leukemic cells in another species and considered mice. It is a rather simple matter to transmit leukemia to inbred mice, and then, a few weeks later, kill them and remove the blood. One can obtain about 1 cc of blood from each mouse, containing about 1/25 cc of leukemic cells. The inbred mice cost about 75¢ each; counting the cost of boarding them and transmitting the leukemia, it was estimated that it would cost about $1.25 to $1.50 to obtain each sample of blood. Since about 1,250 mice would have been needed the cost would have been between $1,500 and $1,900.

Instead of using mice, we called the University of Missouri Veterinary School and asked for help. They informed us that among the animals brought to their clinic there were at times cattle with leukemia, and that they would get us all the leukemic blood we wanted. About three weeks later, a cow brought to the veterinary clinic was found to have leukemia. Since the animal could not be used for food and had lost most of its economic value, the farmer was happy to sell it for $100. The veterinarians then removed about 4,000 cc of blood aseptically, and separated from it more than 50 cc of leukemic cells. The total cost of obtaining the leukemic cells from the cow was less than one-tenth what it would have cost to obtain them from mice, and took less time. The same savings would apply when large masses of a solid cancer were wanted; obviously it is much more economical to obtain large masses from one or two cattle than from several hundred mice.

Cancers in Cattle

Some cancers available to veterinarians are almost ideal for certain research projects. One is an eyelid cancer, which is fairly frequent in Hereford (whiteface) cattle. This cancer, sometimes called "epithelioma" or "cancer eye," begins as a small premalignant outgrowth on the eyelid. It eventually turns into a cancer and gradually invades surrounding tissues; later on, it will metastasize to distant organs (1). Ordinarily, these cancers are not given time to grow. As soon as a farmer sees that one of his cattle has "cancer eye," he takes it to the slaughterhouse. The government veterinarian inspects the animal; if the cancer is not too large and does not seem to have metastasized, he will pass the carcass, except for the head, as being fit for human consumption. If there is evidence that the cancer has metastasized, he will condemn the entire carcass. Since a full-grown animal will bring about $180 to $250, it is easy to see why cattle with early eye cancer are slaughtered quickly. A research facility attached to a veterinary school could purchase these animals at about the market price. A small proportion of cattle with eyelid cancer are being studied in various institutions, but the vast majority are still being slaughtered for beef. Thus, if an adequate national research program were developed, there would probably be no serious shortage of cattle with eyelid cancer for the appropriate studies. According to a study of Brandly and Migaki (2), we can estimate that eyelid cancer develops in about 30,000 to 60,000 cattle in the United States each year. This is considerably more than would be required by the studies suggested here.

Let us consider some of the advantages that the eyelid cancer has for research purposes. The probability that eyelid cancer will develop in an animal can often be determined by a veterinarian even before the cancer itself has developed because usually, a noncancerous growth (keratosis, plaque, or papilloma) develops first. This growth later changes into cancer. Thus, eyelid cancer in cattle can furnish a model for studies of the early development of cancer.

The location of the cancer makes it readily available for biopsy, without the need for any major surgery. If the experimental design requires it, several biopsies can be done at intervals.

The growth rate of an eyelid cancer can be observed, measured, and photographed with no difficulty, at intervals as frequent as may be desired. Thus permanent and accurate data are obtainable. By contrast, measurement of growth of internal cancers is often difficult and confusing, since it involves estimates of size obtained by finger pressure through several layers of normal tissue. For technical reasons, serial photographs of the growth of internal cancers are seldom practical.

The response of the bovine eyelid cancers to experimental treatments can also be readily measured and photographed. This makes them particularly suitable as a test object in evaluating drugs or procedures.

Of particular importance is the similarity between bovine eyelid cancer and cancer in man. Both are spontaneous cancers, and both appear to be similar in anatomy and behavior.

Barron (3) has stated:

Human and bovine ocular squamous cell carcinoma are parallel diseases. The neoplasm in either species may serve as a model for the other.

Bovine eyelid cancer has been rather extensively studied by many investigators (4-16), and a great deal is known about its structure and behavior. Although basic information about this condition is available, it is, unfortunately, not being followed up and exploited in terms of helping develop more effective treatments for human cancer.

In several chapters of this book, potentially valuable experimental studies on bovine eyelid cancer are described. Eyelid cancer as well as other cancers in large animals are particularly suitable for studies on metastases, for studies on the potential value of chemotherapy and radiation as adjuncts to surgery, and in projects for which mice are unsuitable, and that cannot ethically be done on human patients.

Cattle with cancers other than of the eyelid type are usually rejected for food purposes in federally inspected slaughterhouses, and therefore have hardly any residual economic value. If a veterinary school were able to offer a fair price for such animals, it could probably obtain enough cancer specimens to build up a respectable series. The other cancers that occur in reasonable numbers in cattle include cancer of the uterus, malignant melanomas (skin tumors which are usually black), lymphosarcoma and cancer of the bladder (17).

One point of interest is the extreme rarity of mammary cancer in cattle. This is striking in view of the large volume of mammary tissue in the cow. Other domestic animals develop breast cancers much more frequently.

Cancers in Other Farm Animals

A research program in veterinary schools could obtain from the nation's farms, in addition to cattle, a substantial number of farm animals with cancers useful for research, including malignant melanoma in the pig and in the horse (particularly grey horses) (18), kidney cancers (19), and lymphosarcomas (20). In general, the number of these cancers that become available might not be large enough at this time to sustain a comprehensive research program, but the cancers would be useful to check findings on the more common cancers of cattle and dogs. There is also a good possibility that veterinarians could develop special strains of domesticated farm animals with a high incidence of spontaneous cancers. An excellent animal for this purpose would be the so-called miniature pig, which at maturity weighs 150 to 200 pounds—approximately the same as man. Pigs are quite similar to man in some important aspects of physiology and susceptibility to disease (34).

Cancers in Dogs

Dogs have a higher incidence of spontaneous cancers than most animals, and several observers have indicated that, in a given year, about 5 per cent of all mature dogs have cancer (17, 23). The incidence of cancer is about twice as high in purebred as in mixed-breed dogs. The most common cancers in dogs are the mammary gland cancers (17, 22), malignant melanomas (17, 23), mastocytomas (17, 24, 25, 26), bone sarcomas (17, 27), seminomas (17, 30) and lymphosarcomas (28).

Dogs with spontaneous cancer in the United States could be a major resource in cancer research, if appropriate arrangements were made. Today, most dogs found to have cancer are killed at the request of the owners. In a few cases, the owners are able and willing to pay substantial fees for private veterinary surgery. At the present time, facilities do not exist where we could try to cure many of these dogs, even if the owners wished to turn them over to our research hospitals and medical schools. If an appropriate program were to be worked out, centered in the veterinary colleges, it would be quite feasible and economical to provide a therapeutic service to many dogs with cancer, and at the same time obtain invaluable information relating to human cancer (29, 33). Several aspects of such a program require consideration. First, there is the question of the specific care of the animals. In a program as envisioned here, the animals themselves would derive considerable benefit; hopefully, many would be cured. Thus, these studies must be distinguished from those in which the result is not to benefit the dogs, but to benefit man only.

In the proposed studies on dogs with cancers, different types of therapeutic procedures could be tried in order to determine which are most effective. Suppose we wish to know whether surgery preceded by administration of a particular anti-cancer drug would give a higher cure rate than surgery alone. It is difficult to conduct such studies in man, in part, because the doctor is obligated to give each patient the best treatment he can think of. If a surgeon has even a suspicion that a drug would help, he would probably prescribe it for all his patients before surgery. Another doctor who suspects that the drug reduces survival rates would not use it. Furthermore, it would not be feasible to compare the results obtained by the two doctors, since they may be dealing with different kinds of cancers, since their skills may differ, and so forth. On the other hand, it would be both ethical and practical to perform such a study on two fairly evenly matched groups of dogs. It should be emphasized that the study would benefit both groups of dogs, since in the absence of such a program, the dogs would probably not receive any definitive treatment.

Another type of study could be done on new anti-cancer drugs as they are developed, including plant extracts. In our current program, these drugs are tested first in mice, and then those that seem promising may be given to human patients. Our experience has shown, however, that the response of mice with cancer frequently differs from the response of larger animals with cancer. This is probably due in large part to the predominant use of transplanted cancers in mice, while domestic animals and human patients have spontaneous cancers. There may be other reasons for the difference: e.g., species of animals may vary in their ability to handle drugs. As matters stand, it is difficult to know whether a drug that works well in transplanted mouse cancers will work in spontaneous human cancers. Accordingly, patients with early cancer are seldom given the new drugs. They are treated by surgery and radiation, and only if the cancer becomes advanced do they receive the anti-cancer drugs. It is possible, of course, that the drugs are curative only in early cancer. Some scientists believe this to be so. But the risk of giving a relatively unknown drug to a patient with early cancer which might be cured by surgery or radiation seems too high. In this situation, an intermediate step between mouse and man would be of great value. If the new anti-cancer drugs were tested on dogs (or other large animals) with spontaneous cancers we would have this intermediate step. A drug that is as effective in dogs with spontaneous cancers as it is in mice would probably be considered worth giving to human patients. Here, too, it should be noted that all the dogs in the study would benefit; but some would benefit more than others.

Another point to consider is the general care of the dogs. It is proposed that facilities be built in our veterinary schools—initially in a selected five or six schools and, eventually in all 18 schools—to provide optimum general care and comfort for the animals. This includes comfortable quarters with runways and exercise areas, so that owners of dogs could see the facilities and know that their dogs would be comfortable and happy there. Also, there would be an adequate staff of trained attendants, and there would be suitable operating rooms, treatment rooms, and other necessary facilities. All operations would be done with proper anesthetics, and postoperative care would be provided. Dogs with distressing symptoms would be treated appropriately, just as human patients are. For example, a dog that is vomiting would receive anti-vomiting drugs. In effect, the dogs would, and should, receive care comparable to that given to human patients in a hospital. In some cases, it may be feasible, after a treatment has been completed, to allow the dog to return home; the owner would then send in weekly reports on its condition, and the dog would be checked at regular intervals by a cooperating local veterinarian.

A question that may arise is whether a sufficient number of dogs with spontaneous cancers could be obtained by voluntary donations of the owners. I believe that, with the cooperation of local veterinarians, they could and would. Indeed, it is likely that after the program has been in existence for a few years there will be more requests to send dogs to the veterinary school facilities than they can handle.

It is of interest that, in England, Dr. L. N. Owen (33) of the School of Veterinary Medicine at Cambridge University has been conducting a similar program on a small scale, using dogs that are referred to him by practicing veterinarians with the full cooperation of the owners.

Cancers in Cats

Cats also develop spontaneous cancers; if the dog studies described above were to be successful, it might be worthwhile to undertake

272

similar projects using cats. Common cancers of the cat include squamous cell carcinomas (31, 32), which are fairly common on the ear flaps of white cats, and cancer of the mammary gland (33).

Spontaneous Cancers in Mice

Another area in which the veterinary colleges could help the national cancer research program is in supplying mice with spontaneous cancers. Much of the experimental work will still have to be done with mice, but because of the economics of commercial mouse breeding it is difficult to obtain more than a few mice with spontaneous cancers. These occur mainly in elderly mice, and the vast majority of them are mammary cancers. A handful are found in 8-month-old mice, more in 10-month-old mice, and a substantial percentage in 12-month-old animals. At the age of 16 months, from 30 to 90 per cent of a group of female mice will have developed spontaneous mammary gland cancers, depending on the breeding strain. Since the commercial mouse breeders have observed that female mice tend to raise smaller litters after the age of 8 months and since they derive their income mainly from the sales of weanling mice, they have found it economically advantageous to kill female mice at the age of 8 months and replace them with new females. As a result, few female mice in the establishments of commercial breeders become old enough to develop spontaneous cancers. Although a medical scientist may buy, at the minimal price of 15¢ each, the 8-month-old female mice that would otherwise be killed and keep them until they reach an age when many will develop tumors, this would be an expensive undertaking in a medical school or hospital. The mice require not only space that cannot readily be spared but also expert veterinary care.

The story is different for a veterinary college located outside of a large city. Here, elderly female mice could be kept at a reasonable cost until they develop cancers. In general, veterinarians have a clear understanding of the costs of animal care and maintenance, and can do an efficient job more economically than any other group. If the buildings and facilities were supplied by a government agency, a veterinary college could keep large numbers of female mice at a cost of about ½¢ per day per mouse. Thus, a mouse kept from the age of 8 months to 14 months (which should be about the average) would cost 15¢ + 90¢ or $1.05. If 75 per cent of the mice develop cancer, the cost of a mouse with cancer would be $1.40. If substantial numbers of mice with spontaneous cancers of the appropriate size were available at that price, many investigators would wish to use them. If the mice that do not develop cancer could be used in studies of aging and sold to other investigators, the mice with cancer would be available for $1.05.

The initial cost of the buildings and equipment to house these mice would seem to be a legitimate expenditure for the Federal Government, especially since the Government has already paid several million dollars to large drug companies for construction of buildings in which to breed special strains of mice for research purposes.

Again, this phase of the program may be begun in only five or six veterinary colleges, and be expanded as necessary to the others.

Some Financial Considerations

The costs of starting programs in the veterinary colleges would be much lower than is generally realized. The cost of maintaining a cow with cancer, for example, would be less than 1/30 of the cost of maintaining a human patient in a hospital per day. Table 29-1 lists some of the costs of the use of farm animals. Mature cattle can be kept at a cost of less than $1 per day, including feed and general care.

Let us see just how much it would cost to initiate the proposed programs in our veterinary schools. The estimates in Table 29-2 are

Table 29-1. Approximate Costs for Purchase and Maintenance of Large Animals

	Species				
	Cattle	Horse	Pony	Sheep	Swine
Weight in lb. of average mature animal	1200	1400	500	150	400
Cost range	$180–220	$100–300	$50–75	$14–20	$40–75
Daily feed costs	$0.37	$0.32	$0.15	$0.09	$0.21
Man-hours for daily care per animal in herd of 5 or more	0.2	0.5	0.3	0.1	0.2
Cost of daily care at rate of $2.50 per hour	$0.50	$1.25	$0.75	$0.25	$0.50
Area for indoor quarters (sq. ft.)	25–45	120–140	40–50	15–20	35–45

Table 29–2. Estimated Costs of Developing Major Cancer Research Facilities in Veterinary Schools

Year 1	Non-Recurring Costs	Annual Costs
A. Farm Animal Studies per School		
Facilities		
Barns, pens, acreage	$ 800,000	
Laboratory buildings	1,400,000	
Equipment	200,000	
Operations		
Costs of animals		$ 100,000
Cost of animal feed and care		70,000
Salaries of professional and technical personnel		150,000
Total per school	2,400,000	320,000
× 18 schools	43,200,000	5,760,000
B. Studies on Dogs		
Facilities		
Animal quarters, including runways	700,000	
Laboratory buildings	700,000	
Equipment	100,000	
Operations		
Costs of shipping animals		50,000
Cost of animal food and care		80,000
Salaries of professional and technical personnel		150,000
Total per school	1,500,000	280,000
× 6 schools	9,000,000	1,680,000
C. Breeding of Mice with Spontaneous Cancers		
Facilities		
Buildings for mouse breeding	900,000	
Laboratory buildings	400,000	
Equipment	100,000	
Operations		
Cost of procuring mice		30,000
Shipping costs		50,000
Cost of animal feed and care		90,000
Salaries of professional and technical personnel		90,000
Total per school	1,400,000	260,000
× 6 schools	8,400,000	1,560,000
Grand Total	60,600,000	9,000,000

based on discussions with veterinarians, but the author takes full responsibility for them. They are based on the assumption that most of the facilities will be constructed in rural or suburban areas, not within large cities.

As is evident from the table, the program in veterinary schools could be carried out at an estimated cost of just over $60 million for initial construction and equipment, and about $9 million per year in operating expenses for the entire country. This is a modest amount, compared to other government expenditures for programs of less promise and importance. Indeed, after construction of the facilities, the cost of carrying out the program on a nationwide basis per year comes to considerably less than the cost of the space program for a single day!

The construction costs are substantial, but the buildings should be serviceable for perhaps 30 years. If a fully satisfactory cure or control for cancer should be found fairly soon, the buildings could then be used to help find better treatments for other diseases common to man and animals.

In the past, it had been customary for the Federal Government to insist on matching funds for construction of research facilities. That is, a university, college or hospital wishing to construct medical research buildings had to pay for half their cost, and the Federal Government paid the other half. In theory, this may have seemed advisable, but in practice it meant that the wealthier institutions were able to raise much more money than the poorer ones, and thus received the major share of the government monies. By contrast, those institutions that needed funds most received little or no government help. Unfortunately, veterinary colleges are not wealthy, and there is little chance that they could raise funds for half of the construction costs of these research buildings. There is no sound reason why they should be asked to, however. When the Federal Government supports other research programs, such as space exploration, high-energy physics, and some forms of atomic energy, it is willing to pay the entire cost of the buildings needed. Why should cancer research not receive similar consideration? Although the veterinary schools would benefit to some extent, the major beneficiaries would be the people who have cancer and those who will develop cancer—in effect, the general public. It seems perfectly reasonable to expect that the Federal Government, acting in behalf of the general public should be willing to pay the entire cost of these cancer research facilities.

The importance of the potential contribution of the veterinary profession to cancer research should not be underestimated. The conclusion reached by Cotchin (17) seems particularly apt. He stated:

It is hoped that it has been made clear that in veterinary comparative oncology there is a vast and largely unknown field awaiting exploration. If this field is to be adequately and fruitfully explored, then close collaboration of veterinary workers with workers in the field of human and experimental cancer will be necessary, and a bold and imaginative approach cannot fail to produce very important results.

References

1. Russell, W. O., Wynne, E. S. and Loquvam, G. S. Studies on bovine ocular squamous carcinoma ("cancer eye"). *Cancer 9:*1, 1965.
2. Brandly, P. J. and Migaki, G. Types of tumors found by federal meat inspectors in an eight-year survey. Presented at the N. Y. Academy of Sciences, *Conference of Epizootiology of Cancer,* Feb. 11-13, 1963.
3. Barron, C. N. The comparative pathology of neoplasms of the eyelids and conjunctiva with special reference to those of epithelial origin. *Acta Dermato-Venereologica 42:*1, 1962.
4. Loeb, L. and Jobson, G. On carcinoma in cattle. *J. Comp. Med. 21:*385, 1900.
5. French, T. T. A clinical and genetic study of eye cancer in Hereford cattle. *Austral. Vet. J. 35:*474, 1959.
6. Kinsley, A. T. Ocular tumors with case reports. *Am. Vet. Rev. 43:*291, 1913.
7. Sheldon, R. Cancer eye in cattle. *Southwestern Crop and Stock. 5:*36, 1951.
8. Pillay, K. S. Cancer of the eye in cattle. *Indian Vet. J. 8:*129, 1931.
9. Woodward, R. R. and Knapp, B., Jr. The hereditary aspect of eye cancer in Hereford cattle. *J. Animal Sci. 9:*578, 1950.
10. Black, W. L. Survey on the cause of cancer eye in cattle. *Extension Animal Husbandman 33:*9, 1934.
11. Anderson, D. E. Genetic aspects of bovine ocular carcinoma. In *Genetics and Cancer.* Texas, The University of Texas Press, 1959, pp. 364-374.
12. Sykes, J. A., Dmochowski, L. and Russell, W. O. Bovine ocular squamous cell carcinoma. I. Tissue culture studies of plaque. *Proc. Soc. Exptl. Biol. & Med. 100:*527, 1959.
13. Sykes, J. A., Dmochowski, L. and Russell, W. O. Bovine ocular squamous cell carcinoma. II. Tissue culture studies of papilloma. *Proc. Soc. Exptl. Biol. & Med. 101:*192, 1959.
14. Sykes, J. A., Dmochowski, L. and Russell, W. O. Bovine ocular squamous cell carcinoma. III. Tissue culture studies of carcinoma. *Proc. Soc. Exptl. Biol. & Med. 101:*264, 1959.
15. Dmochowski, L., Sykes, J. A., Wynne, E. S. and Russell, W. O. Bovine ocular squamous carcinoma ("Cancer Eye") and its benign precursor lesions in the light of recent tissue culture and electron microscope studies. (Abstract.) *Am. J. Path. 34:*602, 1958.

16. Sykes, J. A., Dmochowski, L., Wynne, E. S. and Russell, W. O. Bovine ocular squamous-cell carcinoma. IV. Tissue-culture studies of bovine ocular squamous-cell carcinoma and its benign precursor lesions. *J. Nat. Cancer Inst. 26:*445, 1961.
17. Cotchin, E. Problems of comparative oncology. *Bull. Wld. Hlth. Org. 26:*633, 1962.
18. Mostafa, M. S. E. A case of malignant melanoma in a bay horse. *Brit. Vet. J. 109:*201, 1953.
19. Sullivan, D. J. and Anderson, W. A. Embryonal nephroma in swine. *Amer. J. Vet. Res. 20:*324, 1959.
20. Monlux, A. W., Anderson, W. A. and Davis, C. L. A survey of tumors occurring in cattle, sheep, and swine. *Amer. J. Vet. Res. 17:*646, 1956.
21. Mulligan, R. M. *Neoplasms of the Dog.* Williams and Wilkins, Baltimore, Maryland, 1949.
22. Smith, H. A. and Jones, T. C. *Veterinary Pathology.* Lee and Febiger, Philadelphia, Pennsylvania, 1961, p. 248.
23. Bloom, F. Spontaneous solitary and multiple mast-cell tumors ("mastocytoma") in dogs. *Arch. Path. 33:*661, 1942.
24. Nielson, S. W. and Cole, C. R. Canine mastocytoma. A report of one-hundred cases. *Amer. J. Vet. Res. 19:*417, 1958.
25. Orkin, M. and Schwartzman, R. M. A comparative study of canine and human dermatology. II. Cutaneous tumors, the mast cell and canine mastocytoma. *J. Invest. Derm. 32:*451, 1959. Also *Vet. Med. 54:*315, 1959.
26. Cotchin, E. Spontaneous sarcomas of bone in dogs: 30 cases. *Brit. Vet. J. 109:* 248, 1953.
27. Huggins, C. and Pazos, R. Studies on tumors of the testis. II. The morphology of testicular tumors of dogs. *Amer. J. Path. 21:*299, 1945.
28. DeMonbreun, W. A. and Goodpasture, E. W. Experimental investigation concerning the nature of contagious lymphosarcoma of dogs. *Am. J. Cancer 21:*295, 1934.
29. Prier, J. E. and Brodey, R. S. Canine neoplasia. A prototype for human cancer study. *Bull. World Health Organ., 29:*331, 1963.
30. Moulton, J. E. *Tumors in Domestic Animals.* University of California Press, Berkeley and Los Angeles, California, 1961.
31. Schaffner, M. H. Squamous cell carcinoma of the pinna of white-eared cats. In: *Current Veterinary Therapy,* 1964-65. Editor: Kirk, R. W. W. B. Saunders Company, Philadelphia and London, 1964, p. 197.
32. Cotchin, E. Neoplasms in cats. *Proc. R. Soc. Med. 45:*671, 1952.
33. Owen, L. N. Treatment of 30 cases of spontaneous tumours in dogs with triethylene glycol diglycidyl ether. *Brit. J. Cancer 16:*441, 1962.
34. Doyle, R. E., Garb, S., Davis, L. E., Meyer, D. K. and Clayton, F. W. Domesticated farm animals in medical research. *Ann. N. Y. Acad. Sci.* In press.
35. McCoy, J. R. Trial of chemotherapeutic agents in spontaneous tumors in dogs. *Ann. N. Y. Acad. Sci. 76:*850, 1958-59.
36. Riggs, C. W. Treatment of canine neoplasm with autogenous vaccinial preparations. *Nature 200:*233, 1963.
37. McKenna, J. M. and Prier, J. E. Some immunologic aspects of canine neoplasms. *Cancer Res. 26:*137, 1966.

The Potential Contributions of Dentists, Pharmacists, Botanists and General Biologists to Cancer Research

Dentists. Some dentists are currently doing research on cancers of the mouth and jaw. The contributions of dental scientists could be much greater, however. In addition to their obvious familiarity with pathological conditions in the mouth, dentists as a group are outstanding in manual dexterity, in the ability to make small, precise objects with great accuracy, and in their knowledge of the reaction of normal tissues to foreign materials. There are two areas in which our dental schools could make major contributions to an expanded national cancer research problem.

First, dentists can make contributions through studies utilizing the hamster cheek pouch. This technique (described in Chapter 14) has considerable potential value in the study of human cancers because the cheek pouch has a special property of tolerating foreign tissue. We must not, however, lose sight of the fact that it is an oral structure, subject to such influences as saliva, food, and bacteria. Some of these influences could substantially modify the results of experiments using the cheek pouch, unless they are understood and considered in the experimental procedure. Since dental scientists, as a group, have a much better understanding of oral physiology and pathology than any other group, it seems sensible to assign to them a major role in studies utilizing the hamster cheek pouch. Although a few dentists are working on the hamster cheek pouch, many more could do so with skill and efficiency.

Second, the ability of dentists to fabricate, and install with great precision, appliances of metal, ceramic and plastic, which are non-irritant to normal tissues, could also be of great value in an expanded cancer research program. For certain studies, it is necessary to enclose a growing cancer in a tiny container with a window—the entire appliance remaining in or on the experimental animal all through the study. The work of Algire and his colleagues (1 to 10) required such a chamber attached to the skin of a mouse. Ide, Baker and Warren (11) used a similar chamber attached to a rabbit's ear, and more recently, Goodall, Sanders and Shubik (12) have designed and used a chamber with transparent window for cancers growing in the hamster's cheek pouch. This seems to be an area in which we could expect significant advance and improvement from dental scientists who would join an expanded national program.

Pharmacists. The colleges of pharmacy are engaged in a certain amount of cancer research work (*see* Chapter 18, Kupchan *et al.*), but here, too, on a much smaller scale than the abilities and training of their staffs warrant. One group of pharmacy scientists, the pharmacognosists, could be of considerable help in an expanded cancer research program. Pharmacognosy is the branch of pharmacy dealing with natural products that are utilized for medicinal purposes. Most of these natural products are of plant origin. The pharmacognosist is trained to recognize the various roots, stems, leaves and so forth from which medicines can be derived. Once considered a vanishing field, pharmacognosy is making a strong comeback, as the value of medicines derived from plants is better understood. In a program of testing plant materials for anti-cancer effects, pharmacognosists would be important members of the research team, helping to insure that the procedures of identifying the raw material are accurate, and that the methods of extraction do not destroy an active material.

Pharmacists are also well versed in the problems of duration of drug action. As pointed out in Chapter 12, a major problem in the use of mice as experimental animals is the rapidity with which they metabolize and excrete almost all drugs. This renders unreliable the usual screening procedures for anti-cancer activity in which an injection is given every 12 or 24 hours. Yet, if the test materials could be injected into the mice in a vehicle that delays absorption, spreading it out over a period of many hours, the reliability and usefulness of the procedure could be greatly increased. When it comes to developing and testing such drug vehicles, research pharmacists are probably the most capable persons, and their help in this area could be critical.

Botanists. There is an excellent chance that effective anti-cancer medications may be found in plants, and, therefore, botanists would be valuable additions to the staff of our cancer research program. The potential importance of plant products to cancer research was described in Chapter 18. It was pointed out that many of our major drugs today still come from plants, and that chemists are unable to synthesize them even though their chemical structures are known. In other cases, synthetic drugs are based on medicines obtained from plants. It is particularly significant that vinblastine and vincristine, anti-cancer drugs obtained from the periwinkle plant, already are curing or controlling some kinds of cancer.

However, the collection of plants to be tested for anti-cancer activity is not being carried out at a rate commensurate with the urgency and importance of the problem, and part of the reason is that many botanists who are able to do such collecting have not been given the financial support needed for the job.

A suitable plant collection program requires a substantial number of trained botanists. It is not enough to have an assortment of plants delivered to a cancer research institute. In order to make effective use of the plants, it is necessary to identify them exactly (genus, species and sometimes variety), to know their age, where, when and how they were collected, how they were handled and stored before delivery to the research facility, and so forth. Such information is important because some plants have much higher concentrations of certain chemicals at different ages or at different seasons of the year. Sometimes one species has a high content of a useful drug, while a closely related species may have such a low content that it is not medically useful. In her popular book, *Green Medicine,* Margaret Kreig describes an occurrence in which this point was not recognized. The Dutch government, trying to grow quinine in the East Indies (now Indonesia), planted a million Cinchona trees, believed to be *Chinchona calisayas* which, in Bolivia, has a high yield of quinine. The Dutch found the quinine content of their million trees to be too low for any practical purposes and had to destroy the entire lot. Either the trees were not *C. calisayas,* but a related species, or they produced quinine only under special conditions. Eventually, the Dutch obtained a high-yielding species, *C. ledgeriana,* which the botanists were able to graft onto hardier Cinchonas and which produced large amounts of quinine.

In the present cancer research program, a few botanists are collecting plants for cancer studies, but they represent a small percentage of the botanists who could make excellent collectors, and who would if they were supported. Many botanists, though now engaged in basic studies, would certainly be willing to defer some of their own projects to aid in a national cancer research program, provided they were given the means to do so.

General Biologists. Many general biologists are thoroughly trained in the fundamentals of the scientific approach, and skilled in general experimental techniques. The term "general biologists" is meant to include biologists whose interests, although sometimes quite specific, are not ordinarily considered to be medically oriented. For example, an expert on the physiology of mollusks might be an invaluable member of a team searching for anti-cancer medications in clams. We may safely assume that many general biologists who are currently doing basic research would be willing to defer these studies for several years to help find a treatment for cancer. Under our present system, there is little opportunity to utilize their services. Only a few general biologists have obtained cancer research grants.

Although most general biologists do not have enough knowledge about the specific field of cancer to initiate and conduct research projects on their own, they could do vital work as members of cancer research teams. It would probably be helpful to offer brief training courses in cancer research to general biologists. This should help increase the number of scientists able to participate in a national cancer research program. It is quite possible that, in some projects, a general biologist might be the leader of the research team.

The ability of general biologists to contribute to cancer research is demonstrated by the work of Sister M. Rosarii Schmeer, whose studies are described in Chapter 26.

References

1. Algire, G. H. and Chalkley, H. W. Vascular reactions of normal and malignant tissue in vivo. I. Vascular reactions of mice to wounds and to normal and neoplastic transplants. *J. Nat. Cancer Inst.* 6:73, 1945-1946.
2. Algire, G. H., Legallais, F. Y. and Park, H. D. Vascular reactions of normal and malignant tissue in vivo. II. The vascular reaction of normal and neoplastic tissues of mice to a bacterial polysaccharide from Serratia marcescens (Bacillus prodigiosus) culture filtrates. *J. Nat. Cancer Inst.* 8:53, 1947.
3. Algire, G. H., Chalkley, H. W. and Earle, W. R. Vascular reactions of normal and malignant tissues in vivo. III. Vascular reactions of mice to fibroblasts treated in vitro with methylcholanthrene. *J. Nat. Cancer Inst.* 11:555, 1951.
4. Algire, G. H. and Legallais, F. Y. Vascular reactions of normal and malignant tissues in vivo. IV. The effect of peripheral hypotension on transplanted tumors. *J. Nat. Cancer Inst.* 12:399, 1951.
5. Algire, G. H., Legallais, F. Y. and Anderson, B. F. Vascular reactions of normal and malignant tissues in vivo. V. The role of hypotension in the action of a bacterial polysaccharide on tumors. *J. Nat. Cancer Inst.* 12:1279, 1952.
6. Algire, G. H., Legallais, F. Y. and Anderson, B. F. Vascular reactions of normal and malignant tissues in vivo. VI. The role of hypotension in the action of components of podophyllin on transplanted sarcomas. *J. Nat. Cancer Inst.* 14:879, 1954.
7. Algire, G. H. Vascular reactions of normal and malignant tissues in vivo. VII. Observations on vascular reactions in destruction of tumor homografts. *J. Nat. Cancer Inst.* 15:483, 1954.

8. Algire, G. H. and Merwin, R. M. Vascular patterns in tissues and grafts within transparent chambers in mice. *Angiology 6:*311, 1955.
9. Merwin, R. M. and Algire, G. H. The role of graft and host vessels in the vascularization of grafts of normal and neoplastic tissue. *J. Nat. Cancer Inst. 17:*23, 1956.
10. Algire, G. H. and Legallais, F. Y. Recent developments in the transparent-chamber technique as adapted to the mouse. *J. Nat. Cancer Inst. 10:*225, 1949.
11. Ide, A. G., Baker, N. H. and Warren, S. L. Vascularization of the Brown-Pearce rabbit epithelioma transplant as seen in the transparent ear chamber. *Am. J. Roentgenol. Radiotherap. 42:*891, 1939.
12. Goodall, C. M., Sanders, A. G. and Shubik, P. Studies of vascular patterns in living tumors with a transparent chamber inserted in hamster cheek pouch. *J. Nat. Cancer Inst. 35:*497, 1965.

The Potential Contributions of the Pharmaceutical Industry to Cancer Research

The pharmaceutical industry has developed many lifesaving drugs; in the field of cancer, industrial scientists have played a major role in developing the vinca alkaloids, vinblastine and vincristine, which are of major value in some cases of cancer and closely related diseases. Accordingly, it is pertinent to consider what the pharmaceutical industry is doing and could be doing in cancer research, and how its contributions may be increased and made more effective.

A pharmaceutical firm can be considered a business that utilizes efficiently the skills and training of many different types of persons in order to produce medicines which will help patients, and profits which will keep the company in business and growing. It is a business that depends upon both imagination and efficiency. It differs from universities and research institutes in many ways, two of which are of particular interest in relation to our subject. First, pharmaceutical firms do not, except in minor and peripheral ways, supply the education and training of the scientists working for them. Thus, they are spared the enormous expense of such education and training, and can afford to pay these scientists high salaries. Consequently, they should share the credit they receive for lifesaving discoveries with the universities that trained the scientists. Furthermore, the pharmaceutical industry is fundamentally dependent upon universities for its continuing process and growth.

Another feature of the pharmaceutical industry is that each of its firms is product-centered. Success is not measured by papers published or by contributions to basic knowledge of life and the universe; it is measured, rather, by profits and growth—and in most cases these depend on patients' lives saved and on distress alleviated. To accomplish these goals, a great deal of central direction is needed within a pharmaceutical company, so that talents are utilized where they can do the most good. The drug industry, therefore, has some important advantages in medical research, and its accomplishments in many fields are superior to those of other research groups. The development of the host of new antibiotics, diuretics, psychoactive drugs, chelating agents, anesthetics and synthetic pain-relievers shows how much the drug industry can contribute.

The pharmaceutical industry has also contributed significantly to cancer research. As pointed out, development of the vinca alkaloids is one such important advance. Also, many of the drugs that are now used for palliation of cancer were developed by the drug industry. Still, it appears that the pharmaceutical industry is not doing all it could in this field. Several large manufacturers seem to have no cancer research programs at all. Others work in cancer research only on the basis of research contracts from the Federal Government; they appear to be unwilling to invest much of their own funds in this area. A few firms maintain and support their own cancer research programs, but not at a level that the seriousness of the problem calls for. It is, therefore, important to try to find out why the drug industry is not pursuing cancer research more vigorously. It is not easy to find out why the drug industry does some things and abstains from others. The over-all research program of any company is usually a well-guarded trade secret.

First, we must understand thoroughly the need for profits in the drug industry. Unless a firm makes profits, it will go out of business. Therefore, before investing the money of the stockholders in a research program, the management of a drug company must have some reasonable expectations that the research will lead to a product that will bring in enough money to pay the costs of research and production and also provide a fair profit. Sometimes, exceptions are made as a "service to humanity," and research is conducted on new drug products that will not have a large market. Such exceptions, however, can involve only relatively small expenditures.

A drug effective against cancer would certainly have a large market, but some drug company officials apparently fear a compulsory licensing law, which would keep them from recouping their expenses. Their reasoning runs about as follows: If a drug company develops an effective, patentable cure for cancer, the demand for the drug would be so great that the original maker probably could not manufacture enough during the first few years. Accordingly, irresistible public pressure would force Congress to pass a law requiring the discovering firm to license all or most of its competitors to

285

produce the drug. To keep the price of the drug low, the licensing law might specify such a low royalty rate, that the first company would not be able to recoup its research investment or, at best, would barely do so. Accordingly, the competing firms that received the licenses would be the ones to make the real profits, not the discoverer.

It might be argued that this attitude is unduly pessimistic, and that Congress would not act unfairly in this sort of situation. We must consider, however, the position and feelings of drug company executives. Many of them believe (and I think wrongly) that Congress has already treated them unfairly by passing the Kefauver-Harris law, and it probably would be futile to try to change their beliefs. On the other hand, this part of the problem could be resolved readily by congressional passage of a fair licensing law now. If the provisions of such a law specified a licensing fee that would enable the original discoverer to make a bigger profit than its competitors, one obstacle to increased cancer research by the drug industry would be removed.

A second problem has to do with the nature of our patent laws. If a drug company synthesizes a new chemical with a useful effect, it can obtain a patent which gives it exclusive rights to that chemical for 17 years. It can also obtain a process patent, which gives it exclusive rights to produce a certain compound in a specified way. A process patent, however, is of limited value because competitors can often find other ways to produce the same material. With regard to naturally occurring products, our patent laws are rather hazy. Suppose a drug manufacturer were to pay for research on a series of plant extracts (Chapter 18), or marine extracts (Chapter 26), and find a cure for cancer in one of them. The firm could not patent the material itself, since it is found in nature. It could get a patent for its process of extracting and purifying the active ingredient, but this is not likely to give the manufacturer adequate protection. For this reason, some drug manufacturers are reluctant to invest in research looking for anti-cancer drugs in plants or marine sources. Yet, with their personnel and facilities, the drug companies are among the best qualified organizations to pursue such research.

One way to solve this problem would be through appropriate modifications in our patent laws, but the patent laws are already so confused and tangled that new modifications might add to litigation rather than to research. A more direct way would be to enact a new law giving an appropriate reward to any drug company that finds a useful anti-cancer drug. The award might be in the form of a specific licensing arrangement, requiring all other firms to pay the finder a royalty for 20 years for the right to produce and sell the product; or it might be in the form of a direct government subsidy. There may be still other suitable arrangements that the drug manufacturers could specify. The important thing is to increase drug industry participation in cancer research, by removing the obstacles, concrete or psychologic, that stand in the way of such research.

PART VI

ORGANIZATION OF A NATIONAL GOAL APPROACH

In earlier chapters, some of the advantages and disadvantages of our present cancer research program were considered. Although some of the advantages of the system under which the present program operates may be declining in relative importance, one advantage remains: it does allow for the development of new ideas and leads in cancer research. Even though we are now engaged in several promising lines of research (which should be followed much more vigorously) we cannot know how long it will take before any one of them will result in practical therapeutic advances. It is quite possible that further development of our present program would open up an approach, not now being considered, that could quickly lead to a cure.

Our present system has also been responsible for the training of about 90 per cent of our cancer research scientists, and we must continue training new generations of scientists. It also makes it possible for some scientists who prefer to work alone to make their contributions to the national effort. Accordingly, it seems essential that, regardless of the inauguration of a new program, the present program be continued with undiminished, and even expanding, support.

Should the present cancer research program become an integral part of the proposed new program, or should it remain separate? There would be some administrative advantages to combining the programs, but the advantages of keeping them separate seem more important.

A small program, combined with a larger one, is likely to be overshadowed. Also, a program designed to develop research leads would hardly receive a fair amount of attention and support from supervisors who are also responsible for exploiting leads and producing practical results at the earliest possible time. It appears likely that a combination of the proposed and present programs would lead to an atrophy of the latter, an atrophy even more pronounced than the one now being caused by budgetary restrictions.

The costs of having the two separate programs would not need to exceed the costs of having their functions combined in a single program. In general, it may be possible to effect savings by consolidating government agencies but there is no reason to believe that any savings would occur in a research program. The costs of the actual experiments would not change. The amount of duplication between a goal-directed program and one designed to develop new leads should be quite small. The costs of central administration of medical research in Washington have always been modest, and should remain so.

If these suggestions are followed, and we should have two separate cancer research programs, one to exploit existing leads and one to develop new ones, the relationship of the investigators to each program will be of interest. There will be some scientists who prefer, or are uniquely qualified for, studies at a more basic level. Their work would be supported by the continuation of the present program. Other scientists, more interested in, or qualified for, goal-directed studies would be supported by the proposed new program. Some of the scientists working in the new program might uncover new leads. If so, the suggested provision (*see* Chapter 33) that they be allowed to spend up to 20 per cent of their budget on related cancer research, not specifically covered by their contracts, should enable them to do enough pilot studies to determine whether or not the new lead holds much promise. If it does, the investigator could apply for a grant from the other program, too. Similarly, a scientist working on basic problems could decide to devote part of his time to goal-directed studies, and contract with the new agency to do so.

University vs. Research Institute

Once a decision has been made to embark on a national program to find a cure or control for cancer, it would be necessary to decide where the research work is to be done—whether in existing universities, medical schools and hospitals, or in new research institutes to be built and staffed by the Federal Government, or in a combination of these.

If the research is to be performed in existing institutions, most of it will be done in universities and those few medical schools that do not have university affiliations. Most of the major hospitals are affiliated with universities, and hospitals that are not so affiliated usually lack the facilities, personnel and space to undertake a major research program.

A few cancer research institutes are already in being and are affiliated with universities. They are doing a good job, but it is doubtful that further expansion is practical for most of them. The National Cancer Institute intramural program is, of course, excellent, but it is already so large that any further increase in size is bound to reduce efficiency. Similar institutes, built in other parts of the country, could be quite practical and effective, however.

Let us consider some of the advantages and disadvantages that might attend a major expansion of the cancer research activities of universities and their affiliated hospitals. Traditionally, the Federal Government has, in almost all cases, provided help for constructing university research facilities on a matching-funds basis. As we have pointed out, this policy has caused the bulk of such Federal funds to be shunted to the wealthier institutions, while those that could not provide half of the building costs could not keep pace. It is doubtful whether many institutions could, in the space of a year or two, raise enough funds to provide half of the cost of constructing new buildings for cancer research. Furthermore, it is difficult to see why they should be asked to do so. The primary beneficiaries of a cancer research program would be the American people, not the universities. The

291

matching-funds requirement for research buildings is an anachronism that has the major effect of impeding our cancer research program.

If, as seems practical and necessary, it were decided that the Federal Government should pay the full costs of new buildings to be used exclusively for cancer research, there would be little difference in the cost of erecting buildings on or near a university campus and those set up as separate research institutes. (There may be a few exceptions involving universities that are located within a large city where land costs are high.)

A major advantage of basing an expanded program in existing universities would be that many of the needed facilities would already be collected there. These facilities would include, in most cases, an excellent medical library, which would be a costly and time-consuming item to replicate in separate research institutes. In addition, several universities include colleges of veterinary medicine, dentistry and pharmacy, which could be major assets in a properly designed national research program. Many cancer researchers prefer a university setting for several reasons. They like the stimulating, broadly based intellectual climate; they consider the presence of bright students, both undergraduate and graduate, an asset in carrying out their research.

As to the disadvantages of basing an expanded national research program in the universities, an allegation frequently made, but one which in reality does not apply to cancer research, is that research programs interfere with teaching of undergraduates. Perhaps this may be the case when the research subject matter is included in the content of courses commonly taught to undergraduates. Most cancer researchers, however, are involved in subjects that are commonly taught to professional, graduate, and postdoctoral students only. At times bright premedical or pre-Ph.D. students are invited to spend the summer working in cancer research laboratories, but this constitutes an addition to, not a deletion from, the total teaching program. Accordingly, there is little if any reason to believe that an expanded cancer research program at universities would in any significant way detract from undergraduate instruction.

Certain difficulties may arise in carrying out cancer research programs in universities where the administrative procedures are geared to running a teaching rather than a research institution. This can result in considerable frustration for investigators who find it hard to work at maximum efficiency if they are required to attend meetings of various faculty committees, or when the working schedules of the supporting departments (animal care, purchasing, and so forth) are based on the academic calendar rather than research needs. This is not an insurmountable obstacle, however.

Space may prove to be a serious problem for some universities. Recent increases in enrollments have required the construction of new dormitories and classrooms on many campuses, and there may not be room for new cancer research buildings. On the other hand, it may be feasible to locate a cancer research facility several miles away from the university campus and still maintain a working affiliation.

A major drawback to the expansion of a national cancer research program at universities is the low salaries that universities pay to technicians. Depending on the particular project, there should be from three to eight technicians for each cancer researcher at the doctoral level. A year or more is generally needed to train these technicians after they have obtained the basic college degree. It is extremely inefficient to have a high yearly turnover of technicians, but this is a rather common occurrence in most universities because of the low salaries paid technicians. Unfortunately, universities are reluctant to raise technicians' salaries to adequate levels even when the funds for these salaries come from outside sources. Since a university employs and pays technicians of various sorts, the administration fears that the university would lose its good technicians to the better paying programs and might be forced, therefore, to raise the salaries of its own employees accordingly. This, of course, would put a serious strain on university finances. It is not at all clear how this problem can be resolved. Hopefully, university administrations that continue to underpay their technicians would be willing to make an exception for technicians working in cancer research.

The advantages and disadvantages of developing new research institutions for cancer research are to a large extent the opposite of the advantages and disadvantages of the expanded university program. For example, the development of new library facilities in new research institutes would require considerable time and money. One important advantage of the new research institutes under direct government control is that the technicians' salary scale would help attract and keep career technicians. Another is that scientists who dislike, or who do not fit into, a university environment could work effectively in the institute. The new institutes need not be built in the vicinity of existing universities. If they were located in areas that are economically depressed or have pockets of unemployment, they would provide a number of job opportunities for unskilled and semi-skilled workers. The influx of professional and technical personnel at reasonable salaries would be a secondary economic benefit. It seems likely that

293

most scientists and technicians would be willing to move their families to such areas, provided the opportunity to accomplish worthwhile research is good.

The most practical arrangement is likely to be one in which both universities and separate research institutes are utilized in an effective balance. A suggested ratio is 2 to 1, with approximately twice as much work and funds allocated to the universities. A substantial part of the universities' share, however, ought to be earmarked for special projects in veterinary medicine, dentistry, pharmacy and the departments of botany. These special projects probably could not be carried out effectively in new research institutes for many years without excessive expenditures.

The Task-Force Approach

The key element in the internal organization of a cancer research program designed to find a cure or control at the earliest possible time is the task force. This would be a group of scientists, properly led, who are working together toward a clearly defined goal. The leadership of each task force would be vested in a specific individual, not a committee. This chief would have authority, financial support commensurate with his responsibilities, and a free hand in recruiting scientists to his task force, within general guidelines that would be laid down by the program director who would be appointed by the President. He might have a committee of advisors, including physicians, scientists, and representatives of the public, but he should have the ability to make the decisions, and the responsibility for those decisions.

The members of the task force could do their work in existing institutes and university laboratories, or in institutes and laboratories still to be built, depending on the nature of the specific project. For scientists working in non-government institutions, the most appropriate form of financial support would be the Federal research contract.

In assigning research projects to scientist teams, it would be advantageous to have each study performed by three different teams, at three different locations. At first, this may seem wasteful, but in the long run, it would probably save money as well as time. The reason lies in the nature of biological research. Findings reported by any individual or group are seldom accepted as accurate by the scientific community unless confirmed by another scientist or team. Often, the time lag between the reports of the initial finding and of the confirmatory findings is two to four years. Frequently, the reports from scientists trying to confirm another scientist's results contradict the original report because of a minor difference in technique. When this happens, the issue is sometimes left in doubt indefinitely; or, if the issue seems interesting to many scientists, several will work on the project. The time and effort spent on these endeavors are substantial.

With three research teams doing the same experiment at three different locations, and making frequent progress reports, several advantages would accrue. In studies using sequential statistical plans, the acquisition of data would proceed much more rapidly. Thus, the chief of the task force could have a good idea of the probable outcome of the study at an early time. This in turn would enable him to plan and assign succeeding experiments quickly. In some studies, the three research teams may show diverging results as an experiment proceeds. This would be a signal to recheck procedures and materials carefully for differences that were not obvious, but that may account for the diverging results. Another advantage of the triplicate plan is that important studies would not be stopped or seriously delayed because of death, illness or transfer of an investigator.

A second element in the research program should be a set of support groups, each with its own chief. These groups would help provide the research teams with materials for their studies. For example, one support group could be responsible for providing large quantities of mice with spontaneous cancers. (This could be done by contractual arrangements with veterinary schools, as described in Chapter 29.) Then, the investigative teams could obtain their animals through the support group rather than compete with each other for scarce animals.

Another support group might be assigned to the clam project (*see* Chapter 26). Let us assume that preliminary studies show clam extract (mercenene) to be effective against spontaneous mouse cancers. It would then be vital to test mercenene against many kinds of cancer in several species of animal. For this, large quantities of clam extract would be needed, and it would obviously be wasteful to have several groups of cancer researchers collecting their own clams and making extracts. Instead, a support group could contract for large quantities of the right species of clam, collected at the right time of year, and could make or arrange to have made adequate amounts of an extract for testing.

Another support group could obtain and prepare plant extracts (Chapter 18). Other support groups could be activated as needed, to provide special assistance to the investigating teams.

Only the broad outlines of a suggested organizational pattern have been given, since the details could be worked out better after the various chiefs of task forces and support groups were appointed. However, an organizational pattern that focuses efforts on a defined goal should be the keystone in this program.

Leadership for a National Program

The leadership of a national program to find a cure or control for cancer could make all the difference between an effective, productive effort and one that routinely expends itself without accomplishing much of practical value.

A thought that is sometimes expressed is that leadership should be given to the person who knows the most about cancer. There are serious drawbacks to such leadership, however. First of all, a particular person may not be equally endowed with knowledge and the ability to lead. A brilliant scientist may have virtually no capacity to lead, or even to work closely with others. History provides examples: Isaac Newton, for all his genius, apparently was not even able to lead students, and Charles Darwin worked virtually alone all through his career.

Then, there is the possibility that a scientist who knows more about cancer than most of his colleagues, in his concentration on known facts, may not be oriented to new approaches and new concepts. An example from the recent past: When the atom bomb was being developed, the Admiral who was our greatest authority on "existing" explosives considered the entire notion of an atom bomb to be unfeasible.

Another idea is that leadership should be given to a committee of experts. Unfortunately, committees, by their nature, can rarely provide effective leadership, even when the individuals on the committee themselves have strong leadership abilities. Our present research program is determined almost entirely by committees, and much of the inefficiency in it can be traced to the committee system in which responsibility is so diffused that it is almost impossible to find out who made certain important decisions. Scientists and professors are often required to serve on committees in their own institutions, but this in no way lessens their aversion to committee decisions. On the other hand, an advisory committee that is truly advisory could be of great value to a good leader.

One way of deciding how to chose a leader for a national cancer research program is to examine the leadership of those national science programs that have been successful in their missions. Thus far, there have been three outstanding examples: the development of the atomic bomb, the development of the Polaris submarine system, and the space program. The leader of the Manhattan project, which developed the atom bomb, was Lieutenant General Leslie Groves; the leader of the Polaris program was Admiral Hyman Rickover; the leader of the space program is Mr. James Webb, a former director of the Bureau of the Budget. These three men have several things in common. First of all, they were and are goal-oriented. They knew exactly what their jobs were and did them in the most direct way available. They could not be diverted, nor did they confuse means with end. They are intelligent men, but none of them was at first an expert in the field he was assigned to lead. They all knew how to utilize, at a high level of efficency, the scientific brains assigned to them; at the same time they retained the respect and goodwill of those scientists. They were able to function effectively with and in government circles, both legislative and executive. Without this essential ability, their projects could have suffered from the kind of financial drought that has affected cancer research since 1962. It would seem sensible to select a leader, or leaders, of this caliber when planning a national program of cancer research.

Budgeting for a National Program

A national program properly designed and executed to find a cure or control for cancer as quickly as possible would not be cheap. Its costs would be considerably greater than those of the present program. However, the eventual gains to the nation, in economic terms alone, would far exceed these additional costs. The income tax paid by people who, instead of dying of cancer, would continue to work and earn would, in a matter of a few years, pay completely the costs of a full-scale, vigorous, effective cancer research program. Furthermore, if cancer did not kill so many people, the costs of life insurance premiums would be much less, and fewer families would need social security and community welfare payments because of loss of a breadwinner.

It has been estimated that, in 1962, cancer cost the United States about 8 billion dollars in reduced earnings. By 1968 this figure will be close to 12 billion per year.

In comparison with other national programs, the proposed cancer research program does not seem excessively expensive. It would cost far less than the space program, which runs about 5 billion per year, and less than the program to develop a supersonic airliner, which will probably cost close to 1 billion dollars a year when it reaches its full growth.

A properly supported cancer research program may cost about 650 million dollars per year—an increase of about 470 million over our present level.

Of this amount, 175 million per year should be allocated to continue our present program, and 25 million per year for purchase of equipment or for needed alterations or additions to the physical plants where research is being carried on. Despite the inefficiences of some of our present efforts, most are developing useful information. Some of our investigators today might be on the right track and it would be wise to keep them there. In addition, our existing program is well suited for developing research leads and accumulating basic data about cancer. These could be useful for other phases of the study. Also, there are many investigators with years of cancer research experience who have permanent positions in universities, hospitals and so forth, and who have developed useful research programs. It would be wasteful as well as impractical to ask them to abandon their own projects and undertake others, perhaps in a different location.

Our present investigator-oriented program is, furthermore, the best we know for utilizing the abilities of the rare genius who might develop a cure or control almost single-handedly. Although we ought not depend on finding such a genius, it would be foolish to structure a research program in such a way that it might exclude him.

We can afford both programs.

The estimated 175 million per year for the continuation of the present investigator-oriented program would actually allow for a reasonable degree of expansion. Some of the investigators currently supported on this program would probably wish to change to the project-oriented program, lessening the competition for funds in the former one.

The remaining 450 million per year should be allocated to a series of goal-oriented projects, as is done in the space program. A certain percentage—say 20 per cent—of each grant ought to be unrestricted funds available to the investigator himself so that he may follow up unexpected results or do cancer research in areas not defined in the grant. Such flexibility would make the entire program much more attractive to scientists.

During the first two or three years, the bulk of the funds should go to pay the costs of construction of new research facilities. Then, as the programs grow, and more scientists and technicians are added, proportionately more funds could be used for operating expenses. Some suggested patterns for cost allocation for the first three years of a national program are presented in Table 33-1.

It should be noted that the suggested budgets of the research programs include salaries of scientists, technicians and other personnel, costs of animals, supplies and incidentals. Where appropriate, overhead payments to existing institutions, not to exceed 20 per cent, should be included.

A suggested—and rather speculative—subdivision of the 450 million for actual research costs, starting in the third year of the program, is presented in Table 33-2.

Table 33–1. Suggested Budgetary Allocations for a National Cancer Research Program

Year 1	In Millions of Dollars
Continuation of existing investigator-centered projects	$175
Construction of 5 cancer research institutes at $40 million each	200
Construction of additional research facilities at 18 veterinary colleges	60
Construction of additional research facilities at universities, medical, dental and pharmacy colleges and hospitals	100
Purchase of equipment	25
Costs of starting project-centered research programs	90
Total	650
Year 2	
Continuation of existing investigator-centered projects	175
Construction of additional research facilities at universities, medical, dental and pharmacy colleges and hospitals	200
Construction of facilities for studies of plants on cancer, including greenhouses in 10 locations	50
Purchase of equipment	25
Cost of project-centered research programs	200
Total	650
Year 3 and thereafter	
Continuation of existing investigator-centered projects	175
Alterations, modifications and additions to existing research facilities	25
Cost of project-centered research programs	450
Total	650

Table 33–2. Suggested Annual Expenditures for Cancer Research Projects in a National Goal Program from Year 3 on (including 20 per cent overhead, but excluding construction)

A.	General projects	In Millions of Dollars
A1.	Improving effectiveness of surgical procedures in cancer (see Chapter 16)	$50
A2.	Studies on effectiveness of chemotherapy as an adjunct to surgical procedures in cancer (see Chapter 16)	20
A3.	Improving radiation therapy for cancer (see Chapter 17)	25
A4.	Testing plant extracts against cancer (see Chapter 18)	60
A5.	Search for agent which induces host blood vessel proliferation, and production of antidote (see Chapter 19)	15
A6.	Studies on effects of vasoconstrictors in shunting of drugs to the cancer (see Chapter 20)	5
A7.	Studies on the invasiveness of cancer (see Chapter 21)	15
A8.	Studies on other cancer cell secretions affecting host (see Chapter 22)	20
A9.	Studies of host defenses and immune responses in cancer (see Chapter 23)	30
A10.	Studies on factors affecting metastases (see Chapter 24)	12
A11.	Bacterial approach to cancer (see Chapter 25)	20
A12.	Search for anti-cancer agents in marine plants and animals (see Chapter 26)	8
A13.	Studies on the effect of massive doses of ascorbic acid in leukemia (see Chapter 27)	3
A14.	Search for exploitable biochemical differences between cancer and normal cells	50
A15.	Search for a cancer vaccine	30
A16.	Studies on cancer and nutrition	5
A17.	In reserve	10
A18.	In reserve	10
A19.	In reserve	10
A20.	In reserve	10

Subtotal—All general projects   408

B. Special projects at colleges of veterinary medicine (in addition to veterinary school participation in general projects)

B1.	Studies on farm animals with cancer (18 schools)	5.8
B2.	Studies on dogs with cancer (6 schools)	1.7
B3.	Breeding of mice with spontaneous cancers (6 schools)	1.6

Subtotal—Special veterinary medical projects   9.1

Table 33–2.—Continued

In Millions of Dollars

C. *Special dental school projects (in addition to dental school participation in general projects)*

C1.	Development of improved chambers for in-vivo study of cancer growth	3.1
C2.	Studies on tumor growth in hamster cheek pouch	4.8

Subtotal—Special dental school projects   7.9

D. *Special pharmacy school projects (in addition to pharmacy school participation in general projects)*

D1.	Comprehensive studies on duration of drug effects and levels in mice	3.0
D2.	Development of techniques to increase duration of effective blood levels of drugs in mice	3.0
D3.	Pharmacognosy of plants with possible anti-cancer actions	2.0

Subtotal—Special pharmacy school projects   8.0

E. *Special botany and agriculture projects (in addition to participation in general projects)*

E1.	Collection of wild plants to be tested for anti-cancer effects	5.0
E2.	Cultivation of plants revealing anti-cancer effects	3.0

Subtotal—Special botany and agriculture projects   8.0

F. *Special services*

F1.	Providing investigators with up-to-date information on current studies	2
F2.	Providing special library and reference services to all investigators	3
F3.	Publication and distribution of several cancer research journals	1
F4.	Meetings, symposia and inspection visits	1
F5.	Consultation costs	1
F6.	Coordination with other research programs	1

Subtotal—Special services   9.0

Total   450.0

CHAPTER 34

Conclusion

In a democracy, the fundamental decisions that affect the lives and well-being of the people are supposed to be based on the wishes of those people. There can be little doubt that the vast majority of American citizens—indeed of all mankind—would like to see a cure or control for cancer developed as soon as possible. It should be clear, however, that in this area our national effort to date has been inadequate. We have not followed through on all the promising research leads. We have not furnished the necessary support to many of our research scientists who want to help. We have not made a determined effort to see that a fair share of our national resources is mobilized for a national cancer research program.

We have not done these things largely because few people have thought of a cure or control for cancer in terms of a major national goal. If the American people can accept the placing of a man on the moon and similar projects as important national goals, surely finding a cure or control for cancer is a reasonable and worthwhile national goal. However, most people's thoughts and opinions on the cancer problem are amorphous; they are confused by optimistic newspaper stories about imminent breakthroughs in cancer research. Members of the health professions know that there were no such breakthroughs in past decades. The death rate from cancer has risen, despite the development of a few anti-cancer drugs—most of which have sharply limited value.

Therefore, in relation to the cancer research problem, the most important function of those in the health professions is the crystallization of the public attitude toward the need for a more effective research program. This can be accomplished without frightening people; indeed, the decision to take positive vigorous action is often an antidote to fear and anxiety. Many citizens need to be helped to understand the potential value of a vigorous national cancer research program. Health professionals can give such help by answering their patients' and friends' questions about medical research or cancer research, or by speaking to various lay groups. Eventually the public will learn about, and understand, the importance of a national cancer research program. Eventually their wishes will become translated into law and into appropriations and projects. How long will it take?

Index

305